T0073410

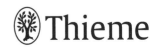

Tinnitus Treatment

Clinical Protocols

Second Edition

Richard S. Tyler, PhD
Professor of Otolaryngology and Professor of Communication Sciences and Disorders
Roy J. and Lucille A. Carver College of Medicine
Department of Otolaryngology–Head and Neck Surgery
University of Iowa
Iowa City, Iowa, USA

Ann Perreau, BA, MA, PhD
Associate Professor of Communication Sciences and Disorders
Audiology Clinic Coordinator
Roseman Center for Speech, Language, and Hearing
Augustana College
Rockland Island, Illinois, USA

83 Illustrations

Thieme
New York • Stuttgart • Delhi • Rio de Janeiro

Library of Congress Cataloging-in-Publication Data is available from the publisher.

Important note: Medicine is an ever-changing science undergoing continual development. Research and clinical experience are continually expanding our knowledge, in particular our knowledge of proper treatment and drug therapy. Insofar as this book mentions any dosage or application, readersmay rest assured that the authors, editors, and publishers have made every effort to ensure that such references are in accordance with **the state of knowledge at the time of production of the book.**

Nevertheless, this does not involve, imply, or express any guarantee or responsibility on the part of the publishers in respect to any dosage instructions and forms of applications stated in the book. **Every user is requested to examine carefully** the manufacturers' leaflets accompanying each drug and to check, if necessary in consultation with a physician or specialist, whether the dosage schedules mentioned therein or the contraindications stated by the manufacturers differ from the statements made in the present book. Such examination is particularly important with drugs that are either rarely used or have been newly released on the market. Every dosage schedule or every form of application used is entirely at the user's own risk and responsibility. The authors and publishers request every user to report to the publishers any discrepancies or inaccuracies noticed. If errors in this work are found after publication, errata will be posted at www.thieme.com on the product description page.

Some of the product names, patents, and registered designs referred to in this book are in fact registered trademarks or proprietary names even though specific reference to this fact is not always made in the text. Therefore, the appearance of a name without designation as proprietary is not to be construed as a representation by the publisher that it is in the public domain. Thieme addresses people of all gender identities equally. We encourage our authors to use gender-neutral or gender-equal expressions wherever the context allows.

© 2022. Thieme. All rights reserved.

Thieme Publishers New York
333 Seventh Avenue, 18th Floor
New York, NY 10001, USA
www.thieme.com
+1 800 782 3488, customerservice@thieme.com

Cover design: © Thieme
Cover image source: © Thieme/Liam Haskill
Typesetting by TNQ Technologies, India

Printed in Germany by Beltz Grafische Betriebe   5 4 3 2 1

ISBN: 978-1-68420-171-6

Also available as an e-book:
eISBN (PDF): 978-1-68420-172-3
eISBN (epub): 978-1-63853-686-4

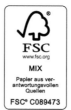

FSC
www.fsc.org
MIX
Papier aus verantwortungsvollen Quellen
FSC® C089473

Contents

Contents

Contents

Videos

Foreword

Audiologists are expected to have the knowledge and skills necessary to provide appropriate care for individuals with a variety of hearing and balance issues. The field of audiology, however, is so rich and diverse that it is inappropriate to assume that audiologists can be experts in every area. For example, an audiologist can specialize in diagnostics, treatment, research, and/or teaching (to name a few), can pick a specific work environment (e.g., health care, private practice, education, manufacturing), and can even select a specific age group for care (i.e., infants, from birth to 3-year-old children, school-aged children, adults, and/or geriatrics). After choosing a specific area of interest, work setting, and/or age group, audiologists are inundated with a variety of different theories, approaches, devices, and techniques, all available to achieve the same goals. Hence, lies the problem. The field is so rich and diverse that it often leaves the audiologists feeling overwhelmed and less confident of their abilities. Historically, audiologists could rely on their graduate programs to provide them with the knowledge and skills needed to feel confident enough to venture out and to begin practice.

Unfortunately, most graduate programs are still not strong or relevant in the area of treating individuals with bothersome tinnitus and/or hyperacusis. This must change. The field of audiology needs to do a better job of providing audiologists with the tools necessary to feel confident in this area. This book does just that! This book and the supplemental online content contain the most comprehensive background and up-to-date strategies and tools for treating individuals with bothersome tinnitus and/or hyperacusis. This textbook should be read by every audiology student not only as an introduction to this area of interest, but as an advanced classroom resource. In addition, any practicing audiologist who feels underprepared in managing tinnitus and hyperacusis should be strongly encouraged to use this textbook and the supplemental materials as a guide. You could not ask for a more talented set of authors who not only contribute to the most current research on tinnitus and hyperacusis, but who are also working in the trenches side by side with their patients providing this much-needed service. Audiologists are the most suitable to work with this patient population. Audiologists need to be providing tinnitus and hyperacusis management services on a much more common basis. This is the textbook to provide the knowledge and confidence that audiologists are lacking. You hold in your hand the only needed resource to begin your work. Read it, watch the online videos, go through the handouts, then have faith in yourself and start implementing these ideas with your tinnitus and hyperacusis patients. If you do this work, you will end up feeling more satisfied in your career than you ever have felt before. If I (along with the authors of this textbook) can do this work, so can you.

Shelley A. Witt, MA/CCC-A
Department of Otolaryngology–Head and
Neck Surgery
University of Iowa
Iowa City, Iowa, USA

Preface

In this second edition, we hope to provide the most comprehensive background and up-to-date strategies for treating tinnitus and hyperacusis patients. The textbook is useful for audiology students as an introduction and as an advanced classroom resource for tinnitus management. Also, because many audiologists and clinicians do not receive sufficient training in assessing and treating tinnitus and hyperacusis, we hope this textbook is valuable in providing additional tools and guidance for practicing clinicians.

Since the first edition of 2005, new developments and areas of interest have emerged that impact treatment. For example, sensory meditation and mindfulness is an approach to treat several chronic health conditions, including tinnitus, which is now included in our second edition. We have also reviewed smartphone apps that have emerged in recent years as a helpful tool for managing tinnitus, but caution is needed. Additionally, hyperacusis, an abnormal sensitivity to sounds, is reported by many patients and is included in this new edition. Although there is now a plethora of "information" available via the Internet and many self-help books for patients to help with tinnitus treatment, this textbook provides helpful information on important topics pertaining to tinnitus that is grounded in years of clinical experience and research. We strive to meet the needs of audiologists and clinicians who guide tinnitus and hyperacusis patients in their journey by providing relevant and updated information, including varied perspectives from authors around the world who are well-respected clinicians and researchers on tinnitus.

This textbook contains 15 chapters. The first three chapters provide an overview of tinnitus models, treatment approaches, and self-treatment options. Chapter 1 reviews neurophysiological and psychological models of tinnitus and therapy approaches including counseling and sound therapy for tinnitus. Chapter 2 provides guidance on treating patients with tinnitus who are diagnosed from otologic pathology such as Meniere's disease, vestibular schwannoma, unilateral sudden sensorineural hearing loss, and middle ear myoclonus. Chapter 3 summarizes an emerging topic of Internet-delivered, self-help treatment, and the research evidence that supports effectiveness of self-help strategies such as apps and self-help books.

The next three chapters, Chapters 4 to 6, summarize counseling approaches for audiologists and psychologists. Chapter 4 on "Tinnitus Activities Treatment" describes our counseling and sound therapy program that has been used in tinnitus management for decades and provides helpful suggestions for audiologists and clinicians to implement this picture-based and customized therapy approach. Chapter 5 introduces the "Three-Track Tinnitus Protocol," a psychological counseling program that outlines the three components of the Patient–Tinnitus Track, the Patient–Life-World Track, and the Clinician–Patient Track in managing tinnitus. Chapter 6 provides an overview of psychological management of insomnia, a common problem among tinnitus patients, and reviews the cognitive behavioral model as it applies to insomnia.

Chapters 7 to 10 describe approaches to managing tinnitus using amplification, sound therapy, and meditation and mindfulness. Chapter 7 describes the benefits of hearing aids in the management of tinnitus for patients who have hearing loss, incorporating research evidence, and outlining new hearing aid technology and fitting strategies. Chapter 8 reviews sound therapy using wearable devices including the mechanisms for sound therapy effectiveness in treating tinnitus and provides a fitting protocol for audiologists and clinicians based on the individual's goals. Chapter 9, a new chapter in the second edition, explores smartphone apps for tinnitus, including apps for assessment and management of tinnitus, and apps for education and wellness, and reviews the limitations associated with apps used for managing tinnitus. Chapter 10, a new chapter, describes several options for relaxation or distraction from tinnitus, including meditation, mindfulness, guided imagery, biofeedback, progressive muscle relaxation, art therapy, music therapy, exercise, and exploration of new hobbies. Many of these relaxation techniques are demonstrated in the chapter, and research and clinical reports are included.

The last five chapters provide guidance on specific topics related to tinnitus management such as treating children with tinnitus, implementing outcome measures, treating hyperacusis, and navigating future directions in tinnitus treatment. Chapter 11 provides a thorough review of etiologies, diagnoses, and treatment options when working with children with tinnitus. Special attention is paid to the prevention of tinnitus through education and awareness on hearing protection and ototoxic medications. Chapter 12 summarizes the methods for measuring tinnitus and reactions to tinnitus, including use of psychoacoustic measures of tinnitus, questionnaires, diaries, and scales on associated problems for depression, anxiety, and sleep. Chapter 13 reviews hyperacusis by introducing its symptoms, causes and mechanisms, and diagnosis and treatment including counseling, sound therapy, medications, and use of hearing protection in noisy situations. Common complaints of patients with hyperacusis are reviewed to illustrate the everyday experiences of patients and ways these complaints can be addressed by the clinician and audiologist. Chapter 14 explores emerging treatments of tinnitus, such as vagus nerve stimulation and transcranial magnetic stimulation, and explains the neural networks for tinnitus to demonstrate the application of these treatments. The final chapter, Chapter 15, provides an overview for audiologists and clinicians who wish to expand their professional services and establish a tinnitus and hyperacusis clinic. We outline group educational and individual counseling sessions, structuring the clinic, and billing for services.

In addition to the textbook, we have developed new supplemental materials to both demonstrate the techniques discussed in the book and to provide helpful tools in tinnitus and hyperacusis management. Some chapters in the book offer appendices, which have been carefully selected to help the audiologist and clinician in implementing treatment protocols and procedures in their clinical practice. Apart from the appendices, there are multiple videos such as interviews of patients with tinnitus and hyperacusis, counseling and sound therapy demonstrations, mindfulness and meditation exercises, psychoacoustic testing, and hearing aid fittings for tinnitus patients. We also included handouts on counseling; relaxation and sound therapy; questionnaires on tinnitus, hyperacusis, and quality of life; and datasheets on psychoacoustic testing for clinicians and audiologists to use in clinical practice. The brochures and slides for Tinnitus Activities Treatment used in our clinics at the University of Iowa and at Augustana College are also available as appendices. All videos are available on Thieme MedOne. We acknowledge the efforts of the reviewers for this book, including researchers, clinicians, and audiology students, who provided valuable inputs for the final product.

Richard S. Tyler, PhD
Ann Perreau, BA, MA, PhD

Acknowledgments

Many have helped with my career and my interest in tinnitus and hyperacusis.

Jim Stouffer helped me appreciate the importance of good science. Bill Yovetich helped me move beyond my stuttering. Arnold Small, David Lilly, Jim Curtis, and Paul Abbas provided a detailed background to the field. Ross Coles opened a switch on tinnitus. Then Johnathan Hazell, Pawel and Margarette Jastreboff, and Jean-Marie Aran opened up the widespread diverse perspectives. Jack Vernon and Mary Meikle showed me how much they cared about their patients. Peter Wilson opened up cognitive behavior therapy for tinnitus for me. Carol Bauer and Bob Dobie brought in the medical perspective. Jay Rubenstein and Paul Van de Heyning convinced me cochlear implants could help. Dick Salvi and Josef Rauschecker searched for mechanisms. Bill Noble and Dennis McFadden helped with the science. Bob Levine opened up somatosensory issues. And Ann and Shelley ... a thoughtful, dedicated team ... WOW ... and there were many more...

Every author in this book has influenced my strategies. We do not have to agree, but listen ... and learn and adapt from our different perspectives; and it is helpful that we all have different perspectives. So many people are moving this forward in so many directions.

Thank You! All of you. I dedicate this book to *You*!

Richard S. Tyler, PhD

This book is shaped by many individuals who have had a hand in my work. To my mentors at the University of Iowa: Carolyn Brown, Paul Abbas, Chris Turner, and Ruth Bentler, thank you for your guidance in my early years. I thank Kathy Jakielski, who has supported me since the day of our first meeting at Augustana College. I appreciate so many colleagues, Shelley A. Witt, Hua Ou, and Smita Agrawal, who have had such a profound impact on me as an audiologist and scholar. To the patients and research participants at the Tinnitus and Hyperacusis Clinic at the University of Iowa and Augustana College Roseman Center for Speech, Language, and Hearing, you give me inspiration and motivation every day! I am grateful for years of mentorship and involvement of students from undergraduates to doctoral candidates in CSD and audiology who have contributed to my work and research over the years. I thank Courtney Baker who assisted with editing and recording of the supplemental videos and was an integral part of creating this new edition. Finally, thanks to Richard S. Tyler for making this dream a reality and helping me achieve this milestone!

I also acknowledge Annette Schneider who assisted with the final proofs of the book.

Ann Perreau, BA, MA, PhD

Contributors

Gerhard Andersson, PhD
Professor
Department of Behavioural Sciences and Learning
Department of Biomedical and Clinical Sciences
Linköping University
Linköping, Sweden

David M. Baguley, BSc, MSc, MBA, PhD
Professor of Hearing Sciences;
Consultant Clinical Scientist (Audiology)
NIHR Nottingham Biomedical Research Centre,
    Hearing Sciences
Division of Clinical Neuroscience,
    School of Medicine
University of Nottingham
Nottingham, UK

Courtney Baker, BA
Doctoral of Audiology Student
Northwestern University
Evanston, Illinois, USA

Manohar L. Bance, MB, ChB, MSc, MM
Professor of Otology and Skull Base Surgery
Department of Clinical Neuroscience
University of Cambridge
Cambridge, UK

Eldre Beukes, PhD
Department of Speech and Hearing Sciences
Lamar University
Beaumont, Texas, USA;
Vision and Hearing Sciences Research Centre
Anglia Ruskin University
Cambridge, UK

Claudia Coelho, MD, PhD
Department of Otolaryngology–Head and
    Neck Surgery
University of Iowa
Iowa City, Iowa, USA;
College of Medicine
Postgraduate Program in Medical Sciences
University of Vale do Taquari
Univates
Lajeado, Rio Grande do Sul, Brazil

Mithila Durai, BSc, MAud (Hons), PhD
Research Fellow (Audiology)
School of Population Health
The University of Auckland
Auckland, New Zealand

Mohamed Salah Elgandy, MD
Department of Otolaryngology–Head and
    Neck Surgery, Zagazig University
Az Zagazig, Ash Sharqiyah, Egypt;
Department of Otolaryngology–Head and
    Neck Surgery
University of Iowa
Iowa City, Iowa, USA

Elizabeth Fetscher, AuD
Communication Sciences and Disorders
Illinois State University
Normal, Illinois, USA

Phillip E. Gander, PhD
Associate Research Scientist
Department of Neurosurgery
University of Iowa
Iowa City, Iowa, USA

Fatima T. Husain, PhD
Professor
Department of Speech and Hearing Science,
    Neuroscience Program
The Beckman Institute for Advanced
    Science and Technology
University of Illinois at Urbana-Champaign
Champaign, Illinois, USA

Tania Linford, BSc, MAud
Professional Teaching Fellow;
Audiologist
Hearing and Tinnitus Clinic
Audiology, School of Population Health
The University of Auckland
Auckland, New Zealand

Patricia C. Mancini, PhD
Associate Professor
Department of Speech-Pathology and Audiology;
Full professor
Speech-Pathology and Audiology Sciences
    Post-Graduate Program
Federal University of Minas Gerais
Minas Gerais, Brazil

Elizabeth Marks, PhD
Clinical Psychologist and Lecturer
Department of Psychology
University of Bath
England, UK

Laurence McKenna, MClin Psychol, PhD
Consultant Clinical Psychologist
Royal National ENT & Eastman Dental Hospitals
UCLH & UCL
London, UK

Anne-Mette Mohr, MA, Candidate of Psychology
Clinical Psychologist;
Director
House of Hearing
Private Practising Clinical Psychologist
Psykologcentret Nordvest
Copenhagen, Denmark

Ann Perreau, BA, MA, PhD
Associate Professor of Communication
    Sciences and Disorders
Audiology Clinic Coordinator
Roseman Center for Speech, Language, and Hearing
Augustana College
Rockland Island, Illinois, USA

Michael Piskosz, BA, BS, MS
Product Manager
Oticon Medical, LLC
Somerset, New Jersey, USA

**Grant D. Searchfield, BSc,
    MAud(Hons), PhD, MNZAS**
Associate Professor;
Director
Hearing and Tinnitus Clinic;
Deputy Director
Eisdell Moore Centre, Faculty of Medical and
    Health Sciences
University of Auckland
Auckland, New Zealand

Alice H. Smith, MA AuD
Professional Teaching Fellow;
Team leader
Hearing and Tinnitus Clinic, Audiology,
    School of Population Health
The University of Auckland
Auckland, New Zealand

Richard S. Tyler, PhD
Professor of Otolaryngology and Professor of
    Communication Sciences and Disorders
Roy J. and Lucille A. Carver College of Medicine
Department of Otolaryngology–Head and Neck
    Surgery
University of Iowa
Iowa City, Iowa, USA

Shelley A. Witt, MA/CCC-A
Department of Otolaryngology–Head and
    Neck Surgery
University of Iowa
Iowa City, Iowa, USA

1 Neurophysiological Models, Psychological Models, and Treatments for Tinnitus

Phillip E. Gander and Richard S. Tyler

Abstract

This chapter provides an overview of different models of tinnitus according to the two major categories of neurophysiological and psychological models. These models lead to different approaches to tinnitus treatment and the implementation of sound therapy and counseling protocols, which are summarized accordingly.

Keywords: neurophysiological, psychological, treatment, sound therapy, counseling

1.1 What Is Tinnitus?

A clear definition of tinnitus is from the study by McFadden.[1] Tinnitus:
- Is a perception of sound (it must be heard).
- Is involuntary (not produced intentionally).
- Originates in the head (not hearing or overly sensitive to an external sound).

The patient's reaction should also be considered. It is helpful to distinguish:
- Tinnitus that is problematic from that which is not.[2]
- How often the tinnitus occurs and how long an episode is (e.g., whether it occurs once a month for 10 s or is present daily).

Tinnitus has been classified in several ways, such as its presumed site of generation and whether it is audible to someone other than the patient (objective tinnitus) or the patient alone (subjective tinnitus). An objective tinnitus, heard by the examiner, may be of middle ear origin or a spontaneous otoacoustic emission arising from the sensorineural system and can occasionally be identified by physical examination to direct treatment options, such as in vascular causes. However, the terms *subjective* and *objective* are not particularly helpful in understanding or treating most forms of tinnitus. Instead, it is more useful to classify tinnitus in a manner analogous to hearing loss according to site of injury or generation[3]; that is, whether it is middle ear, sensorineural, or central tinnitus. A thorough physical examination and treatment of identified ailments, when possible, are important first steps in patients

with tinnitus. However, a physical examination will typically not reveal a clear cause, that is, idiopathic tinnitus. Importantly, in all cases a distinction can be made between (1) the tinnitus and (2) the reaction to the tinnitus, which has become known as the psychological model of tinnitus.[4] Regardless of the classification, the treatments described in this book are applicable to all types of tinnitus. See Appendix 1.1 for an overview of this chapter.

The overall impact of tinnitus on a patient is influenced by the characteristics of tinnitus and of that particular patient.[5] For example, tinnitus is more likely to be annoying if it is louder or has a screeching quality. Some authors have incorrectly suggested that psychoacoustic factors are unimportant or unrelated to tinnitus annoyance. Psychoacoustic factors are indeed relevant,[6,7] although they are only one thing to consider in understanding the effect tinnitus has on a patient. An absence of high correlation between loudness and annoyance does not mean that loudness is not important. Stouffer and Tyler[8] concluded that patients with soft tinnitus are not under as much stress as those who report a loud tinnitus. Also, patients who are under stress or have not had adequate sleep find the tinnitus more annoying.

Tinnitus is not a personality disorder, but psychological factors are involved in the development and maintenance of this problem (see, e.g., Folmer et al,[9] Fowler and Fowler,[10] Nondahl et al[11]). Although patients with severe tinnitus can have clinical depression, in our experience, serious psychological problems are rare among most tinnitus patients. Very few of us, after all, would not be bothered at all if we constantly heard an unwanted sound that we had no control over.

1.2 Neurophysiological Models of Tinnitus

A likely cause for tinnitus is maladaptive plasticity of the central nervous system.[12] In essence, in response to some (typically unknown) causes, mechanisms that keep the nervous system in balance (i.e., homeostasis) lead to changes that result in the perception of tinnitus. In the normal auditory system, increases in neural activity evoked by acoustic stimuli are the basis for sound perception.

Table 1.1 Examples of neurophysiological models of tinnitus

Kiang, Moxon, and Levine[25]	Edge between normal and absent hair cells and subsequent neural activity
Tonndorf[29]	Decoupling of stereocilia between the hair cells and tectorial membrane
Eggermont[26] Moeller[27]	Cross-talk (interneural synchrony) between nerve fibers
Hazell[30]	Tinnitus is a result of automatic gain control system of central nervous system (e.g., normally increasing the sensitivity in quiet), linked to outer hair cells
Penner and Bilger[31]	Spontaneous otoacoustic emissions
Jastreboff[19]	Discordant inner and outer hair cell damage (damaged outer hair cells with reasonably intact inner hair cells)
Salvi et al[20,28]	Increase in central neurons tuned to similar frequencies following reorganization of peripheral hearing loss
Llinás et al[32]	Abnormal neural oscillatory connection between thalamus and cortex
Noreña and Eggermont[33] Eggermont and Roberts[17]	Cochlear damage leads to reduced inhibition in auditory system resulting in increased neural synchrony, spontaneous firing, and burst firing
Kaltenbach, Zhang, and Zacharek[34]	Hyperactivity of dorsal cochlear nucleus
Noreña[35] Schaette and McAlpine[36] Zeng[37]	Homeostatic plasticity after hearing loss results in neural hyperactivity from increased central gain
Leaver et al[38] Rauschecker et al[39]	Failed "noise cancellation" system in frontostriatal network that gates and interprets neural noise
Roberts, Husain, and Eggermont[41]	Basal forebrain cholinergic attention system involved in tinnitus prominence and maintenance
De Ridder, Vanneste, and Freeman[42]	Multiple brain networks that interact with tinnitus "core" subnetwork
De Ridder et al[43]	Hearing loss reduces input and brain fills in missing information to resolve uncertainty
Sedley et al[22]	Brain reinterprets increased neural noise as a sound

Under conditions of a hearing loss, there is a decrease in input to the auditory system in the frequency range of the loss. Normal operation of the nervous system is to restore activity levels that have changed due to this decrease in input, to keep homeostasis.[13] A mechanism for this restoration is modification of the sensitivity of neurons to their input and their resultant output activity by increasing the neural response gain.[14] The increase in gain also leads to an increase in spontaneous activity in the absence of acoustic stimulation. Therefore, neurophysiological models have logically nominated this increase in spontaneous activity as a mechanism of tinnitus. Wherever the site of origin, most probably this activity change is transmitted to and results in an increased spontaneous rate in the auditory cortex. ▶ Table 1.1 reviews a few of the neurophysiological models that have been proposed over the years (for reviews, see Cacace,[15] Eggermont,[16] Eggermont and Roberts,[17,18] Jastreboff,[19] Salvi et al,[20] and Vernon and Moeller[21]). Some of these

are specific to precise anatomic or physiological sites; others are more general models referring to processing principles.

In general, many of these models are insightful and clever. For models to be useful, they should be testable or should lead to a broader understanding and eventually a testable hypothesis. Unfortunately, many of these models are mutually exclusive[22] and so it becomes difficult to separate testable hypotheses that usefully contribute to broader understanding.

Whatever the initial source of tinnitus, it must be perceived in the auditory cortex (see Tyler,[23] p. 136; Vanneste and De Ridder[24]). Broadly, there are three different ways that the mechanism of tinnitus can be coded in the auditory cortex:

- Increased spontaneous activity fed by increase or decrease in activity or edge in activity.[25]
- Cross-fiber correlation with normal or increased spontaneous activity.[26,27]
- More fibers with similar best frequency following hearing loss–induced auditory plasticity.[20,28]

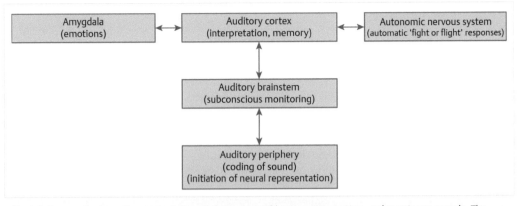

Fig. 1.1 A general schematic representation of the process of hearing, interpreting, and reacting to sounds. The mechanism for the initiation of tinnitus may arise anywhere, but its representation eventually occurs in the auditory cortex. Any emotional responses must involve the amygdala and the autonomic nervous system (known connections between these regions are not shown in the diagram).

► Fig. 1.1 shows a schematic representation of how we hear, interpret, and react to sounds. Sound is transformed from acoustic to electrical information in the cochlea. It is transmitted through the brainstem to the auditory centers of the brain within the temporal lobe of each hemisphere. Other parts of the brain are involved in our memory for sounds and our emotional reaction to them. Such neurophysiological models of hearing have existed for decades and were applied to tinnitus as early as 1988,[44] and later popularized by Jastreboff.[19] Although the mechanism responsible for the source of tinnitus initiation may potentially arise anywhere in the nervous system, its representation in the nervous system must be transmitted to the brain. Wilson[45] (pp. 30, 31) suggested that tinnitus is coded in the auditory cortex "by virtue of the pattern of activity over many cells." Like normal sounds, any reactions patients have to their tinnitus must involve other regions of the brain, such as the amygdala and the autonomic nervous system. Hallam et al[46] (p. 44) discussed "neurophysiological models of habituation" and their importance in understanding and treating the emotional components of tinnitus. This model was widely accepted at the time (e.g., Hazell et al,[47] p. 74).

Noise-induced hearing loss, one of the most common causes of tinnitus, is known to inflict cochlear damage. Early studies of noise-induced hearing loss emphasized that both outer hair cells and inner hair cells are affected (e.g., Liberman and Dodds[48]). More recently, noise trauma has been found to disconnect inner hair cells from sensory neurons before damage to the inner hair cells is observed, a condition called cochlear synaptopathy.[49] This has also been termed "hidden hearing loss" because outer hair cell function, which principally accounts for threshold test results, are unaffected. Importantly, it has been proposed that the change in inner hair cell function could contribute to the generation of tinnitus in some cases.[36]

While cochlear trauma may be an initiating condition, it is clear that tinnitus must also intimately involve the brainstem and cortex (Tyler,[23] p. 136). This can be shown from several observations, including that:

- Sectioning the auditory nerve is often ineffective in reducing tinnitus.[50]
- Masking can be just as effective in the ear ipsilateral to the tinnitus as in the ear contralateral to the tinnitus (e.g., Tyler and Conrad-Armes[51]).
- Observing that a person who is convinced about hearing tinnitus in the right ear can suddenly hear the tinnitus in the left ear when the right ear tinnitus is masked.
- Documenting that disorders of the central auditory pathways can cause tinnitus.[2]

It is of interest, and perhaps a clue, that tinnitus can be influenced by other neurophysiological systems (for reviews, see Cacace,[15,52] Levine et al,[53] Sanchez and Rocha[54]). For example, in some patients, tinnitus can be altered by touches to the hand, jaw movement, pressure to the head, and changes in eye gaze. Whether this is a property of tinnitus in general or just a subgroup can provide important information for treatment approaches.

Of course, because tinnitus can provoke emotional reactions, other neurophysiological systems that are responsible for emotions must also be involved, including the autonomic nervous system

3

and the amygdala. Both Hallam et al[46] and Slater and Terry[55] described how the autonomic nervous system is involved in tinnitus. This unconscious involuntary control system is for "fight or flight." The sympathetic system sets up the body for action, and the parasympathetic system operates after the extra alertness is past, to bring the body from its "highly aroused state to its normal state" (Slater and Terry,[55] p. 177). The authors emphasized how the "dangers" sensed are typically stress related and reviewed in great detail the neurophysiological responses. They suggested coping strategies (e.g., relaxation techniques) as a treatment for the "inappropriate" autonomic response of tinnitus patients. It has been known for decades that a group of cortical and subcortical structures in the center of the brain (the limbic system) are involved whenever emotions are triggered (for reviews, see LeDoux[56] and Mega et al[57]). Jastreboff[19] pointed out that the limbic system, therefore, must be involved in tinnitus patients who have emotional reactions. However, the concept of a single "limbic system" is oversimplified as these structures are involved in different, but related functions.[40] More recent evidence indicates that certain structures, such as the *amygdala*[58,121] may be more important than the whole system.[15]

We like the way Goodey[44] (p. 84) explains tinnitus to his patients:

"Too few messages are passing through the ear to keep the hearing nerve busy and especially in quiet conditions, the electrically active nerve generates its own messages which are heard as tinnitus."

1.3 Psychological Models of Tinnitus

Physiological and psychological models are inherently linked. One cannot have a change in thinking or behaving without some neurophysiological correlate. Studies, and related conceptual frameworks, that focus on thinking and behaving can be considered psychological. ▶ Table 1.2 reviews some psychological frameworks for considering tinnitus treatment.

These models are certainly not mutually exclusive. For example, Hallam et al,[46] in their habituation model, noted that an organism needs to analyze (or attend to) new and potentially important stimuli. How we think about tinnitus influences our inclination to attend to it. External events can reinforce or inhibit our behavior. Learning theory, particularly classical conditioning, has been proposed as an important factor in the reaction to tinnitus (e.g., Jastreboff,[59] McKenna[60]). Hallam et al[46] (p. 44) suggested that "habituation can be delayed by intense, aversive and unpredictable stimuli to which affective significance has been attached by learning."

1.4 Categories of Tinnitus Treatments

We can categorize tinnitus treatments in two ways. First, a treatment can focus on the tinnitus directly, reducing its magnitude or eliminating it completely. This can be approached by medications as described by Baguley in Chapter 2 (also see Dobie,[100] Elgandy and Tyler,[61] and Murai et al[62]) or electrical suppression (e.g., Dauman,[63] Dobie et al,[64] Elgandy et al,[65] Hazell et al,[66] Quaranta et al,[67] Rubinstein and Tyler,[68] Tyler et al,[69] and Zwolan et al[70]) or neuromodulation.[71,72] Important insights in these approaches are discussed by Husain in Chapter 14.

Second, it is possible to treat a patient's reaction to tinnitus. Medications can be used to treat patients with depression and anxiety and to help with sleep problems. Baguley in Chapter 2 highlights how some of the more common medical

Table 1.2 Psychological factors considered in treating tinnitus

Cognitive	Have developed inappropriate ways of thinking about tinnitus	Sweetow[73,74] Andersson and Kaldo (Chapter 8), Hallam and McKenna (Chapter 6), Hallam et al[46]
Habituation	Bothersome tinnitus is failure to habituate	Hallam et al[46] Hallam[75] Hallam and McKenna (Chapter 6)
Attention	Failure to shift attention away from tinnitus	Hallam and McKenna (Chapter 6), Hallam et al[46] Hallam[75]
Learning	Responses to tinnitus are learned	Jastreboff and Hazell[76] Bartnik and Skarz'yn'ski (Chapter 10) also McKenna,[57] Hallam et al[46]
Acceptance	I accept it, is not good or bad	Mohr[77]
Ownership	I own the tinnitus; it is mine	Mohr and Hedelund[78]

conditions influence the counseling strategy. Medications for some patients are important, but they are not specific to tinnitus and will not be reviewed here. Counseling and sound therapy are two treatments that have been in common use since the early 1980s. Appendix 1.1 provides a summary of treatment options.

1.5 Counseling in the Treatment of Tinnitus

Whether we spend 1 minute or 60 minutes with a patient, talking with and listening to the patient are the cornerstones of the current treatment. Counseling for tinnitus patients is often performed by audiologists without a strong theoretical background in the many counseling strategies available. Psychologists frame different counseling approaches (and there are literally hundreds) using very specific guidelines. ▶ Table 1.3 provides a few examples of these frameworks, taken from an excellent summary by Flasher and Fogle.[79]

These theoretical frameworks are also not mutually exclusive, but we suspect that tinnitus counseling would benefit from a deeper understanding of the theoretical background of different counseling approaches. Those clinicians who have some training in these approaches will put themselves in a better position to serve their tinnitus patients.

1.5.1 Be Supportive

We, and others,[80,30,81] have noted how important it is to be supportive and to offer positive encouragement to the tinnitus patient (e.g., Coles and Hallam,[80] Hazell,[30] and Tyler et al[81]).

Whatever counseling strategy is adopted, providing reasonable hope and demonstrating that you are knowledgeable, sympathetic, and sincerely care will likely be helpful. A new and comprehensive approach to this is provided by Mohr in Chapter 5.

1.5.2 Provide Information

Most of the therapies designed for tinnitus provide information. Whichever neurophysiological or psychological model you adhere to, providing information helps patients better understand their problems and feel less victimized and puts them in a position of moving forward in treatment. ▶ Table 1.4 outlines the kinds of information that can be provided.

The relative importance of each of these topics is unclear. It is unlikely that discussing any of them would have a negative impact, and thus, the question really is which to include or exclude, and how much time to spend on each topic. Obviously, too much information can be overwhelming for some patients, and it is possible to provide the information in too much detail or without sufficient clarity. This may prevent a patient from engaging in the other aspects of the treatment. We have proposed using pictures to facilitate the counseling process.[82]

Many of the counseling components of treatment focus primarily on providing information about hearing, hearing loss, and tinnitus (e.g., Bentler and Tyler,[83] LaMarte and Tyler,[84] Sheldrake et al,[85] Tyler and Babin,[3] and Tyler and Baker[86]). Some researchers, such as Hallam,[75] include discussions about habituation and attention in their approaches (see Chapters 3, 4, 5, and 10 of this book), whereas others focus more on brain mechanisms and learning. All of the clinicians writing in this book provide information on their particular counseling approach, and the diversity of topics and emphasis is evident. For example, Chapter 9 shows how Apps can be used by patients to facilitate the transfer of information in conjunction with clinic visits.

1.5.3 Components of Counseling

Briefly, there are three components of most successful counseling programs:
- Changing thoughts.
- Changing behavior.
- Understanding an individual patient's needs.

Changing Thoughts

Providing information can change the way patients think about their tinnitus. However, simply lecturing a patient is not enough, even if the information is useful. Understanding what caused the tinnitus,

Table 1.3 Psychological counseling approaches

Existential therapy	Concerns with individual's overall existence in life, and how one deals with problems. Considers uncertainty, meaning, and isolation (see Chapter 5)
Cognitive therapy	Thoughts influence behavior, erroneous ways of thinking are identified, and steps for coping and correcting thoughts are identified (see Chapters 3 and 4)
Humanistic therapy	Promotes personal growth and positive support in a nondirective fashion (see Chapters 5 and 15)
Behavioral therapy	Focus is on changing the ways in which patients behave (see Chapters 3, 4, and 5)

Table 1.4 General categories of information typically provided to tinnitus patients

Hearing	How we hear
	Anatomy and physiology of hearing
Hearing loss	Anatomy and physiology of hearing loss
	Consequences of hearing loss
Tinnitus epidemiology	Prevalence of tinnitus
	Causes of tinnitus
	Common problems associated with tinnitus
Tinnitus mechanisms	Spontaneous activity of nerves
	Neurophysiological models (see ▶ Table 1.1)
Central nervous system	Role of the brain in perceiving and reacting to sound
Habituation	Effect of repeated exposure to stimuli
	Consequences of fearful stimuli
	Consequences of not habituating to tinnitus
Attention	Factors that contribute to attention
Learning	Factors that contribute to learning
Sleep	Factors that influence sleep
Concentration	Factors that contribute to concentration
Auditory training	Things that influence our hearing and understanding
Lifestyles	How our overall lifestyle, including eating, exercise, and activities, influences our health
Self-image	How our self-image influences our beliefs and reactions
Treatment options	Variety of treatment options available for hearing loss, including hearing aids, cochlear implants, and auditory training
Treatment options for tinnitus	Variety of treatment options available for tinnitus, including coping strategies, relaxation therapy, cognitive behavior therapy, and sound therapies

how the patient learned to react to it, and how the patient can help himself or herself is important. This is a key part of treatments that include aspects of cognitive therapy (see Hallam et al[87]; see also Chapters 3, 4, 9, and 10 in this book), even for young children (see Chapter 11).

Changing Behavior

Sometimes it is possible to change behavior simply by providing information. However, it is usually more effective to practice the desired behavior. Some coping strategies involve changing behavior; others deal with emotional reactions. Providing specific tasks to engage in is part of changing behavior. Chapters 3, 4, 9, and 13 offer numerous examples of engaging the patient in behavior management.

Understanding an Individual Patient's Needs

A broader perspective on tinnitus treatment involves understanding the individual patient, how the person views tinnitus, what support the patient

has, and how tinnitus fits into the bigger picture of the patient's overall life. Listening, as opposed to providing information, is the first step. The Tinnitus Three-Track Tinnitus Protocol, as discussed in Chapter 5, is a wonderful example of this.

1.5.4 Examples of Counseling Treatment Protocols

Several counseling treatment protocols and strategies have been proposed. Most contain some aspect of providing information. Several go beyond that. Tyler and Baker[86] suggest that counseling needs to consider all of the patient's difficulties. They recommend that the major emphasis of counseling address the emotional problems related to tinnitus. Hazell[30] (p. 113) suggests that "it is fruitless and unrealistic to approach the tinnitus in isolation." ▶ Table 1.5 summarizes some of these protocols and strategies.

Cognitive Behavioral Therapy

Cognitive behavioral therapy has been applied to tinnitus for some time, has been discussed in the

Table 1.5 Tinnitus treatment counseling strategies

Tyler and Baker[86] Tyler and Babin[3] Tyler et al[88]	Informational counseling	Providing information Considering emotional problems related to tinnitus
Clark and Yanick[89]	Informational counseling	Understanding individual patient needs
Sweetow[73,74]	Cognitive behavioral therapy	Providing information Sleep Changing attitude and self-esteem Diversionary tactics (attention) Coping strategies Cognitive behavior therapy
Hallam[75]	Habituation therapy	Habituation Attention Relaxation Modifying the environment
Coles[2]	Habituation therapy	Providing information
Coles and Hallam[80]	Habituation therapy	Relaxation Habituation of reaction to tinnitus
Hazell[30]	Masking therapy	Providing information Consideration of all the patient's problems (e.g., business, financial, and domestic) Reassurance Attention Relaxation The use of diaries Modifying the environment
Slater and Terry[55]	Guided therapy	Providing information Attention Activities Habituation Lifestyle changes (being positive and active)
Lindberg et al[90]	Tinnitus behavior therapy	Providing information Coping
Stouffer et al[91]	Informational counseling	Various relaxation procedures Providing information Keeping diaries Changing activities
Jastreboff and Hazell[76]	Retraining therapy	Providing information "Directive" approach
Davis[93]	Living with tinnitus	Providing information Stress management Sleep Changing thinking
McKenna[60]	Habituation therapy	Providing information Habituation Relaxation Reactions to stress Listening to the patient
Henry and Wilson[94,95]	Cognitive behavioral therapy	Providing information Self-help strategies Sleep, depression Attention control Cognitive behavior therapy Relaxation Coping strategies Relapse prevention

(Continued)

Table 1.5 (*Continued*) Tinnitus treatment counseling strategies

Tyler and Erlandsson[96]	Refocus therapy	Three tiers of treatment Attention Engagement in other activities
Tyler et al[97]	Tinnitus Activities Treatment	Group session Individual counseling Thoughts and emotions, hearing, sleep, concentration Hearing aids Sound therapy
Henry et al[98]	Progressive tinnitus Management	Five levels of treatment Triage Audiologic management Group education Tinnitus evaluation Individualized management

literature in great detail, and is arguably the only approach that has been shown to be effective in controlled studies.[99,100,101] Several general concepts are used in many tinnitus counseling protocols, although not always acknowledged. The "providing information" component is intended to change the way individuals think about their tinnitus. The basic premise of cognitive behavioral therapy[94,95,73,74] is the following: Your tinnitus is there. The way that you think about it results in a particular emotional reaction.

Directive Counseling

One approach, directive counseling, or retraining therapy, stands alone, in that it explicitly frowns upon considering individual needs, addressing personal concerns, and providing suggestions for initiating behavioral changes. For example, Jastreboff[102] (p. 291) describes it as a "teaching session": "It is not, and never was, intended to be ... collaborative." Furthermore, it was never intended to "change a patient's perception, attention and emotions towards tinnitus ..., to improve a patient's well-being, everyday life, social interactions and work abilities."

The directive counseling approach prompted some concerns from several clinicians. For example, Wilson et al[103] criticized retraining therapy for its "teaching" approach to counseling, which seemed to disregard standard counseling procedures that include a more interactive approach. Retraining therapy omitted basic principles leading the patient to discover unhelpful thoughts, develop realistic beliefs and attitudes, and modify their emotional response. Kroener-Herwig et al[104] went on to criticize many components of retraining

therapy, one of which was that it "completely neglected" procedures to help the patient modify behavior. They believed that many tinnitus sufferers require more sophisticated strategies than simply teaching information to them. Instead, they felt that some patients should receive intervention programs to change their beliefs about tinnitus, their emotions, and behavior. McKenna[60] questioned the underlying philosophy of Jastreboff's model, noting that its reliance on a classical conditioning perspective ignores the human component of tinnitus. Recent randomized controlled trials of tinnitus retraining therapy (TRT) have found little to no evidence for its effectiveness beyond standard care.[105,106]

1.6 Sound Therapies for Treating Patients' Reactions to Tinnitus

Sound has been used for decades to treat tinnitus (see Searchfield's Chapters 7 and 8). Its role can be understood in terms of:

- Reducing the attention drawn to the tinnitus.
- Reducing the loudness of the tinnitus.
- Substituting a less disruptive noise (background sound) for an unpleasant one (tinnitus).
- Giving the patient some control.[2,107]

Sound therapies include the use of background sound, hearing aids, total masking, partial masking (including retraining therapy), and music therapy. Most of the chapters in this book include sound therapy directly or indirectly. A recent study has documented that sound therapy can indeed help some patients.[108]

1.6.1 Counseling for Sound Therapies

Virtually, all sound therapies are combined with some form of counseling, even if it is just providing information. More typically, in addition to basic information about tinnitus, hearing loss, attention, and habituation, specific counseling is included on the use of sound. This is true whether the sound therapy uses hearing aids or partial masking. Bentler and Tyler,[83] in their discussion of sound therapies, noted that, regardless of the management regimen chosen, counseling needs to be considered an integral component. Coles[2] (p. 395) said that "good counseling will go far toward interrupting the sort of vicious cycles" in addition to the sound therapy. ► Table 1.6 lists some of the topics that are typically covered in counseling for sound therapy.

Occasionally, sound therapies are represented as if they do not include counseling. For example, Henry and Wilson[74] (p. 574) suggest that no specific counseling protocol has been published for partial or total masking. This is at odds with the tinnitus partial masking therapy proposed by Hazell.[30] In Hazell's discussion of masking therapy, detailed counseling strategies are an essential component. In our opinion, no sound therapy should be administered without counseling. Searchfield (Chapter 8) and Perreau et al (Chapter 10) share this perspective.

1.6.2 Use of Hearing Aids

Listening to background sound has been recommended in the treatment of tinnitus for over 50 years.[109] Because most patients with tinnitus also have hearing loss, the use of hearing aids to amplify the background noise is a logical step,[92,110] and many clinicians note the benefit (e.g., Bentler and Tyler[83] and Searchfield et al[111]). Chapter 7 provides an excellent detailed strategy for fitting hearing aids for tinnitus patients.

In the late 1970s and early 1980s, several researchers observed that some patients required high levels of noise to mask the tinnitus, or even could not mask the tinnitus completely. Vernon and Schleuning[110] stressed that the actual level of the noise should be under the control of the patient. Hazell and Wood[113] found that the masking noise can be set so that the patient hears both the masking sound and the tinnitus. They noted

Table 1.6 Components of counseling for sound therapy

Rationale behind the use of background sound
Caution about using noise generators that are too intense; may interfere with speech and everyday sound perception, and may damage hearing
Selecting the type of noise generators
Selecting the ear or ears to receive noise generators
Selecting the ear mold(s) to use, if applicable
Trial periods of the background noise

Sources: After Hazell[30]; Tyler and Bentler.[112]

that the noise provides a distraction that makes patients concentrate less on the tinnitus itself. Other authors reported that the intensity of the tinnitus can be reduced with the use of noise that did not completely mask the tinnitus, or partial masking.

This approach allowed patients to determine the level of noise they could tolerate. Hazell[30] (p. 114) said that the masking sound "is most often effective at an apparent intensity much less than that of the patient's tinnitus."

Partial masking is a term that comes from the psychoacoustic literature, referring to the observation that the loudness of a tone can be reduced in the presence of background noise (e.g., Scharf[114]; ► Table 1.7).

1.6.3 Music Therapy

For many tinnitus sufferers, listening to background music represents a more acceptable and even pleasant alternative to background noise. Slater and Terry[55] found that almost 50% of tinnitus patients they sampled listened to music to help with their tinnitus. We believe that the use of music therapy with tinnitus patients deserves much more attention than it currently gets. The use of background music is recommended by Searchfield in Chapter 8 and by Perreau et al in Chapter 4.

1.6.4 Hyperacusis

Many patients with tinnitus also have hyperacusis.[115] Hazell et al[47] reported that the mean uncomfortable loudness levels in tinnitus patients were 10 to 15 dB lower than in patients with hearing loss without tinnitus (for a review, see Nelting[116]).

The relationship between tinnitus and hyperacusis remains obscure. Loudness is thought to be coded by the number or level of activity of nerve

Table 1.7 Examples of descriptions of partial masking in the literature

Tyler and Babin[3]	"Both the noise and tinnitus are heard, but the tinnitus is reduced in loudness" (p. 3213)
	Patients should "use the lowest level masker that provides adequate relief" (p. 3213)
Coles and Hallam[80]	"A low level background sound against which the loudness of the tinnitus is reduced" (p. 994)
Erlandsson et al[117]	Reduced the noise from the complete masking condition until it was "comfortable enough to listen to" (p. 40)
Hazell[30]	"The masking sound does not completely cover the tinnitus," and it provides a "distracting background sound" (p. 107)
	The "tinnitus tends to 'break through' the masking noise" (p. 112)
Coles[2]	"When the masker is used to provide only a low level of background sound against which the loudness of the tinnitus is reduced" (p. 398)
Tyler and Bentler[112]	"Sometimes a masker can reduce the tinnitus loudness or annoyance, even though the tinnitus remains audible" (p. 55)
	"Partially mask the tinnitus yet produce the lowest SPLs and the least interference with speech" (p. 59)
Bentler and Tyler[83]	"Urge the patient to use the lowest … masker level that provides adequate relief" (p. 30)
Jastreboff and Hazell[118]	"Below the level creating annoyance or discomfort" (p. 210)

fibers. The presence of hyperacusis implies that, for a given intensity, more nerve fibers or a higher rate of activity are produced than would occur normally. Hazell[30] suggested that the central nervous system exerts a "gain control" mechanism to increase peripheral sensitivity affecting outer hair cell activity and tinnitus (see also Jastreboff[19] and Zeng[37]).

Hyperacusis Treatment in Tinnitus Patients

The presence of hyperacusis in tinnitus patients requires some additional counseling and sound therapy considerations, and therefore, this topic is included in Chapter 13. The main difficulty with hyperacusis in the treatment of tinnitus arises because the use of sound therapy can sometimes result in exacerbation of the hyperacusis. Therefore, it is important that clinicians treating tinnitus determine if their patients have hyperacusis and to accommodate this if they are using sound therapy.

Sheldrake et al[85] (cited by Coles[2]) recommended that noise generators be worn for hyperacusis patients for 6 hours per day. The noise should be "audible but comfortable (not necessarily completely masking any tinnitus …)" (p. 399). Sheldrake suggested that hyperacusis patients recovered over a period of a few days to up to 6 months in some cases; many patients gradually regain their tolerance of loud sounds.

1.7 Obstacles to Tinnitus Treatment

1.7.1 Negative Beliefs by Clinicians or Patients

Many clinicians have beliefs that represent obstacles to tinnitus treatment. For example, they believe that:
- They do not have the training.
- They cannot help the patient.
- They will not be reimbursed.

One of the primary purposes of this book is to provide very concrete examples of a variety of treatment strategies. Audiologists, clinical psychologists, and otologists should have the training to implement most of these options. We believe patients can be helped by all the treatments described in this book. Research will eventually determine which are the most helpful and which treatments work best for which patients. Reimbursement should follow studies showing treatment effectiveness; when that happens, more clinicians will make the time to provide tinnitus treatment. It is our job, as clinicians, to show patients how to learn to live with their tinnitus.

Patients also have concepts that are obstacles. They sometimes believe that:
- There is nothing that can be done.
- No one understands their tinnitus.
- Someone, somewhere, has the cure.

Patients who believe nothing can be done to ease the tinnitus often do not seek treatment. This can delay intervention and creates a more problematic case of tinnitus by the time the patient finally seeks help. The beliefs that nothing can be done and that no one understands are distressing to patients. Their crisis deepens, and they may withdraw further. Desperate patients with the financial resources will travel great distances and pay substantial fees if they believe there is hope for them. If they are unsuccessful, this often makes their situation worse. By providing good therapy, measuring clinical effectiveness, and making this information about clinical services public, patients in need will seek help.

Duration and Number of Sessions

The optimal number and duration of treatment sessions will vary across patients. Some patients will require long-term follow-up visits; this should not be viewed as inherently undesirable. For many patients, a simple 5-minute discussion will be sufficient. For others, much longer sessions will be necessary (see Tyler and Erlandsson,[96] for strategies). The clinical psychology literature indicates that most patients will benefit from several short (less than 1 h) visits over several weeks.

Hazell[30] suggested that sound therapy typically requires 2 to 3 months of noise-generator use before any benefit is achieved. Research can be used to determine the optimum treatment duration. This will vary across individuals. The number of sessions and their duration will likely be linked to reimbursement.

Reimbursement

Reimbursement is often available for diagnosing hearing loss and tinnitus. In the United States, there are reimbursement codes for treating central auditory processing disorders and for providing aural rehabilitation. In addition, there are numerous reimbursement codes for providing psychological treatments, including insight-oriented, behavior-modifying, and supportive psychotherapy, interactive psychotherapy, family psychotherapy, biofeedback, behavior modification, and cognitive behavior therapy. These codes are typically used by clinical psychologists and psychiatrists. Research demonstrating clinical effectiveness of tinnitus treatment will facilitate reimbursement.

Psychological Counseling

Flasher and Fogle[79] suggest that audiologists can use basic psychological principles and techniques for which they have knowledge. Clearly, patients who have clinical depression, anxiety disorders, or other psychiatric ailments demand appropriate referrals. This does not mean that audiologists cannot be involved in treating the tinnitus in these cases, however. In our experience, psychiatrists and psychologists often welcome a collaborative effort with an audiologist who has experience in treating tinnitus. Treating tinnitus patients requires a commitment, a plan, and some clinical expertise. You are likely committed if you are reading this book, and if you do not have a plan, this book will offer several options. Clinical expertise comes from training, experience, and certain personal characteristics that can be learned and are often facilitated by personal supervision of real clinical experience. Some of the desirable characteristics are as follows (after Flasher and Fogle;[79] Gladding,[119] and Riley[120]):

- Ability to listen.
- Patience.
- Ability to be encouraging to the patient.
- Ability to talk candidly about depression, anxiety, and other psychological problems.
- Emotional insightfulness.
- Self-awareness.
- Ability to laugh at the bittersweet aspects of life.
- Positive self-esteem.
- Emotional stability.

1.8 Conclusion

Counseling and sound therapy are the fundamental treatments for tinnitus. There are many counseling options, and most include providing information on hearing loss, tinnitus, and attention. We believe that counseling should consider the individual's emotional state. We can learn more from aspects of cognitive and behavioral therapy as they are applied to other problems. A greater emphasis should be placed on improving sleep. Some patients may benefit from systematic therapies covering concentration and relaxation, but these can be offered as optional. The detailed comprehensive therapy plans provided by Henry and Wilson[73,74] are important contributions and supplement the comprehensive therapy protocols of Hallam,[75] Slater and Terry,[55] and Davis.[93] The chapters in this book demonstrate varied approaches to counseling.

Sound therapy, involving wearable and nonwearable devices, should be considered an option. Providing background sound removes some of the annoying characteristics of a piercing tinnitus. Lower levels of partial masking generally are more acceptable. The use of music and other types of nonrandom noise in treating tinnitus should be explored.

To illustrate the experience of patients with tinnitus, this chapter also has two interviews of tinnitus patients, available on the companion website. The interviews describe their reactions to tinnitus, discuss the challenges in having tinnitus, and provide advice for other tinnitus patients.

Acknowledgment

David M. Baguley, Anthony Cacace, Scott Mitchell, Richard Salvi, and Grant D. Searchfield made very helpful suggestions on an earlier draft.

References

[1] McFadden D. Tinnitus: Facts, Theories, and Treatments. Washington, DC: National Academy Press; 1982

[2] Coles RRA. Tinnitus and its management. In: Stephens SDG, Kerr AG, eds. Scott-Brown's Otolaryngology. Guildford, UK: Butterworth; 1987

[3] Tyler RS, Babin RW. Tinnitus. In: Cummings CW, Fredrickson J-M, Harker L, Krause CJ, Schuller DE, eds. Otolaryngology: Head and Neck Surgery. St. Louis, MO: Mosby; 1986:3201–3217

[4] Tyler RS, Aran J-M, Dauman R. Recent advances in tinnitus. Am J Audiol. 1992; 1(4):36–44

[5] Dauman R, Tyler RS. Some considerations on the classification of tinnitus. In: Aran J-M, Dauman R, eds. Proceedings of the Fourth International Tinnitus Seminar. Bordeaux, France: Kugler & Ghedini; 1992:225–229

[6] Hiller W, Goebel G. Factors influencing tinnitus loudness and annoyance. Arch Otolaryngol Head Neck Surg. 2006; 132(12):1323–1330

[7] Hiller W, Goebel G. When tinnitus loudness and annoyance are discrepant: audiological characteristics and psychological profile. Audiol Neurotol. 2007; 12(6):391–400

[8] Stouffer JL, Tyler RS. Characterization of tinnitus by tinnitus patients. J Speech Hear Disord. 1990; 55(3):439–453

[9] Folmer RL, Griest SE, Martin WH. Chronic tinnitus as phantom auditory pain. Otolaryngol Head Neck Surg. 2001; 124(4):394–400

[10] Fowler EP, Fowler EP, Jr. Somatopsychic and psychosomatic factors in tinnitus, deafness and vertigo. Ann Otol Rhinol Laryngol. 1955; 64(1):29–37

[11] Nondahl DM, Cruickshanks KJ, Huang GH, et al. Tinnitus and its risk factors in the Beaver Dam offspring study. Int J Audiol. 2011; 50(5):313–320

[12] Roberts LE. Neural plasticity and its initiating conditions in tinnitus. HNO. 2018; 66(3):172–178

[13] Turrigiano G. Homeostatic synaptic plasticity: local and global mechanisms for stabilizing neuronal function. Cold Spring Harb Perspect Biol. 2012; 4(1):a005736

[14] Sedley W. Tinnitus: does gain explain? Neuroscience. 2019; 407:213–228

[15] Cacace AT. Expanding the biological basis of tinnitus: crossmodal origins and the role of neuroplasticity. Hear Res. 2003; 175(1–2):112–132

[16] Eggermont JJ. Physiological mechanisms and neural models. In: Tyler R, ed. Tinnitus Handbook. San Diego, CA: Singular; 2000

[17] Eggermont JJ, Roberts LE. The neuroscience of tinnitus. Trends Neurosci. 2004; 27(11):676–682

[18] Eggermont JJ, Roberts LE. Tinnitus: animal models and findings in humans. Cell Tissue Res. 2015; 361(1): 311–336

[19] Jastreboff PJ. Phantom auditory perception (tinnitus): mechanisms of generation and perception. Neurosci Res. 1990; 8(4):221–254

[20] Salvi RJ, Lockwood AH, Burkard R. Neural plasticity and tinnitus. In: Tyler R, ed. Tinnitus Handbook. San Diego, CA: Singular; 2000:123–148

[21] Vernon JA, Moeller AR. Mechanisms of Tinnitus. Boston, MA: Allyn & Bacon; 1995

[22] Sedley W, Friston KJ, Gander PE, Kumar S, Griffiths TD. An integrative tinnitus model based on sensory precision. Trends Neurosci. 2016; 39(12):799–812

[23] Tyler RS. Tinnitus. In: Evered D, Lawrenson G, eds. Tinnitus. (Ciba Foundation Symposium 85). London: Pitman; 1981: 136,137

[24] Vanneste S, De Ridder D. The auditory and non-auditory brain areas involved in tinnitus. An emergent property of multiple parallel overlapping subnetworks. Front Syst Neurosci. 2012a; 6:31

[25] Kiang NYS, Moxon EC, Levine RA. Auditory-nerve activity in cats with normal and abnormal cochleas. In: Wolstenholme GEW, ed. Sensorineural Hearing Loss. London: J&A Churchill; 1970:241–273

[26] Eggermont JJ. Tinnitus: some thoughts about its origin. J Laryngol Otol. 1984; 9:31–37

[27] Moeller AR. Pathophysiology of tinnitus. Ann Otol Rhinol Laryngol. 1984; 93(1 Pt 1):39–44

[28] Salvi RJ, Wang J, Powers NL. Plasticity and reorganization in the auditory brainstem: implications for tinnitus. In: Reich GE, Vernon JA, eds. Proceedings of the 5th International Tinnitus Seminar. Portland, OR: American Tinnitus Association; 1996:457–466

[29] Tonndorf J. Stereociliary dysfunction: a case of sensory hearing loss, recruitment, poor speech discrimination and tinnitus. Acta Otolaryngol. 1981; 91(5–6):469–479

[30] Hazell JWP. Tinnitus masking therapy. In: Hazell JWP, ed. Tinnitus. London: Churchill Livingston; 1987:96–117

[31] Penner MJ, Bilger RC. Adaptation and the masking of tinnitus. J Speech Hear Res. 1989; 32(2):339–346

[32] Llinás RR, Ribary U, Jeanmonod D, Kronberg E, Mitra PP. Thalamocortical dysrhythmia: a neurological and neuropsychiatric syndrome characterized by magnetoencephalography. Proc Natl Acad Sci U S A. 1999; 96(26):15222–15227

[33] Noreña AJ, Eggermont JJ. Changes in spontaneous neural activity immediately after an acoustic trauma: implications for neural correlates of tinnitus. Hear Res. 2003; 183(1–2): 137–153

[34] Kaltenbach JA, Zhang J, Zacharek MA. Neural correlates of tinnitus. In: Snow JB, ed. Tinnitus: Theory and Management. London: BC Decker Inc; 2004:141–161

[35] Noreña AJ. An integrative model of tinnitus based on a central gain controlling neural sensitivity. Neurosci Biobehav Rev. 2011; 35(5):1089–1109

[36] Schaette R, McAlpine D. Tinnitus with a normal audiogram: physiological evidence for hidden hearing loss and computational model. J Neurosci. 2011; 31(38):13452–13457

[37] Zeng FG. An active loudness model suggesting tinnitus as increased central noise and hyperacusis as increased nonlinear gain. Hear Res. 2013; 295:172–179

[38] Leaver AM, Renier L, Chevillet MA, Morgan S, Kim HJ, Rauschecker JP. Dysregulation of limbic and auditory networks in tinnitus. Neuron. 2011; 69(1):33–43

[39] Rauschecker JP, May ES, Maudoux A, Ploner M. Frontostriatal gating of tinnitus and chronic pain. Trends Cogn Sci. 2015; 19(10):567–578

[40] Rolls ET. Limbic systems for emotion and for memory, but no single limbic system. Cortex. 2015; 62:119–157

[41] Roberts LE, Husain FT, Eggermont JJ. Role of attention in the generation and modulation of tinnitus. Neurosci Biobehav Rev. 2013; 37(8):1754–1773

[42] De Ridder D, Vanneste S, Weisz N, et al. An integrative model of auditory phantom perception: tinnitus as a unified percept of interacting separable subnetworks. Neurosci Biobehav Rev. 2014; 44:16–32

[43] De Ridder D, Vanneste S, Freeman W. The Bayesian brain: phantom percepts resolve sensory uncertainty. Neurosci Biobehav Rev. 2014; 44:4–15

[44] Goodey R. Tinnitus: When the patient complains of noises in the ear. Patient Management. 1988; 17(9):75–89

[45] Wilson JP. Theory of tinnitus generation. In: Hazell JWP, ed. Tinnitus. London: Churchill Livingstone; 1987:20–45

[46] Hallam RS, Rachman S, Hinchcliffe R. Psychological aspects of tinnitus. In: Rachman S, ed. Contributions to Medical Psychology. Vol. 3. Oxford: Pergamon Press; 1984:31–53

[47] Hazell JWP, Wood SM, Cooper HR, et al. A clinical study of tinnitus maskers. Br J Audiol. 1985; 19(2):65–146

[48] Liberman MC, Dodds LW. Single-neuron labeling and chronic cochlear pathology. III. Stereocilia damage and alterations of threshold tuning curves. Hear Res. 1984; 16(1):55–74

[49] Kujawa SG, Liberman MC. Adding insult to injury: cochlear nerve degeneration after "temporary" noise-induced hearing loss. J Neurosci. 2009; 29(45):14077–14085

[50] House JW, Brackmann DE. Tinnitus: surgical treatment. Ciba Found Symp. 1981; 85:204–216

[51] Tyler RS, Conrad-Armes D. Masking of tinnitus compared to masking of pure tones. J Speech Hear Res. 1984; 27(1):106–111

[52] Cacace AT. The limbic system and tinnitus. In: Snow J, ed. Tinnitus: Theory and Management. Hamilton, Canada: BC Decker; 2004:162–170

[53] Levine RA, Abel M, Cheng H. CNS somatosensory-auditory interactions elicit or modulate tinnitus. Exp Brain Res. 2003; 153(4):643–648

[54] Sanchez TG, Rocha CB. Diagnosis and management of somatosensory tinnitus: review article. Clinics (São Paulo). 2011; 66(6):1089–1094

[55] Slater R, Terry M. Tinnitus: A Guide for Sufferers and Professionals. London: Croom Helm; 1987

[56] LeDoux J. Emotion, Memory, and the Brain. New York: Simon & Schuster; 1994

[57] Mega MS, Cummings JL, Salloway S, Malloy P. The limbic system: an anatomic, phylogenetic, and clinical perspective. J Neuropsychiatry Clin Neurosci. 1997; 9(3):315–330

[58] Husain FT. Neural networks of tinnitus in humans: elucidating severity and habituation. Hear Res. 2016; 334:37–48

[59] Jastreboff PJ. Tinnitus habituation therapy (THT) and tinnitus retraining therapy (TRT). In: Tyler RS, ed. Handbook of Tinnitus. San Diego, CA: Singular; 2000:357–376

[60] McKenna L. Models of tinnitus suffering and treatment compared and contrasted. Audiol Med. 2004; 2:1–14

[61] Elgandy MS, Tyler RS, Coelho C. Help! Our tinnitus patients want a drug? SJO. 2019. DOI: 10.32474/SJO.2019.000147

[62] Murai K, Tyler RS, Harker LA, Stouffer JL. Review of pharmacologic treatment of tinnitus. Am J Otol. 1992; 13(5):454–464

[63] Dauman R. Electrical stimulation for tinnitus suppression. In: Tyler RS, ed. Tinnitus Handbook. San Diego: Singular; 2000:377–398

[64] Dobie RA, Hoberg KE, Rees TS. Electrical tinnitus suppression: a double-blind crossover study. Otolaryngol Head Neck Surg. 1986; 95(3 Pt 1):319–323

[65] Elgandy MS, Tyler R, Dunn C, Hansen M, Gantz B. A unilateral cochlear implant for tinnitus. Int Tinnitus J. 2018; 22:128–132

[66] Hazell JWP, Jastreboff PJ, Meerton LE, Conway MJ. Electrical tinnitus suppression: frequency dependence of effects. Audiology. 1993; 32(1):68–77

[67] Quaranta N, Wagstaff S, Baguley DM. Tinnitus and cochlear implantation. Int J Audiol. 2004; 43(5):245–251

[68] Rubinstein JT, Tyler RS. Electrical suppression of tinnitus. In: Snow J, ed. Tinnitus: Theory and Management. Hamilton, Canada: BC Decker; 2004:326–335

[69] Tyler RS, Owen RL, Bridges J, Gander PE, Perreau A, Mancini PC. Tinnitus suppression in cochlear implant patients using a sound therapy app. Am J Audiol. 2018; 27(3):316–323

[70] Zwolan TA, Kileny PR, Souliere CR, Kemink JL. Tinnitus suppression following cochlear implantation. In: Aran J-M, Dauman R, eds. Tinnitus 91: Proceedings of the Fourth International Tinnitus Seminar. Amsterdam: Kugler; 1992: 423–426

[71] Peter N, Kleinjung T. Neuromodulation for tinnitus treatment: an overview of invasive and non-invasive techniques. J Zhejiang Univ Sci B. 2019; 20(2):116–130

[72] Vanneste S, De Ridder D. Noninvasive and invasive neuromodulation for the treatment of tinnitus: an overview. Neuromodulation. 2012b; 15(4):350–360

[73] Sweetow RW. Cognitive-behavioral modification in tinnitus management. Hearing Instruments. 1984; 35:14–52

[74] Sweetow RW. Cognitive aspects of tinnitus patient management. Ear Hear. 1986; 7(6):390–396

[75] Hallam RS. Tinnitus: Living with the Ringing in Your Ears. New York: HarperCollins; 1989

[76] Jastreboff PJ, Hazell JWP. A neurophysiological approach to tinnitus: clinical implications. Br J Audiol. 1993; 27(1):7–17

[77] Mohr AM. Reflections on tinnitus by an existential psychologist. Audiol Med. 2008; 6:73–77

[78] Mohr AM, Hedelund U. Tinnitus person-centred therapy. In: Tyler RS, ed. Tinnitus Treatment: Clinical Protocols. New York: Thieme; 2006:198–216

[79] Flasher LV, Fogle T. Counseling Skills for Speech-Language Pathologists and Audiologists. Clifton Park, NY: Thomson/Delmar Learning; 2004

[80] Coles RRA, Hallam RS. Tinnitus and its management. Br Med Bull. 1987; 43(4):983–998

[81] Tyler RS, Haskell G, Preece J, Bergan C. Nurturing patient expectations to enhance the treatment of tinnitus. Semin Hear. 2001; 22:15–21

[82] Tyler RS, Bergan C. Tinnitus retraining therapy: a modified approach. Hear J. 2001; 54(11):36–42

[83] Bentler RA, Tyler RS. Tinnitus management. ASHA. 1987; 29 (5):27–32

[84] LaMarte FP, Tyler RS. Noise-induced tinnitus. AAOHN J. 1987; 35(9):403–406

[85] Sheldrake JB, Wood SM, Cooper HR. Practical aspects of the instrumental management of tinnitus. Br J Audiol. 1985; 19 (2):147–150

[86] Tyler RS, Baker LJ. Difficulties experienced by tinnitus sufferers. J Speech Hear Disord. 1983; 48(2):150–154

[87] Hallam RS, Jakes SC, Hinchcliffe R. Cognitive variables in tinnitus annoyance. Br J Clin Psychol. 1988; 27(3):213–222

[88] Tyler RS, Stouffer JL, Schum R. Audiological rehabilitation of the tinnitus client. J Acad Rehabilitative Audiol. 1989; 22: 30–42

[89] Clark JG, Yanick P. Tinnitus and Its Management. Springfield, IL: Charles C Thomas; 1984

[90] Lindberg P, Scott B, Melin L, Lyttkens L. Behavioural therapy in the clinical management of tinnitus. Br J Audiol. 1988; 22 (4):265–272

[91] Stouffer JL, Tyler RS, Kileny PR, Dalzell LE. Tinnitus as a function of duration and etiology: counselling implications. Am J Otol. 1991; 12(3):188–194

[92] Johnson RM, Goodwin P. The use of audiometric tests in the management of the tinnitus patient. J Laryngol Otol Suppl. 1981; (4):48–51

[93] Davis P. Living with Tinnitus. Woolahra, Australia: Gore & Osment; 1995

[94] Henry JL, Wilson PH. The Psychological Management of Chronic Tinnitus: A Cognitive-Behavioral Approach. Boston, MA: Allyn & Bacon; 2001

[95] Henry JL, Wilson PH. Tinnitus: A Self-Management Guide for the Ringing in Your Ears. Boston, MA: Allyn & Bacon; 2002

[96] Tyler RS, Erlandsson S. Management of the tinnitus patient. In: Luxon LM, Furman JM, Martini A, Stephens D, eds. Textbook of Audiological Medicine. Oxford: Isis; 2000:571–578

[97] Tyler RS, Gogel SA, Gehringer AK. Tinnitus activities treatment. Prog Brain Res. 2007; 166:425–434

[98] Henry JA, Zaugg TL, Myers PJ, Schechter MA. The role of audiologic evaluation in progressive audiologic tinnitus management. Trends Amplif. 2008; 12(3):170–187

[99] Andersson G, Lyttkens L. A meta-analytic review of psychological treatments for tinnitus. Br J Audiol. 1999; 33 (4):201–210

[100] Dobie RA. A review of randomized clinical trials in tinnitus. Laryngoscope. 1999; 109(8):1202–1211

[101] Tunkel DE, Bauer CA, Sun GH, et al. Clinical practice guideline: tinnitus. Otolaryngol Head Neck Surg. 2014; 151 (2) Suppl:S1–S40

[102] Jastreboff MM. Controversies between cognitive therapies and TRT counseling. In: Hazell J, ed. Proceedings of the Sixth International Tinnitus Seminar. London: THC; 1999:288–291

[103] Wilson PH, Henry JL, Andersson G, Hallam RS, Lindberg P. A critical analysis of directive counselling as a component of tinnitus retraining therapy. Br J Audiol. 1998; 32(5): 273–286

[104] Kroener-Herwig B, Biesinger E, Gerhards F, Goebel G, Verena Greimel K, Hiller W. Retraining therapy for chronic tinnitus: a critical analysis of its status. Scand Audiol. 2000; 29(2):67–78

[105] Bauer CA, Berry JL, Brozoski TJ. The effect of tinnitus retraining therapy on chronic tinnitus: a controlled trial. Laryngoscope Investig Otolaryngol. 2017; 2(4):166–177

[106] Scherer RW, Formby C, Tinnitus Retraining Therapy Trial Research Group. Effect of tinnitus retraining therapy vs standard of care on tinnitus-related quality of life: a randomized clinical trial. JAMA Otolaryngol Head Neck Surg. 2019; 145(7):597–608

[107] Vernon J. Attemps to relieve tinnitus. J Am Audiol Soc. 1977; 2(4):124–131

[108] Tyler RS, Perreau A, Powers T, et al. Tinnitus sound therapy trial shows effectiveness for those with tinnitus. J Am Acad Audiol. 2020; 31(1):6–16

[109] Goodhill V. The management of tinnitus. Laryngoscope. 1950; 60(5):442–450

[110] Vernon J, Schleuning A. Tinnitus: a new management. Laryngoscope. 1978; 88(3):413–419

[111] Searchfield GD, Kaur M, Martin WH. Hearing aids as an adjunct to counseling: tinnitus patients who choose amplification do better than those that don't. Int J Audiol. 2010; 49(8):574–579

[112] Tyler RS, Bentler RA. Tinnitus maskers and hearing aids for tinnitus. Semin Hear. 1987; 8(1):49–61

[113] Hazell JWP, Wood S. Tinnitus masking: a significant contribution to tinnitus management. Br J Audiol. 1981; 15 (4):223–230

[114] Scharf B. Fundamentals of auditory masking. Audiology. 1971; 10(1):30–40

[115] Tyler RS, Conrad-Armes D. The determination of tinnitus loudness considering the effects of recruitment. J Speech Hear Res. 1983; 26(1):59–72

[116] Nelting M, ed. Hyperakusis. Stuttgart: Georg Thieme Verlag; 2003

[117] Erlandsson S, Ringdahl A, Hutchins T, Carlsson SG. Treatment of tinnitus: a controlled comparison of masking and placebo. Br J Audiol. 1987; 21(1):37–44

[118] Jastreboff PJ, Hazell JWP. Tinnitus Retraining Therapy: Implementing the Neurophysiological Model. New York: Cambridge University Press; 2004

[119] Gladding S. Conseling: A Comprehensive Profession. Upper Saddle River, NJ: Prentice Hall; 2000

[120] Riley J. Counseling: an approach for speech-language pathologists. Contemporary Issues in Communication Sci Disorders. 2002; 29:6–16

[121] Zimmerman BJ, Abraham I, Schmidt SA, Baryshnikov Y, Husain FT. Dissociating tinnitus patients from healthy controls using resting-state cyclicity analysis and clustering. Netw Neurosci. 2018; 3(1):67–89

Appendix 1.1 Tinnitus

Definition and Causes

Tinnitus is a symptom that occurs when you perceive sounds that originate in your head. It is usually accompanied by sensorineural hearing loss. Many people report that their tinnitus sounds like ringing, crickets, or buzzing, but tinnitus can also sound like many different things. The mechanisms that produce tinnitus are not well understood. Anything that causes hearing loss can cause tinnitus, including noise exposure, aging, trauma, and medications.

Prevalence

Approximately 1 person in every 10 has tinnitus. About 1 person in 200 has a very bothersome tinnitus that interferes with their ability to lead a normal life. In about 75% of patients, tinnitus remains the same throughout their life. In about 10% of the patients, the tinnitus gets worse and in about 15%, it improves over time. Most patients learn to adjust to it.

Reactions

People react very differently to their tinnitus. Some find it a little bothersome, but largely ignore it. Others are distressed by their tinnitus and have difficulty concentrating and getting to sleep.

Hyperacusis

Many tinnitus patients find moderately intense sounds very uncomfortable. When present, this "hyperacusis" should be treated with the tinnitus. Treatment usually involves desensitization.

Measurement

Tinnitus can be measured by determining the frequency and level of a tone that has the same pitch and loudness of the tinnitus. In most patients, it is also possible to mask the tinnitus with noise or tones. The amount of noise required to mask the tinnitus can be measured.

Questionnaires

There are now several standardized questionnaires designed to measure the handicapping nature of tinnitus. The patient answers questions like, "Does tinnitus interfere with your ability to talk with someone?"

Treatments

Tinnitus can be a symptom of some other illness. First, have a complete medical examination to determine if you can be treated medically or surgically. There is no magic pill that has been shown to be effective in controlled studies for a large proportion of tinnitus patients. However, there are several treatments that can help people cope with their tinnitus. These include the following.

Psychological Therapies

Cognitive Behavior Modification: This approach helps you to talk about tinnitus in a reasonable fashion, and to plan and carry out trials to change the way you think about and react to tinnitus.

Relaxation Therapy: There are many techniques, for example, using recorded soft music or biofeedback, which can help patients relax when they are particularly bothered by their tinnitus.

Medications

Although medications generally do not cure tinnitus, they can be helpful to reduce stress and facilitate sleep.

Hearing Aids

Most patients with tinnitus also have a hearing loss and may benefit from a hearing aid. Easier communication reduces stress, which could reduce tinnitus. Hearing aids also amplify background noise, and many tinnitus patients report that their tinnitus is better when they listen to low levels of background sound.

Sound Therapy

Most patients report that the presence of background noise or music is helpful.
These sounds can:
- Mask (cover up) the tinnitus.
- Reduce its loudness (while still hearing the tinnitus).
- Distract the patient from attending to the tinnitus.

The types of sound used in Sound Therapy include:

- Broadband noise (heard as "sssshhhh"). Many patients report that it is easier to listen to the noise than it is to listen to their tinnitus.
- Music; usually soft, light, background music (e.g., classical baroque, simple piano music).
- Sound produced particularly for relaxation or distraction (e.g., waves lapping against the shore, raindrops falling on leaves—sometimes these are combined with light music).

There are several different devices that produce these sounds:

- Wearable devices that resemble hearing aid(s).
- Wearable devices with earphones or insert earphones (IPODs or MP3 players).
- Nonwearable devices that include radios, Apps on an IPAD or tablet, or sound generators specifically produced for relaxation or tinnitus. Some devices include different sounds to choose from and many models feature a timer, which can be useful when used at bedside.

Sound therapy does not have to be used all the time. It is possible to obtain a noise generator and a hearing aid in the same wearable device.

Habituation or Retraining Therapy

The brain naturally habituates to sounds that are unimportant. For example, within seconds of entering a room, our brain ignores a noisy refrigerator. Retraining therapy combines counseling and habituation to reduce your fear of tinnitus and structure your environment to ensure that you are frequently in the presence of low levels of background noise. Wearable noise generators may be necessary.

Refocus Therapy

Many patients focus their attention on their tinnitus. They think about their tinnitus much of the day. The more they think about their tinnitus, the worse it gets. The worse it gets, the more they think about it.

Refocus therapy helps you to focus your attention on things in life that you enjoy. It is important to keep yourself busy. Focus your attention on things in life that you enjoy. Try to put tinnitus in the back of your mind.

General Recommendations

- Have a medical examination to be certain that there is no medical treatment for your tinnitus.
- Use hearing protection whenever you are in the presence of intense noise.
- If you are having difficulty communicating, you should use a hearing aid or hearing aids.
- If you are annoyed by loud sounds, this may be related to your tinnitus and you should consider desensitization therapy.
- Try using low-level background sound to reduce the prominence of your tinnitus.
- Try to refocus your attention away from your tinnitus and on something that you enjoy and that occupies your mind.
- If this is not sufficient, consider psychological therapies, medications, sound therapy, retraining therapy, and refocus therapy. Contact an audiologist, otologist, or psychologist who has experience with tinnitus patients.
- Join the American Tinnitus Association for support and information at:
- P.O. Box 424049, Washington, DC 20042–4049
- website: http://www.ata.org

2 Treating Tinnitus in Patients with Otologic Conditions

David M. Baguley and Manohar L. Bance

Abstract

The therapeutic approach required in patients with troublesome tinnitus that is associated with otologic disease is rather different to that for those in whom no pathology can be identified. In this chapter, we consider this issue, using worked examples of Meniere's disease, vestibular schwannoma, sudden sensorineural hearing loss, and middle ear myoclonus. The need for a multidisciplinary team approach is described.

Keywords: tinnitus, otologic, Meniere's vestibular schwannoma

There are guidelines for the treatment of tinnitus in use around the world,[1,2] but little attention is given to the associated otologic disease states, and the treatment of the underlying conditions. In this chapter, we share our perspective on treating patients with tinnitus in whom otologic pathology has been diagnosed, and assert that the tinnitus therapy must be interleaved with treatment of the causative condition. This is of particular importance where the treatment itself may exacerbate tinnitus. For example, the treatment of Meniere's disease with gentamicin ablation therapy carries a risk of both increased hearing loss and more intense tinnitus, as does the translabyrinthine removal of a vestibular schwannoma. When tinnitus treatment is integrated within the overall treatment plan, the overall likelihood of success is increased.

Also implicit within this model is the idea of a multidisciplinary team. The utility of surgical teamwork and collaboration is well established within neuro-otology, but in the case of tinnitus therapy, the medical/surgical team must expand to include the tinnitus therapist, of whichever discipline.[3] The perspectives brought by each individual from his or her own discipline will be invaluable, and it is in such multidisciplinary collaborative models that hope lies for new and effective treatments of tinnitus.[4]

Tinnitus treatment protocols in four specific otologic conditions are described: Meniere's disease, vestibular schwannoma, unilateral sudden sensorineural hearing loss, and middle ear myoclonus. Additional reflection upon tinnitus associated with diagnosis of semicircular canal dehiscence, and benign intracranial hypertension is also undertaken.

Although the treatment approaches to patients with these conditions are described in specific detail, there are insights that will assist the reader in treating patients with other otologic conditions with which tinnitus is associated. These may include otosclerosis, glomus tumors, and conductive hearing loss.

2.1 Treating Tinnitus in Patients with Meniere's Disease

Meniere's disease is defined by the triad of idiopathic recurrent vertigo lasting for minutes to hours associated with tinnitus and hearing loss in the affected ear,[5,6,14] although aural fullness and recruitment for loud sounds is often present as well. Although initially tinnitus may occur only with attacks, and is often low pitched, roaring, buzzing, or ocean-like, later as hearing declines, the tinnitus is often present all the time. The reported incidence of Meniere's disease is highly variable, with estimates of between 4.3 and 100 per 100,000 people; it affects women and men roughly equally, and presents in the fourth decade most often.[5,8] It can often be bilateral, again with very variable estimates from 2 to 73%.[9]

There are some indications that patients with Meniere's disease have specific tinnitus experiences. Stouffer and Tyler[58] noted that patients with Meniere's disease had significantly higher ratings of tinnitus severity and annoyance than patients with other tinnitus etiologies. Douek and Reid[11] found that Meniere's disease patients consistently matched their tinnitus to a low-frequency tone (usually in the range 125–250 Hz), unlike the majority of tinnitus patients, who match tinnitus to a pitch above 3000 Hz.[61] Erlandsson et al[13] noted that those patients with anxiety and depression associated with Meniere's disease found their tinnitus intolerable. The finding that patients with Meniere's disease consider the impact of their symptoms more severe if they are anxious or depressed will not surprise those clinicians who see such patients, and a screen for treatable anxiety or depression, such as the Hospital Anxiety and

Depression Scale (HADS[69]), should be considered. A therapeutic strategy for tinnitus in Meniere's disease should account for these specific issues. The combination of tinnitus and hearing loss should cause the clinician to consider amplification, with a prescription that is mindful of both potential hearing fluctuation and the sometimes marked loudness recruitment. Although the hearing loss will be unilateral in the majority of cases, and thus, may not fall within some traditional amplification protocols, there is qualitative and quantitative evidence that mild unilateral hearing loss may be associated with hearing handicap.[15,16]

Medical and surgical treatments for Meniere's disease primarily are targeted at controlling the vertigo, and may have a risk of exacerbating tinnitus and hearing loss. Vestibular nerve section has been demonstrated to remove input from a labyrinth with Meniere's disease. The ablation of the medial efferent auditory input to a cochlea when the inferior vestibular nerve is sectioned, containing medial efferent fibers,[17] which then join the cochlear nerve at the anastomosis of Oort,[18] has a hypothetical risk to frequency selectivity and to the coding of tinnitus intensity by the efferent system. Scharf et al[19] found, however, that the performance of 16 patients on psychoacoustic testing was not degraded following vestibular nerve section. Baguley et al[20] have reviewed the effect of vestibular nerve section on tinnitus and found that tinnitus remains at preoperative levels or improves in the majority of patients.

Medications used for Meniere's disease such as betahistine or diuretics are not ototoxic at doses used for this indication. However, almost all medications can have tinnitus as a side effect, if only there is exacerbated anxiety about side effects or sleep disturbance. Perhaps the most widely used invasive intervention is the use of intratympanic steroids.[21] Although these steroids are not ototoxic, the risk of perforation to the tympanic membrane, albeit low, can result in a mild conductive hearing loss, exacerbating tinnitus. Another common alternative is the use of intratympanic gentamicin to perform a chemical labyrinthectomy for vertigo control. Reports of the effect of this procedure on tinnitus are variable. Several authors have reported that tinnitus may improve or even abate after treatment using intratympanic delivery of gentamicin,[22,23] but because the procedure involves a potential risk to cochlear function,[24] one should be mindful of the possibility of tinnitus exacerbation.

A note of caution is offered by Vernon et al[25] who reported that following the successful control of vertigo, some patients with Meniere's disease focus more on their tinnitus, and hence are more distressed by the tinnitus. This provides supporting evidence for the approach described herein, where tinnitus therapy is coincident with interventions for the vestibular and hearing symptoms of Meniere's disease.

2.1.1 Treatment Protocol

There are several elements of tinnitus treatment specific to patients with Meniere's disease, addressing the issues just described, as summarized in ▸ Table 2.1.

Association with Vertigo

In many patients, increased tinnitus may be an element of the prodrome to an attack of vertigo. As such, the strong association of tinnitus with disabling rotary vertigo can be a factor in the persistence of distress and needs to be addressed in counseling. Medical or surgical treatment may reduce the incidence and severity of such attacks, but the psychological association with tinnitus may well persist beyond the physical link. As already mentioned, an observation has been made that when vertigo resolves, tinnitus may apparently worsen.[25] As such, a patient with Meniere's disease who is vertigo free may be in urgent need of intervention for tinnitus.

Table 2.1 Elements specific to tinnitus treatment in Meniere's disease

Specific therapy	When undertaken?
Counseling regarding association between tinnitus and debilitating vertigo	Ongoing
Hearing aid prescription with multiple programs	Second session if appropriate
Relaxation therapy	Second/third session as appropriate
Onward referral for anxiety and/or depression	As indicated by HADS score
Hearing rehabilitation (speech reading, hearing tactics, auditory training)	Ongoing
Abbreviation: HADS, Hospital Anxiety and Depression Scale.	

Sound Therapy and Fluctuating Hearing Loss

The hearing loss associated with Meniere's disease is typically unilateral and low frequency, and as such, is not commonly associated with a significant impact on daily functions. It does, however, have significant consequences for the use of sound therapy for tinnitus. If a noise generator is to be used, one should be mindful of the fact that the lower frequency element of the noise will be attenuated in the perception of the patient, and that this may well be the frequency region where the tinnitus is matched. As such, the fitting of a device that produces sufficient energy in the low frequencies to be effective in reducing the starkness of the tinnitus is indicated. A multiprogram device, with one program producing more low-frequency noise, also may be helpful.

More commonly undertaken in our clinic is the unilateral fitting of a multiple memory hearing aid or patients with unilateral Meniere's disease. Amplification is almost always essential in bilateral Meniere's disease. The hearing aids fitted should be carefully programmed to the most usual audiometric configuration, and one should be mindful of the need to use appropriate compression in these patients who are likely to experience recruitment. Where there is evidence of threshold fluctuation, programs within the aid should be utilized to meet amplification needs at times of exacerbation or improvement in hearing, and the patient should be carefully instructed on their use. In addition, instruction in speech reading, hearing and communication strategies, and auditory training may be indicated.

Stress, Tinnitus, and Meniere's Disease

The relationships between stress, tinnitus, and Meniere's disease are complex and require some skill on the behalf of the clinician for any given individual.[5] Careful history taking in this regard is essential. Although progressive muscle relaxation therapy has a role, a proportion of patients may need to use biofeedback to facilitate learning to reduce chronic sympathetic autonomic arousal. In addition, sleep hygiene tactics may be introduced as an element of relaxation therapy.[26]

Onward Referral for Depression and Anxiety

Given the well-established incidence of stress and anxiety in the Meniere's disease population, there is the possibility that these symptoms may be evident in the history taken in the tinnitus clinic and may also have an association with tinnitus. Careful use of a screening tool such as the HADS[27,69] may be useful with tinnitus patients.[28,29]

2.2 Treating Tinnitus in Patients with a Vestibular Schwannoma

Vestibular schwannoma, sometimes mislabeled as acoustic neuroma, is a benign neoplasm on the vestibular nerve. Its incidence is approximately 1 to 2/100,000.[30] It can be bilateral in conditions such as neurofibromatosis type 2 (NF2) (▶ Fig. 2.1).

Tinnitus is a common symptom reported in patients diagnosed with vestibular schwannoma, having been stated as being present in 73% of cases ($n = 473$)[31] and being the principal presenting symptom in 11%. There are several hypotheses regarding the generation of tinnitus by this benign tumor arising from the vestibular nerve: the first hypothesis is ephaptic coupling (cross-talk of fibers within a compressed cochlear nerve[32]). This cochlear lesion is due to ischemia caused by the tumor compromising blood flow in the labyrinthine artery, which runs through the internal auditory canal, or by biochemical degradation of the cochlea.[33] The second hypothesis relates to the potential dysfunction of the medial auditory efferent pathway within the inferior vestibular nerve due to compression in the internal auditory

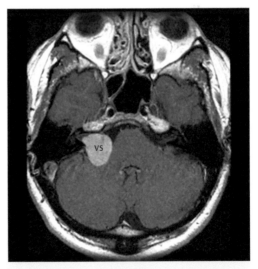

Fig. 2.1 Vestibular schwannoma (VS) on right side.

canal.[34] Intriguingly, in many cases, the tinnitus persists after surgical removal of the tumor[34] and is persistently present in 83% of patients undergoing surgical removal.[35] Reports indicate that this postoperative tinnitus is severe in a proportion of cases ranging from 2.5%[36] to 6%,[37] although in a web-based survey, 27% of 143 participants indicated that postoperative tinnitus was "a very big problem."

As with preoperative tinnitus, the mechanism of postoperative tinnitus remains unclear. Of the hypotheses mentioned earlier, ephaptic coupling could also be applied to the postoperative situation because cross-talk has been demonstrated in damaged peripheral nerves.[38] Tumor removal necessitates section of the inferior and superior vestibular nerves, and thus, efferent dysfunction will result due to the ablation of efferent fibers within the inferior vestibular nerve. However, an argument against this representing a significant factor in tinnitus persistence is found in studies that indicate that patients undergoing successful hearing preservation surgery to remove a vestibular schwannoma are less likely to have postoperative tinnitus than those undergoing translabyrinthine surgery.[39] When such hearing preservation surgery is successful, cochlear nerve function in theory is preserved, though there may be a slight effect on hearing. Of course, the vestibular nerve is sectioned (and thus, efferent input ablated) once the tumor is removed.

Treatment of a vestibular schwannoma with stereotactic radiosurgery is an alternative to traditional surgery. Scant attention has been paid to the impact upon tinnitus, with some reviews not mentioning tinnitus at all (e.g., Mahboubi et al[40]). Hebb et al[41] reported that tinnitus handicap reduced in a cohort of patients with a vestibular schwannoma undergoing stereotactic radiosurgery, but did not report the extent of that improvement.

Although previous studies have demonstrated that severely distressing tinnitus is not common following vestibular schwannoma treatment,[41] there are indications[42] that patients with severe and distressing tinnitus preoperatively may choose to begin tinnitus therapy while awaiting surgery (or is enrolled in a watch, wait, and rescan program), in the knowledge that tinnitus persists for such patients. There is evidence that intense or intrusive preoperative tinnitus may be more likely to be troublesome postoperatively.[43] It may be, however, that after diagnosis and discussion as to the intended surgical or other treatment of the tumor, the patient is able to cope better knowing

the cause of the tinnitus; the flip side is that the tinnitus could be exacerbated.

The use of questionnaires such as the Tinnitus Handicap Inventory[44,45] or the Tinnitus Functional Index[46] at diagnosis would allow the therapist to identify those patients in whom the tinnitus symptom is associated with significant distress and justifies therapy.[47] In those patients in whom preoperative tinnitus abates (15–18% of patients undergoing translabyrinthine removal[37,36]), this therapy will have made the wait for surgery more bearable. In those patients in whom the tinnitus persists, such therapy will facilitate habituation to tinnitus in the postoperative period. We should also be mindful of patients who do not experience tinnitus preoperatively, but might report tinnitus following surgery (27–35%[37,36]). These patients should undergo careful counseling about the possibility of tinnitus postsurgery to lessen fears if it does emerge after surgery.

2.2.1 Treatment Protocols

In this protocol, patients with vestibular schwannoma and troublesome tinnitus will receive a consultation in the tinnitus clinic after treatment in the neuro-otology clinic, and tinnitus has been identified as a problem. Treatment elements specific to patients with a vestibular schwannoma and tinnitus are summarized in ▶ Table 2.2.

Information about Mechanisms

Even if information about tinnitus is given to patients diagnosed with a vestibular schwannoma, few patients seem to be able to assimilate it. This result is not surprising, given the impact of tumor diagnosis and a possible neurosurgical procedure pending. There is an opportunity to inform patients reporting tinnitus about the mechanisms that may be implicated in having tinnitus associated with a vestibular schwannoma, which may occur either pre- or postoperatively, or as part of a watch, wait, and rescan program.

Preoperatively, and in the watch, wait, and rescan group, this can include discussion of cochlear involvement (either by ischemia or biochemical degradation) and, postoperatively using phantom limb analogies. These mechanisms are briefly reviewed above and in detail elsewhere.[34] Patients with gaze-modulated tinnitus may find explanation of this phenomenon particularly beneficial, although one must acknowledge that there are many unanswered questions.

Table 2.2 Elements specific to tinnitus treatment in vestibular schwannoma

Specific therapy	When undertaken?
Counseling regarding the association between the tinnitus and vestibular schwannoma, and any treatment	Within 1 month postdiagnosis, and posttreatment (when undertaken)
Hearing aid prescription, considering CROS, BiCROS, transcranial CROS, or contralateral BAHA	Patient preference for timing and strategy
Relaxation therapy (progressive muscle relaxation)	First session
Onward referral for anxiety and/or depression	As indicated by HADS score
Hearing rehabilitation (speech reading, hearing tactics, auditory training)	Ongoing

Abbreviations: BAHA, bone-anchored hearing aid; BICROS, bilateral contralateral routing of sound; CROS, contralateral routing of signal; HADS, Hospital Anxiety and Depression Scale.

Watch, Wait, and Rescan

With the increased popularity of the watch, wait, and rescan strategy,[48] specific consideration should be given to tinnitus and the need for timely therapy. There is a tendency for such patients not to be considered for tinnitus treatment (nor indeed for auditory or vestibular rehabilitation), though this may be very beneficial. Tinnitus has been identified as a factor in reduced quality of life in patients with a conservatively managed vestibular schwannoma.[49] Of specific note is that some patients in the watch, wait, and rescan group become very concerned about the changes (e.g., pitch and loudness) noticed in their tinnitus, fearing that this may signal a sudden growth in tumor volume. More frequent monitoring of the tumor using magnetic resonance imaging is indicated in such situations.

Sound Enrichment Is Contraindicated

Patients who undergo a translabyrinthine removal of a vestibular schwannoma, or indeed a failed hearing preservation approach, have a permanent unilateral, profound, sensorineural hearing loss. As such, the often used strategy of sound enrichment from a source of low-level, continuous background noise is contraindicated because such patients will find it markedly harder to discriminate any other sound against that background. This exacerbation of hearing handicap should be avoided. In addition, in some patients, sound exposure in the contralateral (good) ear may exacerbate tinnitus.[50]

Postoperative Hyperacusis

It has been noted anecdotally that patients who undergo vestibular schwannoma removal in which hearing is sacrificed in the tumor ear may experience hyperacusis in the contralateral ear in the immediate postoperative period, which then resolves. This has not been empirically verified, and indeed this would be problematic to accomplish, but an explanation may be helpful for some patients. A reasonable discussion would involve the effect on the auditory system of sudden deafferentation, and of the efferent pathways that may then be adversely affected. CROS (contralateral routing of signal), BICROS (bilateral contralateral routing of sound), Transcranial CROS, and contralateral BAHA (bone-anchored hearing aid) hearing aid devices offer the possibility of some awareness of sound presented to an ear with significant hearing loss. Detailed protocols for the fitting of such devices are readily available (see Dillon[51]). Little evidence is available regarding the efficacy of such devices in the vestibular schwannoma patient group, though evidence is emerging that benefit may be achieved with the use of a contralateral bone-anchored hearing aid in speech recognition in some tasks.[52,53,54,55] Even less evidence is available regarding the effect of such devices on tinnitus. Given the phantom limb analogy with tinnitus following vestibular schwannoma removal, it is possible that providing sound input that appears to derive from an ear with severe to profound hearing loss may reduce tinnitus. The potential analogy being that a visual input appearing to derive from a phantom hand reduces phantom pain.[57] Further work is needed in this area, but a trial of CROS devices in such patients may be cautiously attempted.

In NF2 patients and in patients with a unilateral vestibular schwannoma with severe tinnitus, an emerging option is the use of cochlear implants with the vestibular schwannoma still in place that can be used to help suppress the tinnitus with sound input.[58]

2.3 Treating Tinnitus in Patients with Unilateral Sudden Sensorineural Hearing Loss

A sudden sensorineural hearing loss is considered to be an otologic emergency[56,57] to preserve hearing, and necessitates urgent investigation and treatment particularly when steroids are used orally or intratymanically.[60,61] Also, the clinician must consider imaging to rule out an underlying vestibular schwannoma as the cause of the sudden hearing loss. The vast majority are idiopathic, but unilateral sudden hearing loss can also arise from barotrauma (e.g., diving, flying, and blowing nose), head trauma, surgical trauma, blast injury, or ototoxic damage as might follow from chemotherapy. However, little attention has been paid to the consequence to daily functions when patients experience a sudden sensorineural hearing loss.

The perceived hearing handicap of patients with unilateral hearing loss has been considered.[16] A series of 43 patients with unilaterally normal hearing completed the Hearing Handicap Inventory for Adults.[62] It was noted that almost three-quarters (73%) reported mild or greater hearing handicap, which was indicative of "communication and psychosocial problems," despite the normal contralateral ear. The patients were recruited from otolaryngology outpatients, but it was not recorded how long the patients had experienced the unilateral hearing loss, or if the loss had been gradual or sudden. It might be expected that the sudden and possibly traumatic onset of a unilateral hearing loss involves more handicap than a loss of insidious onset. Another study[63] investigated the tinnitus handicap associated with sudden sensorineural hearing loss in a group of patients utilizing the Hearing Handicap Inventory for Adults and the Tinnitus Handicap Inventory as outcome measures. Tinnitus was reported by 14 of the 21 patients who responded to the mailed questionnaires from a total of 38 patients identified as having undergone a sudden sensorineural hearing loss in the years 1988 to 1997. The median total Tinnitus Handicap Inventory score for those with tinnitus was 20 (interquartile range 52), and in 4 patients of the 14 with tinnitus (28.6%), the tinnitus handicap was moderate or severe. The onset of tinnitus was coincident with sudden sensorineural hearing loss in 8 patients (57% of the 14 with tinnitus) and occurred within 48 hours in the remaining 6 (43%). In 18 patients (or 86% of the 21 patients), a significant hearing handicap was demonstrated. Thus, it may be inferred that distressing tinnitus is not unusual following a sudden sensorineural hearing loss, and that therapy for both hearing and tinnitus is recommended for such patients on a systematic basis in conjunction with medical treatment of the condition at the time of admission for a sudden hearing loss (▶ Table 2.3).

2.3.1 Early Intervention

After medical treatment with steroids, the patient may well be anxious and upset. In addition, the patient may not yet be aware of the potential handicap associated with a unilateral sudden sensorineural hearing loss due to the structured and limited conversations that occur in a hospital or during medical appointments. However, attendance for medical treatment represents an opportunity for early discussion and support that may prove beneficial.

2.3.2 Information Regarding Mechanisms

As with the other otologic pathologies already described, clear and modern explanations of tinnitus mechanisms are beneficial. In the case of sudden sensorineural hearing loss, reference could be made to phantom limb analogies.

Table 2.3 Elements specific to tinnitus treatment in sudden sensorineural hearing loss

Specific therapy	When undertaken?
Early audiologic intervention	At completion of salvage treatment (e.g., systemic or intratympanic steroids)
Information regarding mechanisms	At completion of salvage treatment (e.g., systemic or intratympanic steroids)
Hearing aid prescription, considering CROS, BiCROS, transcranial CROS, or contralateral BAHA	Patient preference for timing and strategy
Onward referral for anxiety and/or depression	As indicated by HADS score

2.3.3 Hearing Therapy

For many patients, the tinnitus handicap following sudden sensorineural hearing loss is intimately bound up with hearing handicap. As such, instruction in hearing tactics, speech reading, and structured practice in auditory discrimination is of significant potential benefit for these patients. An emerging option is the use of cochlear implants for severe tinnitus in unilateral hearing loss, which has been reported with good results[64] for tinnitus suppression.

2.3.4 Treating Tinnitus Associated with Middle Ear Myoclonus

Middle ear myoclonus (MEM) is a condition characterized by a repetitive (though rarely regular) sound sensation or perception of movement within the ear. The auditory percept can be clicking or buzzing, and in the majority of cases, the condition is unilateral. MEM can be associated with or exacerbated by stress. The diagnosis of MEM is largely based on the patient's history; although in some cases, the myoclonic activity can be recorded as deflections on long-time base tympanometry (▶ Fig. 2.2), and rarely physical movement of the tympanic membrane can be observed on otoscopy.

Although MEM presents rather differently than subjective tinnitus, patients with MEM may well be referred to tinnitus services by clinicians when these patients are unsure of how to proceed. Patients are often very troubled by the condition, which may be maddening or irritating, saying things like "it feels like there is a crazy insect stuck in my ear!" It can be elicited sometimes with blowing air on the closed eyelids, facial stroking, or a tuning fork held up to the ear.[65] Differential diagnoses include temporomandibular joint clicking, hearing Eustachian tube sounds during opening and closing of the tube with swallowing, and having palatal myoclonus, a hair or other foreign body next to the eardrum, or an actual insect in the ear!

Following history taking, otoscopy, audiometry, and diagnostic tympanometry, patients appreciate an explanation of their condition, and this can be underpinned using an anatomical diagram of the ear that includes the middle ear muscles.

In some cases, pressure in the external auditory meatus can alleviate the symptom. The diagnostic indicator of this would be a patient who regularly places an index finger in their ear, or who tells the tester that the clicking has ceased during tympanometry. This effect can be replicated in the long term by a tightly fitting custom silicone earmold, such as those used to protect the ear during swimming. In other cases, section of either the tensor tympani (TT) or the stapedius muscle, or both, may be undertaken. This management option raises the issue of how a clinician may reliably distinguish between the muscles involved. Some guidelines on how tympanometry can help with this are found in Aron et al.[66] Briefly, with the external ear canal at ambient pressure, both the TT and stapedius cause an increase in stiffness (decrease in input admittance), although the TT to a greater extent than the stapedius muscle. With the external ear canal negatively pressurized, TT contractions reverse to cause an increase in admittance, and stapedius contractions still cause a decrease in admittance. It should be noted that both tympanic muscles can co-contract (▶ Table 2.4).

2.4 Other Relevant Conditions

There are many otologic, and neurologic, conditions where tinnitus is a feature. In a patient with a complaint of autophony and/or pulsatile tinnitus,

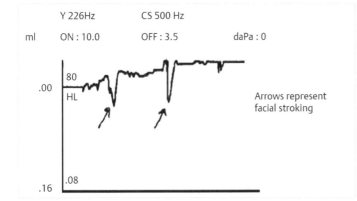

Fig. 2.2 Long time-base tympanometry in subject whose middle ear myoclonus (MEM)-associated tinnitus was provoked by loud sounds or facial stroking.

Table 2.4 Elements specific to tinnitus treatment in middle ear myoclonus

Specific therapy	When undertaken?
Trial of occlusive earmold	At diagnosis
Relaxation therapy (progressive muscle relaxation)	First session
Selective tenotomy	Patient/Otologist decision

a potential diagnosis of semicircular canal dehiscence should be considered.[67] A feature of benign intracranial hypertension (BIH) can be pulsatile tinnitus (often cardiac synchronous) with a marked exacerbation on lying down.[68] In both these conditions, the management of intrusive tinnitus is an essential component of the care of the patient.

2.5 Conclusion

This chapter has discussed the specific strategies indicated in tinnitus therapy in four otologic pathologies. In all cases, teamwork to manage these conditions is key, and it is important to be aware that the treatment of the health condition may affect or even produce tinnitus. Counseling the patient about tinnitus and providing tinnitus treatment early and often when necessary are vital to the overall success of the patient's care.

Acknowledgment

David M. Baguley is supported by the NIHR but the views herein are his own, and do not represent those of the NIHR or the UK Department of Health and Social Care.

References

[1] Cima RFF, Mazurek B, Haider H, et al. A multidisciplinary European guideline for tinnitus: diagnostics, assessment, and treatment. HNO. 2019; 67 Suppl 1:10–42

[2] Tunkel DE, Bauer CA, Sun GH, et al. Clinical practice guideline: tinnitus. Otolaryngol Head Neck Surg. 2014; 151 (2) Suppl:S1–S40

[3] AAO-HNS. Guidelines for the diagnosis and evaluation of therapy in Meniere's disease. Otolaryngol Head Neck Surg. 1995; 113(3):181–185

[4] Henry JL, Wilson PH. The psychological management of chronic tinnitus. Boston, MA: Allyn & Bacon; 2001

[5] Basura GJ, Adams ME, Monfared A, et al. Clinical practice guideline: Meniere's Disease. Otolaryngol Head Neck Surg. 2020; 162 2_suppl:S1–S55

[6] Lopez-Escamez JA, Carey J, Chung WH, et al. Classification Committee of the Barany Society, Japan Society for Equilibrium Research, European Academy of Otology and Neurotology (EAONO), Equilibrium Committee of the American Academy of Otolaryngology-Head and Neck Surgery (AAO-HNS), Korean Balance Society. Diagnostic criteria for Meniere's disease. J Vestib Res. 2015; 25(1):1–7

[7] Wazen JJ, Spitzer JB, Ghossaini SN, et al. Transcranial contralateral cochlear stimulation in unilateral deafness. Otolaryngol Head Neck Surg. 2003; 129(3):248–254

[8] da Costa SS, de Sousa LC, Piza MR. Meniere's disease: overview, epidemiology, and natural history. Otolaryngol Clin North Am. 2002; 35(3):455–495

[9] Huppert D, Strupp M, Brandt T. Long-term course of Meniere's disease revisited. Acta Otolaryngol. 2010; 130(6):644–651

[10] Stouffer JL, Tyler RS. Characterization of tinnitus by tinnitus patients. J Speech Hear Disord. 1990; 55(3):439–453

[11] Douek E, Reid J. The diagnostic value of tinnitus pitch. J Laryngol Otol. 1968; 82(11):1039–1042

[12] Svedlund J, Zoger S, Holgers K-M. (2002). The Hospital Anxiety and Depression Scale as an instrument in tinnitus. In: Patuzzi R, ed. Proceedings of the VIIth International Tinnitus Seminar. Perth: University of Western Australia

[13] Erlandsson SI, Eriksson-Mangold M, Wiberg A. Meniere's disease: trauma, distress and adaptation studied through focus interview analyses. Scand Audiol Suppl. 1996; 43 Suppl 43:45–56

[14] Wright T. Meniere's disease. BMJ Clin Evid. 2015; 2015:505

[15] Harford E, Barry J. A rehabilitative approach to the problem of unilateral hearing impairment: the contralateral routing of signals (CROS). J Speech Hear Disord. 1965; 30:121–138

[16] Newman CW, Jacobson GP, Hug GA, Sandridge SA. Perceived hearing handicap of patients with unilateral or mild hearing loss. Ann Otol Rhinol Laryngol. 1997; 106(3):210–214

[17] Rasmussen GL. The olivary peduncle and other fiber projections of the superior olivary complex. J Comp Neurol. 1946; 84:141–219

[18] Oort H. Uber die Verastellung des Nervus Octavus bei Sautetieren. Anat Anz. 1918; 51:272–280

[19] Scharf B, Magnan J, Chays A. On the role of the olivocochlear bundle in hearing: 16 case studies. Hear Res. 1997; 103(1–2): 101–122

[20] Baguley DM, Axon P, Winter IM, Moffat DA. The effect of vestibular nerve section upon tinnitus. Clin Otolaryngol Allied Sci. 2002; 27(4):219–226

[21] Patel M, Agarwal K, Arshad Q, et al. Intratympanic methylprednisolone versus gentamicin in patients with unilateral Meniere's disease: a randomised, double-blind, comparative effectiveness trial. Lancet. 2016; 388(10061): 2753–2762

[22] Atlas JT, Parnes LS. Intratympanic gentamicin titration therapy for intractable Meniere's disease. Am J Otol. 1999; 20 (3):357–363

[23] Silverstein H, Arruda J, Rosenberg SI, Deems D, Hester TO. Direct round window membrane application of gentamicin in the treatment of Meniere's disease. Otolaryngol Head Neck Surg. 1999; 120(5):649–655

[24] Berryhill WE, Graham MD. Chemical and physical labyrinthectomy for Meniere's disease. Otolaryngol Clin North Am. 2002; 35(3):675–682

[25] Vernon J, Johnson R, Schleuning A. The characteristics and natural history of tinnitus in Meniere's disease. Otolaryngol Clin North Am. 1980; 13(4):611–619

[26] McKenna L. Tinnitus and insomnia. In: Tyler RS, ed. The Tinnitus handbook. San Diego, CA: Singular; 2000

[27] Bjelland I, Dahl AA, Haug TT, Neckelmann D. The validity of the Hospital Anxiety and Depression Scale. An updated literature review. J Psychosom Res. 2002; 52(2):69–77

[28] Andersson G, Kaldo-Sandström V, Ström L, Strömgren T. Internet administration of the Hospital Anxiety and Depression Scale in a sample of tinnitus patients. J Psychosom Res. 2003; 55(3):259–262

[29] Svedlund J, Zoger S, Holgers K-M. (2002). The Hospital Anxiety and Depression Scale as an instrument in tinnitus. In:

Patuzzi R, ed. Proceedings of the VIIth International Tinnitus Seminar. Perth: University of Western Australia

[30] Driscoll CLW. Vestibular schwannoma. In: Jackler RK, Driscoll CLW, eds. Tumours of the ear and temporal bone. Philadelphia: Lippincott Williams & Wilkins; 2000:172–218

[31] Moffat DA, Baguley DM, Beynon GJ, Da Cruz M. Clinical acumen and vestibular schwannoma. Am J Otol. 1998; 19(1):82–87

[32] Møller AR. Pathophysiology of tinnitus. Ann Otol Rhinol Laryngol. 1984; 93(1 Pt 1):39–44

[33] Schuknecht HF. Pathology of the ear. 2nd ed. Philadelphia, PA: Lea & Febiger; 1993

[34] Baguley DM, Chang P, Moffat DA. Tinnitus and vestibular schwannoma. Semin Hear. 2001; 22:65–77, 88

[35] Bell JR, Anderson-Kim SJ, Low C, Leonetti JP. The persistence of tinnitus after acoustic neuroma surgery. Otolaryngol Head Neck Surg. 2016; 155(2):317–323

[36] Baguley DM, Moffat DA, Hardy DG. What is the effect of translabyrinthine acoustic schwannoma removal upon tinnitus? J Laryngol Otol. 1992; 106(4):329–331

[37] Andersson G, Kinnefors A, Ekvall L, Rask-Andersen H. Tinnitus and translabyrinthine acoustic neuroma surgery. Audiol Neurotol. 1997; 2(6):403–409

[38] Seltzer Z, Devor M. Ephaptic transmission in chronically damaged peripheral nerves. Neurology. 1979; 29(7):1061–1064

[39] Catalano PJ, Post KD. Elimination of tinnitus following hearing preservation surgery for acoustic neuromas. Am J Otol. 1996; 17(3):443–445

[40] Mahboubi H, Sahyouni R, Moshtaghi O, et al. CyberKnife for treatment of vestibular schwannoma: a meta-analysis. Otolaryngol–Head and Neck Surg. 2017; 157(1):7–15

[41] Hebb ALO, Erjavec N, Morris DP, et al. Quality of life related to symptomatic outcomes in patients with vestibular schwannomas: a Canadian Centre perspective. Am J Otolaryngol. 2019; 40(2):236–246

[42] Baguley DM, Stoddart RL, Moffat DA. What is the demand for audiological and vestibular rehabilitation after surgery for vestibular schwannoma? In: Sanna M, et al. eds. Acoustic neurinoma and other CPA tumors. Bologna: Monduzzi; 1999:1101–1105

[43] Wang JJ, Feng YM, Wang H, et al. Changes in tinnitus after vestibular schwannoma surgery. Sci Rep. 2019; 9(1):1743

[44] Newman CW, Jacobson GP, Spitzer JB. Development of the tinnitus handicap inventory. Arch Otolaryngol Head Neck Surg. 1996; 122(2):143–148

[45] Newman CW, Sandridge SA, Jacobson GP. Psychometric adequacy of the Tinnitus Handicap Inventory (THI) for evaluating treatment outcome. J Am Acad Audiol. 1998; 9(2):153–160

[46] Meikle MB, Henry JA, Griest SE, et al. The tinnitus functional index: development of a new clinical measure for chronic, intrusive tinnitus. Ear and Hearing. 2012; 32: 1–24

[47] Baguley DM, Andersson G. Factor analysis of the tinnitus handicap inventory. Am J Audiol. 2003; 12(1):31–34

[48] Bashjawish B, Kılıç S, Baredes S, Eloy JA, Liu JK, Ying Y-LM. Changing trends in management of vestibular schwannoma: a national cancer database study. The Laryngoscope. 2019; 129:1197–1205

[49] Lloyd SK, Kasbekar AV, Baguley DM, Moffat DA. Audiovestibular factors influencing quality of life in patients with conservatively managed sporadic vestibular schwannoma. Otol Neurotol. 2010; 31(6):968–976

[50] Cope TE, Baguley DM, Moore BC. Tinnitus loudness in quiet and noise after resection of vestibular schwannoma. Otol Neurotol. 2011; 32(3):488–496

[51] Dillon H. Hearing aids. 2nd ed. New York: Thieme; 2012

[52] Bosman AJ, Hol MK, Snik AF, Mylanus EA, Cremers CW. Bone-anchored hearing aids in unilateral inner ear deafness. Acta Otolaryngol. 2003; 123(2):258–260

[53] Finbow J, Bance M, Aiken S, Gulliver M, Verge J, Caissie R. A comparison between wireless CROS and bone-anchored hearing devices for single-sided deafness: a pilot study. Otol Neurotol. 2015; 36(5):819–825

[54] Niparko JK, Cox KM, Lustig LR. Comparison of the bone anchored hearing aid implantable hearing device with contralateral routing of offside signal amplification in the rehabilitation of unilateral deafness. Otol Neurotol. 2003; 24(1):73–78

[55] Wazen JJ, Spitzer JB, Ghossaini SN, et al. Transcranial contralateral cochlear stimulation in unilateral deafness. Otolaryngol Head Neck Surg. 2003; 129(3):248–254

[56] Arts H. Differential diagnosis of sensorineural hearing loss. In: Cummings C, Fredickson J, Harker L, eds. Otolaryngology head and neck surgery. Volume 4 Ear and cranial base. St Louis: Mosby. 1998.

[57] Ramachandran VS, Rogers-Ramachandran D. Synaesthesia in phantom limbs induced with mirrors. Proc Biol Sci. 1996; 263(1369):377–386

[58] Harris F, Tysome JR, Donnelly N, et al. Cochlear implants in the management of hearing loss in Neurofibromatosis Type 2. Cochlear Implants Int. 2017; 18(3):171–179

[59] Hughes GB. Sudden hearing loss. In: Gates GA, ed. Current therapy in otolaryngology: head and neck surgery. 6th ed. St. Louis, MO: Mosby; 1998

[60] Fishman JM, Cullen L. Investigating sudden hearing loss in adults. BMJ. 2018; 363:k4347

[61] Plontke SK. Diagnostics and therapy of sudden hearing loss. GMS Curr Top Otorhinolaryngol Head Neck Surg. 2018; 16: Doc05

[62] Newman CW, Weinstein BE, Jacobson GP, Hug GA. The Hearing Handicap Inventory for Adults: psychometric adequacy and audiometric correlates. Ear Hear. 1990; 11 (6):430–433

[63] Chiossoine-Kerdel JA, Baguley DM, Stoddart RL, Moffat DA. An investigation of the audiologic handicap associated with unilateral sudden sensorineural hearing loss. Am J Otol. 2000; 21(5):645–651

[64] Cabral Junior F, Pinna MH, Alves RD, Malerbi AF, Bento RF. Cochlear implantation and single-sided deafness: a systematic review of the literature. Int Arch Otorhinolaryngol. 2016; 20 (1):69–75

[65] Bance M, Makki FM, Garland P, Alian WA, van Wijhe RG, Savage J. Effects of tensor tympani muscle contraction on the middle ear and markers of a contracted muscle. Laryngoscope. 2013; 123(4):1021–1027

[66] Aron M, Floyd D, Bance M. Voluntary eardrum movement: a marker for tensor tympani contraction? Otol Neurotol. 2015; 36(2):373–381

[67] Ward BK, Carey JP, Minor LB. Superior canal dehiscence syndrome: lessons from the first 20 years. Front Neurol. 2017; 8:177

[68] Wall M. Update on idiopathic intracranial hypertension. Neurol Clin. 2017; 35(1):45–57

[69] Andersson G. The role of psychology in managing tinnitus: a cognitive behavioral approach. Semin Hear. 2001; 22: 65–76

[70] Hoistad DL, Melnik G, Mamikoglu B, Battista R, O'Connor CA, Wiet RJ. Update on conservative management of acoustic neuroma. Otol Neurotol. 2001; 22(5):682–685

[71] Stangerup SE, Tos M, Thomsen J, Caye-Thomasen P. True incidence of vestibular schwannoma? Neurosurgery. 2010; 67(5):1335–1340, discussion 1340

[72] Valente M, Valente M, Enretto J, Layton KM. Fitting strategies for patients with unilateral hearing loss. In: Valente M, ed. Strategies for selecting and verifying hearing aid fittings. 2nd ed. New York: Thieme; 2002

3 Internet-Delivered Guided Self-Help Treatments for Tinnitus

Gerhard Andersson and Eldre Beukes

Abstract

This chapter describes the development and evaluation of Internet-delivered cognitive behavior therapy for tinnitus. The chapter covers different aspects of the treatment including how to support the treatment and the effects in research studies. Some problems that may occur have also been discussed.

Keywords: tinnitus, Internet-delivered, cognitive behavior therapy, guided self-help

3.1 Background

3.1.1 Tinnitus and Self-Help Material

Numerous barriers exist to accessing health care, including the area of hearing health care.[1] This has led to many people with debilitating conditions to not seek or obtain specialized help.[2] Some patients may attempt to treat themselves without the involvement of health care professionals and hospital facilities. To increase access to health care, self-help approaches have been promoted in recent years. Although self-help is not a replacement for assessments and treatment, it may be the only option when professional help is inaccessible or considered too expensive. Self-help approaches provide information and resources for individuals to do in their own time. See Appendix 3.2 for example of a leaflet used for information. Self-help materials include information leaflets, self-help books (bibliotherapy), Internet resources, smartphone apps, or a combination of these approaches.

Self-help materials are often suggested for patients with tinnitus, a prevalent disorder that can be very distressing. Although specialty tinnitus clinics are in high demand, numerous geographical and service constraints, such as a lack of trained professionals, often limit access to appropriate tinnitus care.[26] Due to the challenges associated with the provision of tinnitus therapy, numerous self-help resources have been developed (see also appendix).[1] One example is information leaflets regarding tinnitus and its treatment. These have been developed by national organizations, for example, the American Tinnitus Association, Swedish Hard of Hearing Association, and the British Tinnitus Association. Such leaflets, or those produced and distributed by the local tinnitus clinics in the form of information packs, have been instrumental in spreading accurate information regarding tinnitus and its treatment.[3]

For those requiring more input, tinnitus self-help books are frequently recommended. There are surprisingly few self-help books dealing with tinnitus, compared with those available for related conditions such as depression and insomnia. It is beyond the scope of this chapter to review all the self-help literature and information on tinnitus, so we will comment on just a few examples. An early influential self-help book for tinnitus was published by the psychologist Richard Hallam[4] that has been translated into at least two other languages (Swedish and German). Most of its content is still relevant, except the section on masking therapy that is now outdated. Davis[5] published a self-help book, *Living with tinnitus*, which includes good advice. The format of this book makes it highly accessible to most individuals who want to learn more about tinnitus. Henry and Wilson[6] published a self-help cognitive-behavioral treatment approach book: *Tinnitus: a self-management guide for the ringing in your ears*. Another self-help book was published by McKenna et al,[7] *Living with tinnitus and hyperacusis*.

Although there is empirical support for the use of self-help books for many conditions such as headaches, sleep problems, and anxiety, only two controlled studies have been conducted with tinnitus patients on the efficacy of self-help books for tinnitus.[8,9] Malouff et al[9] studied the book by Henry and Wilson,[6] and Kaldo et al[8] assessed the Swedish self-help Cognitive Behavioral Therapy (CBT) book,[10] which has also been translated into German.[11] Results have varied but in the Kaldo et al trial, moderate to large effects were seen.[8] There is a later Swedish self-help book that is based on acceptance-oriented CBT.[12] This has only been tested in the form of an Internet program.[13]

Due to the increased access to the Internet over the last 25 years, the Internet has been increasingly used as a major low-cost source for informal help-seeking. It has also become commonly used to search for health-related information[14] such as advice when experiencing tinnitus.[15] Information about tinnitus can be found on many Internet platforms such as YouTube videos[16] and social media such as tinnitus Facebook groups.[17] Help for tinnitus in the form of information and sound enrichment is also available through numerous downloadable smartphone apps[18] (see Chapter 9). Such self-help resources may also be consulted prior to or concurrent to receiving treatment.[19] There are two factors regarding Internet self-help materials that need consideration. One is that there is great variability regarding the quality of online health care information for tinnitus.[15] The other factor is that self-help on its own is rarely as effective as when some form of guidance or professional support is provided. Professional guidance supports patients as they pursue self-help treatment, provides feedback to the patient about their progress, and monitors progress closely throughout treatment.[20] Even with the provision of only minimal support that is not in real time (e.g., by emailing), better outcomes are found compared with when no support is provided.[21] These barriers associated with some self-help interventions can be addressed by providing standardized self-help material in a structured manner via the Internet together with minimal professional support.

The Internet is a global computer network, providing electronic communication facilities and a platform to share information. The use of the Internet has dramatically changed the ease of access to and the spread of information worldwide. As the Internet now reaches most of the world's population, guided Internet-based self-help programs for tinnitus have been developed. Providing treatment via the Internet has advantages over other self-help resources as the advice can be given continuously without delay. In comparison with ordinary treatment, it is cost-effective and it makes the treatment accessible to those who are geographically remote from a specialty tinnitus center.[22] Online tinnitus interventions show real potential in decreasing the difficulties associated with accessing tinnitus care and in reducing tinnitus-related problems.[23] Due to the potential for these interventions as a form of tinnitus self-help, this chapter focuses on considerations for the delivery of online tinnitus interventions.

3.2 Internet-Delivered Guided Self-Help

In essence, Internet self-help treatment is a translation of a regular clinical treatment protocol, with alterations to the format. It consists of three main elements: assessment, provision of the intervention materials, and guidance by a professional while undertaking the intervention. The intervention format differs from traditional care, in that online interactive features enable the user to complete assessments, quizzes, worksheets, diaries, and exercises online for the professional to provide feedback. For the intervention to be effective, many aspects need consideration. Two of the most important aspects are the theoretical foundation of the intervention and the second is the platform that will be used for the intervention. The main elements of guided self-help are discussed in the sections that follow.

3.2.1 Technical Functionality of the Internet Platform

Of essence is careful consideration of the actual Internet platform that will be used. The platform provides the intervention materials via webpages that are accessible on most electronic devices, for example, laptops, tablets, and smartphones. Enhanced technical and functional capabilities are required to ensure that it is user-centric and promotes engagement with the intervention. The ePlatform, iTerapi, was designed in Sweden and has been used for various conditions,[22] and tested in over 100 behavior intervention trials, including several trials on tinnitus and other audiological conditions.[23] The platform has been custom developed with the required data security measures and technical capabilities in place. It enables communication between a therapist and a user of the intervention. This interaction can be either synchronous (e.g., real-time live chats on skype) or asynchronous (e.g., e-mail) or using a blended approach (e.g., email supplemented with telephone calls). The specific technical and functional aspects of the iTerapi research treatment platform are described by Vlaescu et al,[24,25] whereas aspects specific to tinnitus interventions are described by Beukes et al.[17] There are several other existing solutions in clinical practice that are similar to iTerapi.

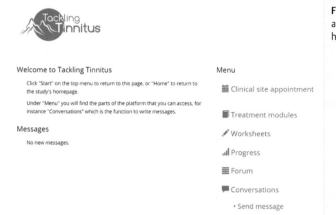

Fig. 3.1 Example of an online assessment form or example of the homepage.

To be able to do the intervention, individuals need to have access to the Internet via a computer, a smartphone, or a tablet. Before starting the intervention, access to the Internet and an electronic device should be evaluated, as well as computer user experience. Extensive Internet and computer technical experience should not be required as the platform is designed to be user-friendly without technical complications (see ▶ Fig. 3.1). For a patient, the online environment resembles systems that are used to pay bills online, that is, the systems are encrypted and often use a double authentication procedure at login. In cases when the Internet fails to work, or when individuals have problems with their connection, the possibility to contact their therapist by phone is an option.

3.2.2 Conducting Assessments

Individuals initially register for the intervention online. Before starting treatment, a comprehensive medical and audiological screening is recommended. Self-reported questionnaires should also be included in the screening to assess the severity of the tinnitus and associated problems. This may take place online or in a clinic before starting, with additional checks that no new conditions such as a major health concern (e.g., cancer) have been discovered. Completing questionnaires online is preferred for ease of use and convenience in storage of the data. Further, studies have shown that online administration does not affect the psychometric properties of the questionnaires (e.g., Andersson et al[34]). Once the screening has been completed, it is recommended that the individual be contacted, either for an assessment session in a clinic or for a phone call. Personal contact is also recommended

after completing the intervention. Although this personal contact is not consistently included in online interventions (e.g., Rheker et al[27]), the personal contact enhances the experience of the patient undertaking the intervention.[28] Questionnaires for follow-up assessments are recommended once the intervention is completed to assess the intervention effects. Weekly monitoring is also possible by providing weekly short questionnaires to be completed to assess progress.

3.2.3 Theoretical Foundation of the Intervention

The theoretical foundation of an intervention is essential to promote long-term effectiveness. Many tinnitus interventions exist, although not all are based on strong empirical research. CBT for tinnitus was developed due to the relationship between tinnitus and psychological distress. It is directed toward altering unhelpful thoughts about tinnitus through behavior modifications and thereby changing an individual's reaction toward their tinnitus. The use of CBT for managing tinnitus has been researched over several years in controlled trials and longitudinal studies.[29,30,31] Results from many studies highlight the effectiveness of CBT at decreasing tinnitus distress and annoyance, anxiety, and improving daily life functioning. Due to the strong evidence base, current practice guidelines[32] globally recommend that CBT be offered to individuals with tinnitus. Despite these recommendations, there is a sparse provision of CBT for tinnitus globally and it is often the least recommended tinnitus treatment.[26]

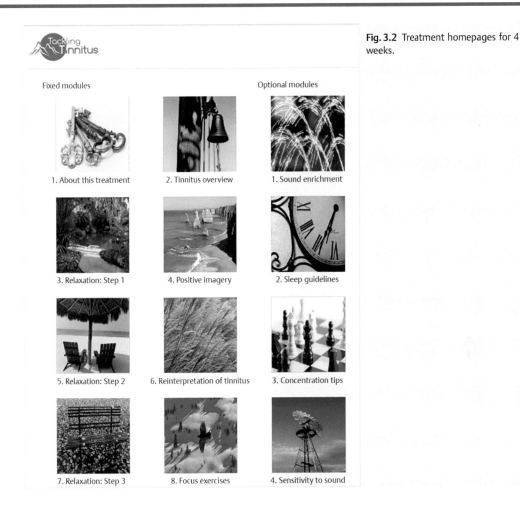

Fig. 3.2 Treatment homepages for 4 weeks.

Due to the limitations regarding access to CBT for tinnitus, a CBT manual for those with tinnitus was developed in Sweden.[10] This program has a strong theoretical base, as is founded on a cognitive rationale[6] and a learning theory approach.[33] It has been used for over 20 years and been evaluated in numerous randomized controlled trials, with the first publication by Andersson et al.[34] This program has undergone many developments and is available in four languages. It has also been provided as regular health care in Sweden since 1999 (see Kaldo-Sandström et al[35]). The provision of such evidence-based programs should be prioritized during the development of any Internet-based intervention.

3.2.4 The Intervention Content

The content contains several modules that mirror face-to-face treatment, some of which are tailored to the needs of the clients (e.g., insomnia management; see Chapter 6). These sections are generally provided systematically over a 6- to 10-week period during which two to three modules are released weekly (see ▶ Fig. 3.2). CBT principles such as goal setting, a clear structure, active participation, relapse prevention, and setting a time-frame for completing the intervention are incorporated. In its current English version, there are 22 modules, 17 of which are recommended for everyone, together with 5 optional modules (see ▶ Table 3.1). The modules are divided into six sections, namely, (1) an overview, (2) a progressive applied relaxation guide, (3) CBT strategies, (4) sound enrichment advice, (5) optional modules to deal with the effects of tinnitus, and (6) relapse prevention and maintaining the results. The text is furthermore supplemented with diagrams (e.g., how thoughts, emotions, behaviors, and physical sensations are linked) and

Table 3.1 Example modules used in Internet-based CBT for tinnitus

Module	Content	Intervention load	
		Reading time	Daily practicing
Part 1: Overview			
Program rationale and explanation of the content	Explanation and introduction to the content	15 min	Setting goals
Tinnitus overview	Explanations to aid understanding tinnitus	15 min	Reading the module
Part 2: Progressive relaxation guide			
Step 1: Deep relaxation	The rationale for using relaxation and the difference between tense and relaxed muscles	15 min	Twice a day for 10–15 min
Step 2: Deep breathing	Using diagrammatic breathing, using a relaxation word, and relaxing without tensing first	10 min	Twice a day for 10 min
Step 3: Entire body relaxation	Relaxing the entire body at once instead of individual muscle groups	10 min	Twice a day for 10 min
Step 4: Frequent relaxation	Incorporating sorter relaxation frequently during daily activities	10 min	5–10 times 1–2 min
Step 5: Quick relaxation	Using relaxation following stressful events	10 min	7–15 times a day for up to 1 min
Step 6: Relaxation routine	A routine to incorporate deep and quick relaxation every week	10 min	Deep relaxation twice a week, Frequent relation 8 times a day, Rapid relaxation during, before, or after difficult situations
Part 3: CBT techniques			
Positive imagery	The use of positive metal images to aid relaxation and reduce stress	10 min	Twice a day for 5 min
Changing views of tinnitus	Reinterpreting the tinnitus to associate it with a different more neutral or positive sound	10 min	Once a day for 5 min
Shifting focus	Ways of moving focus from the tinnitus to other tactile, auditory or visual stimuli	10 min	4 times a day for 2 min
Thought patterns	Understanding the influence of thoughts on emotions and behaviors	15 min	3 times a week for 10 min
Challenging thoughts	Addressing negative thought patterns	15 min	4 times a week for 5 min
Being mindful	Focusing on the present moment	10 min	2–5 times a day during normal activities
Listening to tinnitus	Graded exposure to reduce the avoidance of and fear associated with tinnitus	10 min	Once a day
Part 4: Sound enrichment			
Sound enrichment*	Using background sounds to distract from tinnitus and hearing aids when hearing loss is present	10 min	As required
Part 5: Dealing with the effects of tinnitus			
Sleep guidelines*	Strategies to improve sleep	15 min	As required
Improving focus*	Tips to improve concentration and task management	10 min	Implement daily
Listening tips*	Communication tactics to aid listening difficulties	15 min	As required
Part 6: Maintenance and relapse prevention			
Summary	Key messages for each chapter	15 min	Reading the module
Future planning	Maintenance and relapse prevention planning	15 min	Future plan

Abbreviation: CBT, cognitive behavioral therapy.
* Tailored according to the expressed needs.

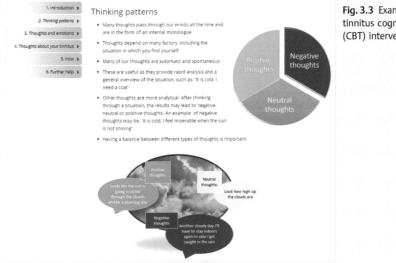

Fig. 3.3 Example of a page in the tinnitus cognitive behavioral therapy (CBT) intervention.

video explanations (e.g., relaxation demonstrations) as seen from ▸ Fig. 3.3. An overview of the modules on the iTerapi system is provided below.

Part I: An Overview

The intervention starts with an overview that provides information on several topics including how to navigate the program, how psychological mechanisms might affect tinnitus, and how to set goals for therapy. To increase understanding and knowledge about tinnitus and clarify common myths, a module about tinnitus is included.

Part II: Applied Relaxation

A progressive relaxation program is delivered to aid quick relaxation and relaxation during everyday life as outlined in ▸ Table 3.1. It starts with applied relaxation step 1, addressing the difference between tense and relaxed muscles. This involves tensing and relaxing each muscle group in turn. Step 2 progresses to relax without first tensing the muscles together with controlled breathing. Step 3 progresses to relaxing all the muscle groups at the same time. Step 4 encourages frequent relaxation in everyday situations to establish the habit of relaxation. Step 5 discusses relaxation during stressful events and step 6 covers a weekly relaxation routine. The Internet-administration provides a flexible approach to what information is presented, including information about possible obstacles and problems when practicing relaxation techniques. Instruction on how to use positive imagery techniques is included in association with the relaxation. The relaxation

program has been found to be very helpful and unproblematic as patients find it fairly easy to learn relaxation via the Internet (e.g., Beukes et al[36]). More information about these techniques is described later in Chapter 10.

Part III: The CBT Tools

The CBT content includes thought analysis, cognitive restructuring, and positive imagery techniques. The cognitive therapy part of our self-help program explains the "situation-cognition-emotion" perspective of understanding tinnitus distress. It also introduces common cognitive "errors" (e.g., overgeneralization), and ways to find alternatives to negative automatic thoughts. Because it is a text-based self-help approach, information is presented clearly with diagrams (refer to ▸ Fig. 3.3) and video instruction. If there are questions or misunderstandings, there is the possibility to contact the therapist at any point throughout the therapy.

Next, attention shifting is reviewed. For example, the patient is given exercises on how to shift attention from tinnitus to other sounds, or from tinnitus to other bodily sensations or positive images. Techniques such as reinterpretation of tinnitus and gradual exposure to tinnitus/quiet environments are also presented.

Part IV: Sound Enrichment

Sound-based approaches, including the use of hearing aids for hearing loss and sound therapy to reduce the tinnitus percept and facilitate habituation, are also included in the intervention. The purpose of sound enrichment, which sounds to use, the level of the sounds, and ways of delivering the sounds are covered. The role of sudden changes, or contrasts, is explained, and it is suggested that sudden changes in background sound (e.g., from music to silence) are likely to increase the salience of tinnitus. Although annoying, it is explained that this contrast effect is not dangerous and is not a sign that tinnitus loudness has increased permanently. Regarding which sounds to use, the most important principle is that patients should not completely mask their tinnitus. Patients may vary in terms of attention-grabbing properties (interest). For example, often a meaningless background sound (e.g., traffic from the street) is good when the patient is concentrating on other things, but there are also situations for which an interesting sound (e.g., a podcast) is preferable.

Part V: Dealing with the Effects of Tinnitus

Optional modules are included to add an element of tailoring, and participants can choose whether or not to do these modules. These modules address practical difficulties associated with tinnitus. For example, suggestions and strategies are provided to address insomnia[37] and listening difficulties.[38] Information on hyperacusis is presented and advice on how to manage it through gradual sound enrichment and exposure is offered. Because tinnitus can make focusing on tasks more difficult, advice on how to minimize concentration difficulties that are often experienced is included. These strategies include encoding and ways to facilitate retrieval from memory.

Part VI: Relapse Prevention and Maintenance

The last modules review the intervention and goal achievement. The final section addresses the long-term maintenance of the strategies. For example, this module includes planning, or the implementation of these exercises for the future. Relapse prevention is minimized as the program encourages continuing useful techniques, relaxation, and regular physical exercise.

3.2.5 Supporting Patients

While undertaking the intervention, it is recommended that patients be minimally guided by a professional. The professional can provide feedback on work done, introduce new weekly materials, answer questions, encourage them, and provide clarification. Although therapeutic alliance in Internet interventions has been highly rated from the patients' perspective, more research is still needed regarding the role of online guidance.[39] Providing optimum guidance in terms of the communication mode, the quantity of guidance, and who provides the guidance has not been fully established.[40] Psychologists, with expertise in the provision of CBT, are optimally placed to provide this guidance, but few psychologists are involved in tinnitus rehabilitation.[41] Where studied, the level of experience and qualification of the e-Health therapist has not appeared to affect treatment efficacy.[21] Clinician-guided self-help, thus, represents a promising alternative in combination with other forms of management. We have also recently found that audiologists can serve as supporting therapists,[42] as the treatment is delivered via the program and the main part of the support is in the form of encouragement and answering questions regarding the program.

When guidance is online, there are potential disadvantages, as there is no way of observing if techniques, such as relaxation training, are practiced properly. Hence, tracking homework compliance and reviewing weekly report cards are very important as well as monitoring progress and encouraging patients to send in their questions. Potential problems with applying the techniques and doing the relaxation exercises can be covered when providing guidance.

3.2.6 Fostering Adherence

As with any self-help intervention, treatment compliance and adherence depends on the individual undertaking the intervention. Although Internet treatment can follow existing clinical protocols, as done using the Uppsala Treatment Program,[43] certain practical aspects must be detailed to avoid misunderstanding the purpose of Internet-based self-help of tinnitus. Self-help treatment is not a quick fix and does not consist of only information. Patients should be aware of the fact that they need to devote time each day to the treatment exercises. This time depends on the strategy used; it could be at least 20 to 45 min/d. For the program to have any effect, it is crucial that the patients move through the exercises regularly and that they contact their therapist if there are any questions or technical problems. Most of the modules provided involve homework assignments and practice logs (or diaries) in the platform that should be

Monitor your progress

Record when you use this technique, using the form and example below:

DATE	How good I am at this before this session Rate from 1-10 with 10 being very successful	ACTIONS e.g. Changing your view of tinnitus	COMMENTS These may include when, where and for how long something was done. You can also note what you can do differently next time or change.	How well this went Rate from 1-10 with 10 being very successful
7/7	0	Changing views of tinnitus	Sound: leaves rustling Image: a quiet lake at sunset Volume: The wind blowing to mask the sound Comments: I thought this was going to be hard, but it really worked very effectively. Will try a different image tomorrow to compare. Spent 5 min	2
7/8	2	Changing views of tinnitus	Sound: clock ticking Image: sitting comfortably inside a warm wooden log cabin Volume: fire crackling Comments: I found the rhythmic ticking of the clock did not work as well although I was able to explore this image well. I may try to replace	3

Fig. 3.4 Example of a worksheet or diary used in the tinnitus Internet intervention.

completed and submitted on an ongoing basis (see ▶ Fig. 3.4). When submitting practice logs, the therapist can respond with feedback on treatment progress, focusing on the positive aspects. Moreover, misconceptions about immediate treatment effects and, for some patients, a desire to adhere too strictly to the instructions given are addressed. For example, patients may believe that the treatment will not be of any help if they are unable to practice as many times as instructed. Another use of the feedback is to help the patient go through the treatment within a reasonable amount of time. Some patients may need to be encouraged to fill in the diary and to move onto the next module.

3.3 Evaluation of Internet-Interventions for Tinnitus and Potential Problems

3.3.1 Effects of the Internet-Based Self-Help for Tinnitus

The effects of Internet treatments for tinnitus have been tested in controlled efficacy trials, effectiveness studies, and also summarized in meta-analyses. The first trial was on the Swedish original program, with promising outcomes, but high dropout rates.[43] The program was then updated and tested against the provision of face-to-face group CBT.[44] Subsequently, the program was translated into English and tested in a cluster randomized trial.[45] Uncontrolled effectiveness trials were also published on the Swedish program.[46,35] The Swedish researchers also developed a program based on acceptance and commitment therapy that was tested in a further randomized controlled trial.[13] Then, a collaboration with German researchers was initiated that led to three controlled trials.[47,48,49] Another German research group developed and tested a program of their own.[50] The latest addition is an English and updated version of the Internet CBT program that has been tested in an open trial,[51] a controlled efficacy trial,[42] and a controlled effectiveness trial.[52]

When summarizing the controlled effects, Beukes et al[23] reported a medium overall controlled effect size for tinnitus distress (d = 0.50). However, as expected effects are larger when compared against no treatment ($d = 0.61$) versus active controls ($d = 0.35$). It is important to note that there are substantial differences in effects, with the most recent trials from Germany and the United Kingdom generally showing larger effects. Overall, Internet CBT has indicated potential in improving tinnitus distress and the associated comorbidities such as depression, anxiety, and depression, both immediately after intervention and in the long term (e.g., Beukes et al[53] and Weise et al[11]).

33

3.3.2 Problems Related to Dropouts and Compliance

Perhaps because of the nature of the Internet, and selective recruitment in our first controlled trial, we initially had problems with what we first thought was dropouts from the treatment. Later, this turned out to be problems caused by lack of time. In the clinic, it will be immediately apparent if patients decline treatment because of time constraints. Dropout rates were high in a further study[45] due to limitations of the protocol followed. The dropout rates in later trials improved with a mean dropout rate of 14% (range 4–51%), indicating that such interventions are viable.[23]

Intervention compliance can be problematic, but no more than in regular clinical practice. Interestingly, when implementing the Internet-based treatment in clinical practice, we have found a higher adherence to the treatment by those patients who have been referred from counties outside of our own. Most likely, this is explained by their efforts in getting a referral from their home counties (which often is restricted in Sweden). Thus, many factors may be associated with compliance that should be considered, beyond simply the format of intervention.

3.3.3 Security and Technical Concerns

The risk of revealing sensitive information data security is important to consider in any Internet intervention. Secure and encrypted communication is used to reduce the probability of identity theft. Not only by demanding a personal password to log in, but also by using a unique single-use password that is sent automatically to the client's cell phone (or via a separate card reader). As the Internet is increasingly used and technology is improved, issues regarding security become less difficult to solve. However, for the time being, there is no 100% guarantee for protection against intrusion. Rarely, if ever, is this mentioned as a problem by our patients. However, security matters should be discussed with the patient, especially if they share a computer and e-mail account with family members. Problems need not arise if they are discussed before the patient starts treatment. For example, personal feedback should be sent via the internal messaging system in the platform which is encrypted. This is preferred instead of via e-mail which has greater risks for security

breaches. We have yet to experience any security breaches in our system.

Because we see all patients face-to-face at their first assessment session, the risk of having a faked response decreases. In contrast with our previous research studies in which participants could remain anonymous (e.g., Andersson et al[43]), unrealistic responses regarding questionnaires and noncompliance (while still sending in homework assignments) should be monitored.

3.4 Conclusion

The Internet is now widely spread and the majority of people in the world use the Internet to access information, including health-related information. It is increasingly an accepted medium for clinician-patient interaction, given that security measures are in place. The Internet is also widely used by tinnitus patients to access information regarding their condition, as attested by the numerous web pages, Facebook groups, and other social media dealing with the condition.

The Internet has changed the way health care is provided to some extent, and this is likely to continue. However, there are also changes in technology, and further research is needed on the topic of Internet interventions so we can learn more about the mechanisms of change in addition to the treatment effects of these interventions.

In conclusion, it is necessary to develop and test self-help approaches for the management of tinnitus. The vast majority of the online information (e.g., apps) and self-help books have not been evaluated empirically and it is very likely that much self-help material can be used as an adjunct to the care provided at the clinic. The Internet is promising in its capacity to reach many people who are unable to access interventions and do so at a lower cost.

References

[1] Barnett M, Hixon B, Okwiri N, et al. Factors involved in access and utilization of adult hearing healthcare: a systematic review. Laryngoscope. 2017; 127(5):1187–1194

[2] Mahboubi H, Lin HW, Bhattacharyya N. Prevalence, characteristics, and treatment patterns of hearing difficulty in the United States. JAMA Otolaryngol Head Neck Surg. 2018; 144(1):65–70

[3] Zarenoe R, Bohn Eriksson T, Dahl J, Ledin T, Andersson G, & on behalf of the Östergötland tinnitus team. Multidisciplinary group information for patients with tinnitus: an open trial. Hear Balance Commun. 2018; 16:120–125

[4] Hallam RS. Living with tinnitus: dealing with the ringing in your ears. Wellingborough: Thorsons; 1989

[5] Davis P. Living with tinnitus. Woollahra: Gore & Osment Publications; 1995

[6] Henry JL, Wilson PH. Tinnitus: a self-management guide for the ringing in your ears. Boston, MA: Allyn & Bacon; 2002

[7] McKenna L, Baguley D, McFerran DJ. Living with tinnitus and hyperacusis. London: Sheldon Press; 2010

[8] Kaldo V, Renn S, Rahnert M, Larsen H-C, Andersson G. Use of a self-help book with weekly therapist contact to reduce tinnitus distress: a randomized controlled trial. J Psychosom Res. 2017; 63(2):195–202

[9] Malouff JM, Noble W, Schutte NS, Bhullar N. The effectiveness of bibliotherapy in alleviating tinnitus-related distress. J Psychosom Res. 2010; 68(3):245–251

[10] Kaldo V, Andersson G. Kognitiv beteendeterapi vid tinnitus [Cognitive-behavioral treatment of tinnitus]. Lund: Studentlitteratur; 2004

[11] Weise C, Kleinstäuber M, Kaldo V, Andersson G. Mit Tinnitus leben lernen. Ein manual für therapeuten und betroffene. Berlin: Springer Verlag; 2016

[12] Zetterqvist V, Andersson G, Kaldo V. Leva med tinnitus [Living with tinnitus]. Stockholm: Natur och Kultur; 2013

[13] Hesser H, Gustafsson T, Lundén C, et al. A randomized controlled trial of Internet-delivered cognitive behavior therapy and acceptance and commitment therapy in the treatment of tinnitus. J Consult Clin Psychol. 2012; 80(4):649–661

[14] Jiang S, Street RL. Pathway linking Internet health information seeking to better health: a moderated mediation study. Health Commun. 2017; 32(8):1024–1031

[15] Manchaiah V, Dockens AL, Flagge A, et al. Quality and readability of English-language Internet information for tinnitus. J Am Acad Audiol. 2019; 30(1):31–40

[16] Basch CH, Yin J, Kollia B, et al. Public online information about tinnitus: a cross-sectional study of YouTube videos. Noise Health. 2018; 20(92):1–8

[17] Manchaiah V, Ratinaud P, Andersson G. Representation of tinnitus in the US newspaper media and in Facebook pages: cross-sectional analysis of secondary data. Interact J Med Res. 2018; 7(1):e9

[18] Sereda M, Smith S, Newton K, Stockdale D. Mobile apps for management of tinnitus: Users' survey, quality assessment, and content analysis. JMIR Mhealth Uhealth. 2019; 7(1):e10353

[19] Tan SSL, Goonawardene N. Internet health information seeking and the patient-physician relationship: a systematic review. J Med Internet Res. 2017; 19(1):e9

[20] Barak A, Klein B, Proudfoot JG. Defining internet-supported therapeutic interventions. Ann Behav Med. 2009; 38(1):4–17

[21] Baumeister H, Reichler L, Munzinger M, Lin J. The impact of guidance on internet-based mental health interventions—a systematic review. Internet Interv. 2014; 1(4):205–215

[22] Andersson G. Internet-delivered psychological treatments. Annu Rev Clin Psychol. 2016; 12:157–179

[23] Beukes EW, Manchaiah V, Allen PM, Baguley DM, Andersson G. Internet-based interventions for adults with hearing loss, tinnitus, and vestibular disorders: A systematic review and meta-analysis. Trends Hear. 2019; 23:2331216519851749

[24] Vlaescu G, Carlbring P, Lunner T, Andersson G. An e-platform for rehabilitation of persons with hearing problems. American Journal of Audiology. 2015;24: 271–275

[25] Vlaescu G, Alasjö A, Miloff A, Carlbring P, Andersson G. Features and functionality of the Iterapi platform for internet-based psychological treatment. Internet Interventions. 2016; 6:107–114

[26] Bhatt JM, Lin HW, Bhattacharyya N. Prevalence, severity, exposures, and treatment patterns of tinnitus in the United States. JAMA Otolaryngol Head Neck Surg. 2016; 142(10):959–965

[27] Rheker J, Andersson G, Weise C. The role of "on demand" therapist guidance vs. no support in the treatment of tinnitus via the internet: a randomized controlled trial. Internet Interv. 2015; 2:189–199

[28] Beukes EW, Manchaiah V, Davies ASA, Allen PM, Baguley DM, Andersson G. Participants' experiences of an Internet-based cognitive behavioural therapy intervention for tinnitus. Int J Audiol. 2018; 57(12):947–954

[29] Fuller T, Cima R, Langguth B, Mazurek B, Vlaeyen JWS, Hoare DJ. Cognitive behavioural therapy for tinnitus. Cochrane Database Syst Rev. 2020; 1(1):CD012614

[30] Hesser H, Weise C, Westin VZ, Andersson G. A systematic review and meta-analysis of randomized controlled trials of cognitive-behavioral therapy for tinnitus distress. Clin Psychol Rev. 2011; 31(4):545–553

[31] Hoare DJ, Kowalkowski VL, Kang S, Hall DA. Systematic review and meta-analyses of randomized controlled trials examining tinnitus management. Laryngoscope. 2011; 121(7):1555–1564

[32] Fuller TE, Haider HF, Kikidis D, et al. Different teams, same conclusions? A systematic review of existing clinical guidelines for the assessment and treatment of tinnitus in adults. Front Psychol. 2017; 8:206

[33] Hallam R, Rachman S, Hinchcliffe R. Psychological aspects of tinnitus. Contr Med Psychol. 1984; 3:31–53

[34] Andersson G, Kaldo-Sandström V, Ström L, Strömgren T. Internet administration of the Hospital Anxiety and Depression Scale in a sample of tinnitus patients. J Psychosom Res. 2003; 55(3):259–262

[35] Kaldo-Sandström V, Larsen HC, Andersson G. Internet-based cognitive-behavioral self-help treatment of tinnitus: clinical effectiveness and predictors of outcome. Am J Audiol. 2004; 13(2):185–192

[36] Beukes EW, Manchaiah V, Baguley DM, Allen PM, Andersson G. Process evaluation of Internet-based cognitive behavioural therapy for adults with tinnitus in the context of a randomised control trial. Int J Audiol. 2018; 57(2):98–109

[37] Morin CM. Relief from insomnia: getting the sleep of your dreams. New York: Doubleday; 1996

[38] Andersson G. Hearing impairment. In C. Radnitz (Ed.), Cognitive-behavioral interventions for persons with disabilities. Northvale, NJ: Jason Aronson. 2000; 183–204

[39] Sucala M, Schnur J B, Constantino M J, Miller S J, Brackman E H, Montgomery, G H. The therapeutic relationship in e-therapy for mental health: a systematic review. J Med Internet Res. 2021; 14(4):e110

[40] Berger T. The therapeutic alliance in internet interventions: a narrative review and suggestions for future research. Psychother Res. 2017; 27(5):511–524

[41] Gander PE, Hoare DJ, Collins L, Smith S, Hall DA. Tinnitus referral pathways within the National Health Service in England: a survey of their perceived effectiveness among audiology staff. BMC Health Serv Res. 2011; 11:162

[42] Beukes EW, Baguley DM, Allen PM, Manchaiah V, Andersson G. Audiologist guided Internet-based cognitive behaviour therapy for adults with tinnitus in the United Kingdom: a randomised controlled trial. Ear Hear. 2018; 39(3):423–433

[43] Andersson G, Strömgren T, Ström L, Lyttkens L. Randomized controlled trial of internet-based cognitive behavior therapy

for distress associated with tinnitus. Psychosom Med. 2002; 64(5):810–816

[44] Kaldo V, Levin S, Widarsson J, Buhrman M, Larsen HC, Andersson G. Internet versus group cognitive-behavioral treatment of distress associated with tinnitus: a randomized controlled trial. Behav Ther. 2008; 39(4):348–359

[45] Abbott JA, Kaldo V, Klein B, et al. A cluster randomised trial of an internet-based intervention program for tinnitus distress in an industrial setting. Cogn Behav Ther. 2009; 38(3):162–173. Add Andersson 2000

[46] Kaldo V, Haak T, Buhrman M, Alfonsson S, Larsen H-C, Andersson G. Internet-based cognitive behaviour therapy for tinnitus patients delivered in a regular clinical setting: outcome and analysis of treatment dropout. Cogn Behav Ther. 2013; 42(2):146–158

[47] Jasper K, Weise C, Conrad I, Andersson G, Hiller W, Kleinstäuber M. Internet-based guided self-help versus group cognitive behavioral therapy for chronic tinnitus: a randomized controlled trial. Psychother Psychosom. 2014; 83(4):234–246

[48] Weise C, Kleinstäuber M, Andersson G. Internet-delivered cognitive-behavior therapy for tinnitus: a randomized controlled trial. Psychosom Med. 2016; 78(4):501–510

[49] Rheker J, Andersson G, Weise C. The role of "on demand" therapist guidance vs. no support in the treatment of tinnitus via the internet: a randomized controlled trial. Internet Interventions. 2015;2:189–199

[50] Nyenhuis N, Zastrutzki S, Weise C, Jäger B, Kröner-Herwig B. The efficacy of minimal contact interventions for acute tinnitus: a randomised controlled study. Cogn Behav Ther. 2013; 42(2):127–138

[51] Beukes EW, Allen PM, Manchaiah V, Baguley DM, Andersson G. Internet-based intervention for tinnitus: outcome of a single-group open trial. J Am Acad Audiol. 2017; 28(4):340–351

[52] Beukes EW, Andersson G, Allen PM, Manchaiah V, Baguley DM. Effectiveness of guided internet-based cognitive behavioral therapy vs face-to-face clinical care for treatment of tinnitus: a randomized clinical trial. JAMA Otolaryngol Head Neck Surg. 2018; 144(12):1126–1133

[53] Beukes EW, Allen PM, Baguley DM, Manchaiah V, Andersson G. Long-term efficacy of audiologist-guided Internet-based cognitive behavior therapy for tinnitus. Am J Audiol. 2018; 27 3S:431–447

[54] Vlaescu G, Carlbring P, Lunner T, Andersson G. An e-platform for rehabilitation of persons with hearing problems. Am J Audiol. 2015; 24(3):271–275

Appendix 3.1 Suggested Self-Help Resources for Tinnitus

Books on Tinnitus:

- *Tinnitus: A Self-Management Guide for the Ringing in Your Ears* (Henry and Wilson 2002).
- *The Consumer Handbook on Tinnitus* (Tyler 2016).

Support Networks for Tinnitus:

- American Tinnitus Association: www.ata.org
  - *Support Group.*
  - *Telephone/Email Support.*

Sound Therapy:

- Sound Pillow: www.soundpillow.com ($50–150).
- Sound Generators: www.amazon.com ($40 +):
  - SNOOZ White Noise Sound Machine ($80).
  - Marpac Dohm White Noise generator ($45).

Smartphone Apps:

- ReSound[GN] Tinnitus Relief.
- Tinnitus Balance by Phonak.
- Starkey Relax.
- Widex Zen, Tinnitus Management.

Resources for Anxiety:

Books

- *The Anxiety & Phobia Workbook* (Bourne 2015).
- *Mastery of Your Anxiety and Panic III* (Craske and Barlow 2006).
- *Feel the Fear and Do it Anyways* (Jeffers 1992).
- *Don't Panic: Taking Control of Anxiety Attacks* (Wilson 1996).
- *Worry: Controlling it and Using it Wisely* (Hollowell 1997).

Online

- The Anxiety Panic Internet Resource: www.algy.com/anxiety/anxiety.php
- Anxiety Disorders Association of America: www.adaa.org

Resources for Depression:

Books

- *The Mindful Way Through Depression* (Williams et al 2007).
- *Feeling Good: The New Mood Therapy* (Burns 1999).
- *Mind over Mood: Change How You Feel by Changing the Way You Think* (Greenberger and Padesky 1995).
- *Understanding and Overcoming Depression: A Common Sense Approach* (Bates 1999).

Online

- National Alliance on Mental Illness: www.nami.org
- Depression. Org: www.depression.org

Resources for Stress Management and Relaxation[2]:

Books

- *The Relaxation and Stress Reduction Workbook* (Davis et al 2008).
- *Wherever You Go, There You Are* (Kabat-Zinn 1994).
- *The Stress and Relaxation Handbook: A Practical Guide to Self-Help Techniques* (Madders 1997).
- *The Wellness Book: A Comprehensive Guide to Maintaining Health and Treating Stress Related Illness* (Benson and Stuart 1992).
- *A Mindfulness-Based Stress Reduction Workbook* (Stahl and Goldstien 2010).

Appendix 3.2 Tinnitus Self-Treatment Brochure

If you have tinnitus, you should be able to get a very worthwhile degree of relief with the approaches suggested in this brochure. This self-treatment can be done either before or after seeking professional advice from the audiologists at (**Insert your clinic name here**). However, we recommend that you visit an otologist to reassure you that there is no underlying health condition causing the tinnitus for you to worry about. If you are not reassured, you could ask to be referred to your physician or another specialist to make sure. It is possible that you may have to wait for an appointment—so why not start to help yourself manage your tinnitus now?

By following the advice in these notes, you can actually treat your tinnitus yourself and possibly achieve a gradual reduction of tinnitus to something that will eventually no longer matter much or at all.

What Is Tinnitus?

Tinnitus is the experience of hearing a sound from within one or both of your ears, or your head. It is often described as a ringing, buzzing, or whistling noise. It is usually due to minor disorder of your hearing system and is often associated with aging or exposure to loud noise. It is a symptom, not a disease.

Although tinnitus can sometimes be very distressing, it is usually not life-threatening, and the quality of your life can be recovered. You may not be able to get rid of your tinnitus noise completely, but you can gradually reduce or eliminate the way tinnitus affects you, so that you hardly notice it. Most people who are upset by their tinnitus learn to manage it through doing things for themselves to improve their tinnitus. However, it may take several months—this is quite normal, so don't feel disheartened.

Your Hearing System

When you hear outside sounds, those sounds travel in waves in the air and are converted by your inner ear (cochlea) into nerve signals that are like tiny electrical currents. These signals pass up your hearing nerve to the base of your brain. Your brain then sorts out what is immediately important. It usually ignores meaningless sounds, and it can learn to do the same with the internal sound of your tinnitus.

We can distinguish particular sounds in a great hubbub of other sounds. For example, most people can probably pick out the sound of their name uttered by someone in a room of chattering people and can detect a single musical instrument in a full orchestra. Unfortunately, many people with tinnitus tend to do this with their tinnitus when it starts—we naturally home in on that new, unfamiliar, and unwanted noise.

Selectivity and Attention

Your hearing system has an automatic property of selectivity. That is, parts of the hearing system within your brain increase the degree to which they select out certain important, strange, or worrying sounds (including tinnitus) for special attention, and filter out the hearing of other sounds. Also, as you get older, your ability to hear external sounds reduces, and the resulting lack of contrasting sound makes you become more aware of internal tinnitus noises. Any other form of hearing disorder or damage, such as from repeated exposure to loud noise (for example, gunshots, noise at work, or very loud music), can add to this natural hearing loss and make tinnitus even more noticeable.

Habituation

Imagine you have a new refrigerator. At first you can't help but hear its hum, but after a while you find you are no longer aware of it. Other people hearing your new fridge for the first time say how loud it is, but you are habituated to it—you are no longer conscious of it, your brain has decided to stop monitoring its constant, meaningless, nonthreatening ticking. This is a natural process, called habituation that your brain uses to stop overloading itself with the need to monitor all sorts of harmless information—and that applies to tinnitus, too.

Tinnitus naturally subsides over time. It isn't a progressive condition that gets worse the longer you have it or the older and the more hard of hearing you become—it's quite the opposite! But you can do things to speed up this habituation process, and to alleviate some of the effects of tinnitus until it subsides.

Anxiety, Tension, and Learning How to Relax

It is very common to worry about tinnitus and for this to cause tension, so learning how to relax is part of the relief process. Tinnitus often creates a vicious cycle of tension and worry that keeps the tinnitus worse than it could be. The following figure shows how this works.

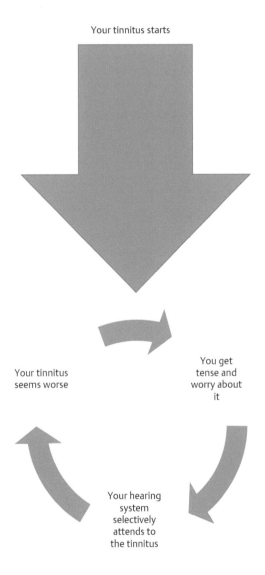

Your tinnitus starts

Your tinnitus seems worse

You get tense and worry about it

Your hearing system selectively attends to the tinnitus

But you can break this cycle! If you break it, the chain of events will reverse.

As a first step, read these notes again to make sure that you understand how worrying about your tinnitus and constantly listening to it will feed this vicious cycle. Monitoring your tinnitus and worrying about it will only make it worse.

Relaxation Exercises

To help relieve the tension in your body, you can use simple relaxation exercises that involve training your body to relax. You can read about exercises in books, listen to them via podcasts or YouTube, or learn how to do them from participating in our Tinnitus Activities Treatment, whichever you prefer.

Here are some simple examples of relaxation exercises:

1. Imagine you are taking a tour of your body. Find a comfortable position and bring your attention to your breath and the part of your body you are focusing on. Starting with your feet, breathe and scan your feet. Once you have scanned your feet, let your awareness go from that body part and move to the next. You can extend to your legs, to your back and belly, then to your hands, arms, your neck, jaw, and face. If your mind wanders from your breath, just bring your attention back to your breath without judging your thoughts.
2. Breathe slowly and deeply, hold your breath a moment, relax, then let it out, wait a moment, then breathe slowly and deeply again, and so on.

Once you have learned such breathing and muscle relaxation exercises, you can do them regularly, wherever and whenever you can find the time and space. It will take a bit of practice, but you should quickly start to feel the benefits, and you will gradually learn how to relax your body without having to do the exercises. As you learn to relax your body, you will also find it easier to relax your mind.

Some people find that aromatherapy, improved posture, massage, meditation, pilates, and yoga have similar relaxing benefits, as can simply resting in a relaxing environment, perhaps with dim lights and soft music. The key is to find what helps you relax the most and easiest, and practice it often.

Sound Therapy

The normal natural history of tinnitus is for it to gradually recede into the background so that you eventually become hardly aware of it—the habituation process described earlier. You can speed up this process by increasing the amount of background sound near you, what some audiologists call "sound therapy." This reduces the contrast between the level of your tinnitus and the tension it causes, thus promoting the habituation process and interrupting the vicious cycle described above. These principles and procedures involved are similar to those used in most forms of sound therapy.

Additional background sounds can come from:

- Pleasant low-level sounds from a television, radio, or music, from a fan, or from outside through an open window.
- Sound conditioners—tabletop devices or smartphone apps that play natural sounds (such as the sound of gentle waves, the rain, or a stream), or "white" noise (a continuous "shhh"-like sound).
- A wearable noise generator—a device that looks like and is worn like a hearing aid, but which makes its own "shhh" sound.
- Wearing and using a hearing aid, even if you have only slight difficulty in hearing.

Exactly what is the best level of additional sound to use varies, but we have found that most patients prefer a volume level just below that of their tinnitus that decreases the prominence of their tinnitus. However, if that is too loud for you, then use the loudest level you can put up with. But if you want to use more noise and drown out (mask) your tinnitus, do so if you find it suits you.

The key is to avoid quiet rooms and situations. In the quiet, your brain will try to hear any sound more clearly, and that will include the sound of your tinnitus. You should reinforce your background sound whenever the background is rather quiet, as often and for as long as you can.

If increasing background sound annoys other people around you, use a personal listening device such as a smartphone and headphones. You may find that using "in-ear" earphones delivers the sound into your ears better than headphones.

Most importantly, you also need sound therapy in bed, whether asleep or awake. It is particularly harmful if you lie in the quiet of the night listening to your tinnitus when you can't get to sleep, or when you wake up during the night. You could try sleeping with the window open, or have a gently ticking clock in your room, or use a sound pillow attached to the sound source of your choice. You are less likely to disturb others this way.

Recreation and Health

Having active interests and hobbies can enhance the quality of your life. They can put your tinnitus into a better perspective so you can still enjoy life to the full. It's never too late to learn or to get involved!

Some people have seen the positive side of their tinnitus and have welcomed the push it gave them to do something new, to rekindle old interests, or to take on the challenge of working for a tinnitus support group.

How is your general health? Are you getting a good, varied diet, plenty of exercise and rest, and some enjoyable social activity? If you find that certain foods or drinks, or activities or situations aggravate your tinnitus, you could cut down a little, cut them out, or find alternatives. With just a few adjustments, you will find that tinnitus won't stop you carrying on with life the way you want to.

Hyperacusis (Pronounced hyper-a-KOO-sis)

This means a condition of oversensitivity to loud sounds, even moderately loud sounds. It is found in many people with troublesome tinnitus and might be caused by a similar brain mechanism. Like tinnitus, hyperacusis can usually be improved using sound therapy procedures already described, although for hyperacusis the level of added sound is gradually increased, step by step, over a period of weeks or months. This treatment process is called "desensitization."

Earplugs

If you have tinnitus, you should not wear any kind of earplugs that make it more difficult to hear, except when you are in a very loud noise. They will not help your tinnitus: indeed they will probably make it seem louder while you wear them. Generally, it is not a good idea to wear earplugs if you have hyperacusis (unless you are using earplugs temporarily in a noise that is unbearably loud to you) as they can prevent your ears from getting accustomed to sounds. On the other hand, you should always use ear protection when you are exposed to very loud sounds, whether or not you have tinnitus or hyperacusis.

Temporary Deafness and Temporary Tinnitus

If you have been exposed to a particularly loud sound, for example, a loud music or fireworks or working around loud noise, you may often experience dullness of hearing or tinnitus, or both, immediately afterwards. Provided you don't let yourself get into a state of great anxiety about it, this will usually disappear after a few minutes or hours. These temporary effects should be taken as a warning, though—there is risk of permanent damage if you expose your ears repeatedly to such loud sounds.

Further Information and Help

With this insight into tinnitus, you may feel you can now learn to ignore yours. At our clinic, we offer tinnitus treatment, including sound therapy and counseling using the Tinnitus Activities Treatment that individualizes therapy for each patient. If you want to know more about tinnitus or schedule an appointment, contact us.

Source: Adapted from Sizer DI, Coles RRA. Tinnitus self-treatment. In Tyler RS, Tinnitus Treatment: Clinical Protocols, 1st ed. Thieme Publishers. 2006.

4 Tinnitus Activities Treatment

Ann Perreau, Richard S. Tyler, Patricia C. Mancini, and Shelley A. Witt

Abstract

Tinnitus Activities Treatment (TAT) was developed at the University of Iowa in the 1980s to help patients manage their bothersome tinnitus. Three goals are targeted in TAT: (1) to provide counseling on tinnitus and related problems, (2) to suggest coping strategies, and (3) to recommend partial masking using sound therapy. TAT is unique because it uses picture-based counseling materials with images and charts that are helpful illustrations of complex concepts and ensure sessions proceed in an orderly manner. We suggest using the Tinnitus Primary Functions Questionnaire to determine the sessions that are relevant for the patient and to document treatment effectiveness. TAT offers content for the four areas that are impacted by tinnitus including thoughts and emotions, hearing and communication, sleep, and concentration and includes an introduction and summary session. We include homework and practice activities with each session to allow patients to practice the suggested strategies. Through TAT, we advocate for a collaborative and holistic approach to helping patients manage their tinnitus by listening to the patient, understanding their needs, and providing directive counseling to address their concerns. Nurturing patient expectations and providing hope are essential to the therapeutic process.

Keywords: tinnitus, counseling, sound therapy, audiologists

4.1 Introduction

Tinnitus Activities Treatment (TAT), our counseling and sound therapy program, was created in the 1980s to provide structure to helping tinnitus patients, which included coping strategies and total and partial masking.[1,2] An essential component of our treatment is to determine problems experienced by patients that are associated with their tinnitus. This can be accomplished by administering tinnitus questionnaires, as described later in Chapter 12. We recognize the importance of considering all difficulties experienced by the patient,[1] and refrain from considering tinnitus as an isolated problem. For example, we ask patients about their general outlook on life during treatment to gauge their emotional well-being. Informational counseling on tinnitus is incorporated at all stages of activities treatment to lessen fears, unknowns, and misconceptions about tinnitus, to promote better expectations for tinnitus treatment, and to empower patients to accept their tinnitus. We suggest coping strategies throughout treatment that target the unique problems faced by each patient using activities and techniques guided by the audiologist. Finally, activities treatment combines sound therapy, specifically partial masking, to reduce the prominence of the patient's tinnitus.[3,4] Our general recommendation is to use the lowest level of masker such that the tinnitus and the background sound will both be audible.[5] We demonstrate partial masking to patients by comparing it to candle in a dark room (e.g., tinnitus in a quiet room) versus brightly lit room (e.g., partial masking). As shown in ▶ Fig. 4.1, tinnitus is more noticeable in a quiet room and less noticeable when a low-level background sound is present. Sound therapy is not appropriate for all patients, especially those with hearing loss who experience diminished speech perception with sound therapy. Many patients will have tried sound therapy on their own, so providing guidance to patients is an important part of treatment. Refer to Chapters 7 and 8 on sound therapy for specific details.

The counseling approach implemented in TAT has been influenced by a number of significant studies and contributions.[6,7,8,9,10,11,12] More recent descriptions of our treatment are available in the literature.[13,14] Our experience in treating tinnitus patients and our discussions with other experts led us to group the problems faced by tinnitus patients into four broad categories[2]:
• Thoughts and emotions.
• Hearing and communication.
• Sleep.
• Concentration.

Functional impairments in these areas can lead to additional social and work problems. We believe that a complete therapy program should address all of these categories. Any area not of concern for the patient can be omitted from counseling. The counseling provided in each of these areas is described in more detail later in this chapter.

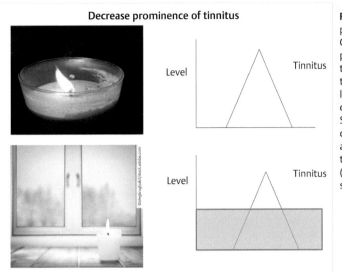

Decrease prominence of tinnitus

Fig. 4.1 Illustration demonstrating partial masking of light and sound. On the *left*, a candle in a dark room is partially masked by the bright sunlight through a window. On the *right*, tinnitus is partially masked by a low-level background sound. Small candle in dark room = very noticeable. Similar to tinnitus in a quiet room. Put candle in front of brightly lit window and it is not as noticeable. Similar to tinnitus with low-volume noise. (Source: *Bottom left*: ©olegkruglyak3/stock.adobe.com)

Some of the key principles of TAT include nurturing patient expectations, providing counseling using pictures on areas that are impacted by tinnitus, and implementing a patient-centered approach to care.

4.1.1 Patient Expectation Nurturing

First, we have emphasized the importance of audiologists to nurture patient expectations and provide a positive outlook[15] as opposed to a negative prognosis (nothing can be done). The specific attributes of nurturing patient expectations include:
- Be perceived as a knowledgeable professional.
- Be sympathetic.
- Demonstrate that you understand tinnitus.
- Provide a clear therapy plan.
- Show that you sincerely care.
- Provide reasonable hope.

4.1.2 Picture-Based Counseling

TAT also uses picture-based counseling that was introduced in 2001 for tinnitus patients.[16] Using this approach, the illustrations are shared by the patient and audiologist in a collaborative manner to facilitate discussion on various topics related to tinnitus and its treatment. The picture-based approach has several advantages because:
- The sessions proceed in an orderly fashion.
- The clinician does not overlook important concepts.
- It is easier for the patient to understand concepts.

- Treatment can be easily utilized by other audiologists and therapists.
- It is easy to control counseling across conditions and therapists when comparing tinnitus treatments.

4.1.3 Patient-Centered Approach to Care

We have emphasized the importance of adapting tinnitus counseling to the needs and interests of the patient using a collaborative approach. Because activities treatment includes multiple sessions, sessions can be selected that are most relevant and helpful for the patient. We begin our tinnitus counseling by typically identifying three goals of therapy with the patient. Then, we administer the Tinnitus Primary Functions Questionnaire (TPFQ; see Appendix 4.1)[14] to document the problems associated with their tinnitus and use these results to determine the areas that require treatment. In addition, we provide an introduction to activities treatment where we encourage audiologists to listen to their patient and ask questions to determine what is important for the patient. Why is the patient here? What does he or she expect from therapy? Is the patient alone, or does he/she have support?

Because we cannot assume that we know what is best for the patient, probing questions help the audiologist to learn the patient's motivations and expectations for seeking treatment. This information is crucial to creating a patient-centered plan for tinnitus counseling. The introduction session to

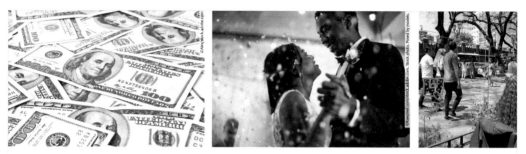

When your tinnitus began, what was your life like (home, work, etc.)?

Fig. 4.2 Illustration used to ask patients about their life situation when tinnitus began. Ask the patient to describe what their life was like when tinnitus began. Are other important things going on in their life (i.e., sickness/illness, problems at work or in the home) in addition to tinnitus? These answers can influence the direction of counseling. (Source: *Left*: ©Alex/stock. adobe.com; *center*: ©Rawpixel.com/stock.adobe.com. Stock photo. Posed by models.)

activities treatment is intended to be a brief overview in the first session with patient, lasting about 15 minutes. Some of the topics in our introduction to activities treatment include:

• What caused tinnitus?
• When tinnitus began, what was your life like? (▶ Fig. 4.2)
• How has tinnitus influenced your life?
• How do you think we can help?

After the introduction session, the audiologist will have a better understanding of the whole patient and their difficulties experienced by tinnitus and will be well equipped to initiate counseling. In some cases, a referral may be needed to other professionals (i.e., psychologists, physicians) who can also assist the patient. An initial counseling session also provides an opportunity to determine if more tinnitus counseling is warranted. A description of the sessions for activities treatment follows.

4.2 Discussion

4.2.1 Thoughts and Emotions

Tinnitus patients, like most people, have concerns and problems that affect their emotional well-being. As we have previously discussed, we begin by learning from the patient what general concerns are important for them. Occasionally, it will become evident that these problems are beyond our expertise, and a referral to a clinical psychologist or psychiatrist should be made. In the thoughts and emotions session, we aim to provide basic information about hearing loss and tinnitus, how our thoughts are influenced by tinnitus, and how to change our reactions to tinnitus. Providing

basic information about hearing loss and tinnitus often alleviates patient's concerns and fears about tinnitus and provides tools to refocus their thoughts away from tinnitus and concentrate on other aspects of life (see Appendix 4.2 for a patient handout on things to do for tinnitus).

Providing Information about Hearing, Hearing Loss, Tinnitus, and Attention

To educate patients on hearing loss and tinnitus, we begin by providing a general description of how we hear and the spontaneous activity of hearing nerves (▶ Fig. 4.3). This neural activity is used to code the presence of acoustic sound. However, even without sound, there is random spontaneous activity in the nerves and brain. Later, we explain how tinnitus is likely coded by the spontaneous activity of the hearing nerve (▶ Fig. 4.4).

We also address a few common concerns directly with patients, including that tinnitus does not make a person deaf, senile, or imply a state of mental illness. Often, reassuring patients that tinnitus is not an indication of a life-threatening disease, and educating them on the common occurrence of tinnitus in the general population removes some of these concerns. If negative thoughts about tinnitus predominate one's thoughts, it is easy to become preoccupied with them.

To explain the influence of tinnitus on one's thoughts, we discuss how conscious attention works.[7] Hallam,[7] who emphasized the importance of hearing and attention, noted that we can only attend to one stimulus at a time (▶ Fig. 4.5). Other

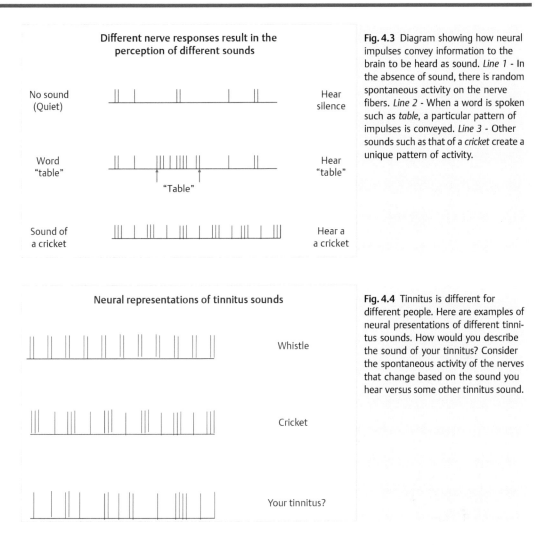

Different nerve responses result in the perception of different sounds

No sound (Quiet) — Hear silence

Word "table" — "Table" — Hear "table"

Sound of a cricket — Hear a a cricket

Fig. 4.3 Diagram showing how neural impulses convey information to the brain to be heard as sound. *Line 1* - In the absence of sound, there is random spontaneous activity on the nerve fibers. *Line 2* - When a word is spoken such as *table*, a particular pattern of impulses is conveyed. *Line 3* - Other sounds such as that of a *cricket* create a unique pattern of activity.

Neural representations of tinnitus sounds

Whistle

Cricket

Your tinnitus?

Fig. 4.4 Tinnitus is different for different people. Here are examples of neural presentations of different tinnitus sounds. How would you describe the sound of your tinnitus? Consider the spontaneous activity of the nerves that change based on the sound you hear versus some other tinnitus sound.

stimuli will remain in our subconscious until they grab our attention and move into our conscious attention, or be ignored. As humans, we notice important stimuli and ignore unimportant stimuli (▶ Fig. 4.6). Hallam provided the helpful analogy, the background sound of a refrigerator hum, to illustrate our ability to ignore certain stimuli. The hum is repetitive, and though the sound of a new refrigerator may be loud at first, the repetitive sound will not activate the amygdala and autonomic nervous system with continued exposure. It will not attract our conscious attention and will eventually be deemed unimportant. Likewise, if we decide tinnitus is unimportant, we will not attend to it, it becomes less noticeable, and we can habituate to the sound, though this may take some time. Hallam suggested that most people can learn to ignore tinnitus in about 18 months.

Change the Emotional Reaction to Tinnitus

Our activities treatment is designed not only to change how patients think about tinnitus, but also how they react to tinnitus. One of the first steps to change the reaction to tinnitus is to change how we interpret the importance of tinnitus. Moreover, recognizing several facts about tinnitus will lessen its importance: (a) tinnitus is likely the result of increased neural activity, (b) tinnitus is common and affects nearly 15% of adults, and (c) tinnitus is not threatening our health or hearing. Cognitive therapy separates the tinnitus from the patient's reaction to it. Thus, we emphasize that having tinnitus and a patient's reaction to tinnitus are two different things.

Next, we explain the connection between our thoughts and emotions in a general sense, and then as applied to tinnitus. Tinnitus is a sound—neither

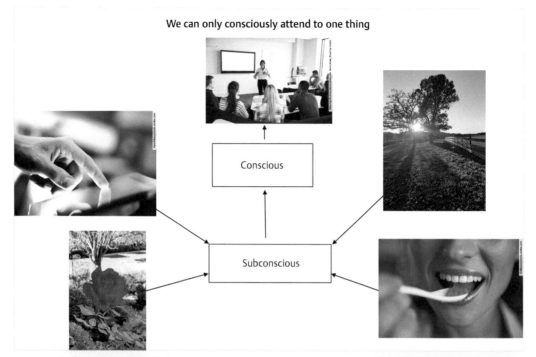

We can only consciously attend to one thing

Fig. 4.5 Diagram representing how many sensory stimuli are received subconsciously, yet we can usually attend to only one thing consciously. We can only consciously attend to one stimuli at a time. We receive many stimuli at a given time. All other stimuli will remain in our subconscious until it grabs our attention and moves to conscious attention, or is ignored. (Source: *Top left*: ©peshkova/stock.adobe.com; *top center*: ©Monkey Business/stock.adobe.com. Stock photo. Posed by models; *bottom right*: ©Alliance/stock.adobe.com)

We notice important things and ignore unimportant stimuli

Refrigerator: Ignore

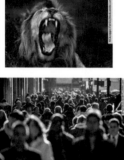

Lion: Cannot ignore

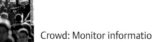

Crowd: Monitor information automatically

Fig. 4.6 Diagram displaying how neutral sounds that do not carry any significant information will be ignored and important sounds (e.g., an alarm, a lion roar) that carry with them an emotional reaction will not be ignored. Some sounds like crowd noise will be monitored automatically and not attended to consciously. (Source: *Center*: ©Giuseppe D'Amico/stock.adobe.com; *bottom*: ©Von blvdone/stock.adobe.com)

good nor bad. It is just a sound. When tinnitus enters a patient's life, personal thoughts are attached to this sound. It is important to help patients understand that these personal thoughts have a direct connection to emotions, and emotions create physical reactions. We address this explaining that: (1) positive thoughts = positive emotions; (2) negative thoughts = negative emotions; and (3) neutral thoughts = no emotions. The brain can learn a different response (e.g., negative) to the same doorbell

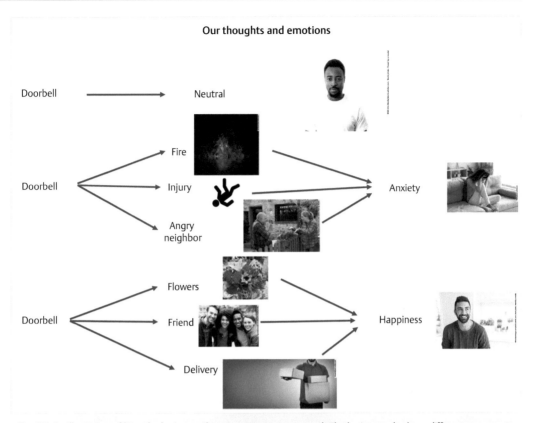

Fig. 4.7 An illustration of how the brain can "learn" a response to a sound. The brain can also learn different response to same sound. The brain automatically attaches an emotional reaction to doorbell depending on the consequence. Same sound produces opposite reactions of the body depending on the context and the interpretation of what is going on. In a similar fashion, exactly the same sound of tinnitus might produce an entirely different reaction depending on the context. (Source: *Neutral*: ©SB Arts Media/stock.adobe.com. Stock photo. Posed by a model; *fire*: ©Victor/stock.adobe.com; *angry neighbor*: ©JackF/stock.adobe.com. Stock photo. Posed by models; *friend*: ©goodluz/stock.adobe.com. Stock photo. Posed by models; *delivery*: ©ronstik/stock.adobe.com; *anxiety*: ©fizkes/stock.adobe.com; *happiness*: ©Krackenimages.com/stock.adobe.com. Stock photo. Posed by a model.)

sound, and we attach an emotional reaction (i.e., anxiety) to the doorbell depending on the consequence (▶ Fig. 4.7).

Even subconscious negative thoughts can make the situation worse; so, it is important to help patients identify underlying negative thoughts. Helping patients reframe negative thoughts to more constructive ones can help minimize negative emotions and, ultimately, make the tinnitus less prominent. Please note that this is a good, but very simplistic way to think about thoughts and emotions. The human psyche is much more complex than this. Sometimes it can be difficult to reconstruct negative thoughts to more neutral or positive ones, and that not all patients are successful at this. However, replacing negative thoughts with more constructive and/or positive thoughts can help reduce and/or neutralize negative emotions, making it easier to manage the tinnitus sound (▶ Fig. 4.8).

We also encourage patients to refocus their attention on other activities, such as joining new clubs or learning new tasks. We often discuss their hobbies, what activities are helpful to ignore tinnitus, and the possibilities of new activities that bring intrinsic value and enjoyment. It is important for patients to know that many people who have tinnitus are able to lead happy, productive lives. Group counseling (Chapter 15) can be very effective with tinnitus patients to demonstrate involvement in activities and ways to refocus away from tinnitus.

Patients often benefit from having a specific assignment to work on to assist them in changing their reactions to tinnitus. We sometimes encourage use of a "tinnitus diary" for the first weeks of treatment (see Appendix 4.3a for a tinnitus diary). Patients can log their thoughts and worries about tinnitus, and then challenge these thoughts with more constructive ways of thinking. Patients can also

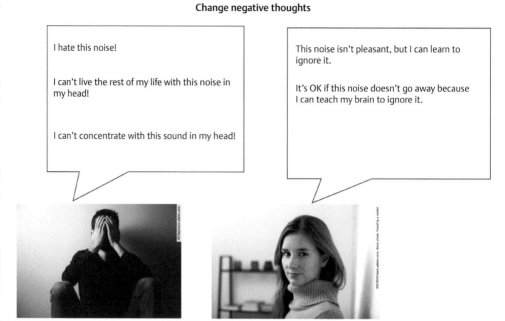

Fig. 4.8 Illustration showing different ways of thinking about tinnitus. One person "hates" the tinnitus. The other person doesn't like it but is prepared to learn different ways of reacting to it. When engaging in negative thoughts, encourage the patient to challenge these thoughts. Examples: "I hate this noise!" This is a negative thought that will elicit negative emotions (anger, frustration). "I can't live the rest of my life with this noise in my head!" This is also a negative thought that will lead to negative emotions such as worry, anxiety, and hopelessness. Recommend that they engage in constructive thoughts and help them feel the physiological/emotional difference. For example, "This is okay." Less emotionally charged. (Source: *Left*: ©Tiko/stock.adobe.com; *right*: ©RFBSIP/stock.adobe.com. Stock photo. Posed by a model.)

list the situations and activities where their tinnitus is worse and situations where it was better. This will provide helpful information to discuss with the patient about how to change their reaction to tinnitus, how to modify the environment, and what sounds could be added to decrease the prominence of their tinnitus. Appendix 4.3b shows an example tinnitus diary from a patient. We recommend that the diary be used for only a few weeks because we want the patients to move away from thinking about their tinnitus and refocus on other activities that they enjoy.

Finally, the use of background sound at a low level (or partial masking) can be beneficial for many patients to reduce the prominence of tinnitus and change their reaction to it. Because Chapters 1 and 8 discussed masking in depth, we will focus on providing patient education about use of background sound. For most patients, providing a rationale for the use of background sound in decreasing tinnitus and the activities related to background sound is typically helpful. Specifically, low-level background noise makes tinnitus difficult to detect and interferes with the detection of tinnitus-related neural activity (▶ Fig. 4.9). In addition, background sounds can partially mask the

unwanted sound we hear (▶ Fig. 4.10). A great exercise is to have the tinnitus patient take some time to "sound search," or search for sound(s) that will mix well with the tinnitus, making the tinnitus less noticeable. In our experience, most patients will have done this already, but it can be helpful to revisit the sounds that are most effective in reducing tinnitus. It may be important to remind the patient that they are not looking for a sound to make the tinnitus to go away, but a more neutral sound that might make the tinnitus less noticeable.

4.2.2 Hearing and Communication

The goal of this therapy is to help patients understand how tinnitus affects hearing and provide approaches for improving hearing abilities. Many patients are not aware of what can be done to help. By improving hearing and communication in different situations, we hope to:

- Alleviate difficulties that might be experienced due to hearing loss.
- Alleviate difficulties that might be experienced due to tinnitus.
- Reduce stress.

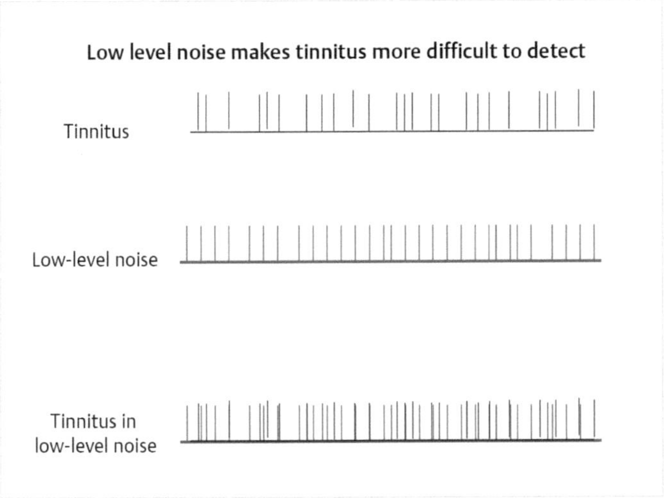

Low level noise makes tinnitus more difficult to detect

Tinnitus

Low-level noise

Tinnitus in
low-level noise

Fig. 4.9 In quiet, the tinnitus signal is enhanced and the brain has nothing else to distract it from "hearing" the tinnitus. If put low-volume noise in environment, it becomes harder for the brain to keep track of or detect the tinnitus. The low-volume sound is used to interfere with the detection of the tinnitus-related neural activity. We are consciously aware of only a small portion of incoming sounds because these sounds are filtered out before they reach the level of conscious perception. As your emotional reaction to the tinnitus is reduced, the brain will interpret the tinnitus the same way it does other insignificant background noise and filter it out.

Background sound masks unwanted sounds

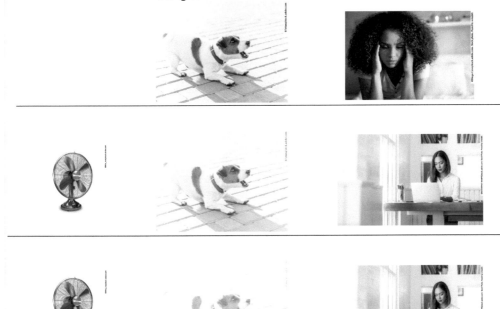

Fig. 4.10 An example of how background noise can partially mask an annoying barking dog while someone is trying to concentrate on work. The background sound can partially mask the unwanted sound we hear. Here, a barking dog is the unwanted sound, and the fan is the background sound that helps minimize the barking dog sound. (Source: *Left*: ©Wire_man/stock.adobe.com; *center*: ©Tetiana/stock.adobe.com; *top right*: ©Diego Cervo/stock.adobe.com. Stock photo. Posed by a model; *center and bottom right*: ©NATHAPHAT NAMPIX/stock.adobe.com. Stock Photo. Posed by a model.)

Further, there are many factors that affect communication such as hearing loss, the amount of background noise, the ability to see talker, familiarity with talker, familiarity with topic, and stress level (▶ Fig. 4.11) that are incorporated into activities treatment. Many of these topics can be demonstrated, not simply discussed.

Factors that affect communication

- Hearing loss

- Background noise

- Ability to see the talker

- Familiarity with talker

- Familiarity with topic of discussion

- Stress level

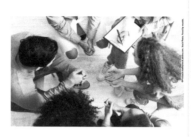

Fig. 4.11 There are many different factors that affect communication. Many of these can be actually demonstrated, not simply discussed. (Source: ©Prostock-studio/stock. adobe.com. Stock Photo. Posed by models.)

Hearing and Hearing Loss

One way to reduce difficulties associated with hearing loss is to help the patients better understand hearing and hearing loss. First, we briefly explain to our patients how the auditory system works by reviewing basic anatomy and physiology of the ear. Second, we talk to them about how the auditory system is affected by hearing loss. We review the patients' audiograms so that they understand if they have hearing loss and the severity of the hearing loss in detailed manner. Finally, we ask that the patient share the difficulties they face as a result of their hearing loss. Particularly, we help them understand the perceptual consequences of hearing loss and that some sounds that they once heard well may be difficult to distinguish, or may not be audible to them at all. For example, if the patients have a high-frequency hearing loss, we would explain to them why they perceive people talking to them as "mumbling," or why sounds with mostly high-frequency energy like /s/ are more difficult to hear. We also explain to them how noise can affect their hearing and the importance of the signal-to-noise ratio.

Hearing Difficulties due to Hearing Loss and Tinnitus

It is important to help patients understand and distinguish difficulties that they may be experiencing due to hearing loss versus those that they may be experiencing as a result of tinnitus. We explain to patients that hearing loss will make some sounds they hear seem distorted and other sounds almost completely inaudible. We also explain that tinnitus does not cause hearing loss, but it can produce hearing difficulty by distracting one from listening. The ringing, buzzing, or roaring sound of tinnitus can also produce a masking of environmental sounds.[17] In addition, we explain that tinnitus can cause difficulties in distinguishing one sound from another because the tinnitus sound can be confused with external sounds especially if they have the same pitch. For example, sometimes people with tinnitus may hear a sound, like a fan, and later discover that it was actually their tinnitus.

Strategies to Improve Hearing and Communication

There are three main areas that we discuss in detail to help patients better manage their hearing loss. See Appendix 4.4 for a handout on these strategies. These consist of the following.

Use of Amplification

The first step in managing hearing loss is to make sure that patients are fit with an appropriate hearing device (refer to Chapter 7). This may consist of fitting the patient with a hearing aid, cochlear implant, or an assistive listening device. First, we explain to the patient how hearing devices function. Next, we discuss the goals of amplification appropriate for their hearing loss and personal life, such as improved audibility of environmental sounds, improved communication and conversational abilities, and reduced listening effort. We also emphasize importance of binaural hearing aids over monaural fittings, not only for hearing ability but also for tinnitus reduction. Finally, if the patients are already wearing hearing devices, we check the appropriateness of the fit using real ear measures, and answer any questions that they may have about their current hearing device.

Environment

Patients are often unaware of how the environment influences their hearing performance. We teach patients that environments with the following characteristics are more suitable for facilitating a conversation.[18]

- Good lighting:
  - Make sure there is adequate light to illuminate the communication partner's face without shadowing it.
  - Move away from light that is shining directly in the listener's eyes and making it difficult to see communication partner's face.
- Positioning:
  - Be close to the communication partner to enhance the signal-to-noise ratio.
  - Make sure that the face of the communication partner is visible and not in profile.
  - Move away from the noise, or reposition yourself so that the noise source is away from the talker.
- Minimizing visual distractions:
  - Turn off the TV, cell phone, tablet, or other electronic devices.
  - Close a door to eliminate movement from another room.
  - Close a window to eliminate blowing curtains or outside distractions.
- Minimizing noise:
  - Turn off extraneous noise sources (TV, radio, kitchen noises, etc.).
  - Close doors and windows to minimize background noise.

Communication

One of the most important things we do with our patients is to empower them to take charge of their hearing loss by using an effective communication style. First, we define assertive communication and compare that with passive and aggressive styles.[19] We also discuss with patients the communication style that they typically use. Then we demonstrate, regardless of their personality type, how to become an assertive rather than a passive or aggressive communicator. Finally, we demonstrate and discuss the following:

- Use of repair strategies to repair communication breakdowns (i.e., ask for individuals to slow down, use of clear speech, repeat, rephrase, reduce, or elaborate sentences).
- Use of anticipatory strategies prior to communication interactions (i.e., anticipate what the topic of conversation, learn key vocabulary words, practice the dialogue that will likely occur, use relaxation techniques to remain calm when you feel you are lost in the conversation).
- How to disclose hearing loss to potential conversation partners, when appropriate.

- Speech reading strategies (watch lips, facial expressions, and body movements).

Finally, we encourage patients to keep track of what repair and anticipatory strategies they use, and how use of the strategies might have helped them to hear and communicate better.

4.2.3 Sleep

Sleep disturbances are very common in tinnitus patients (e.g., McKenna[20]; Tyler & Baker[2]; see Chapter 6). Some patients have trouble falling asleep, others wake up during the night, but many patients report that being fatigued or tired makes tinnitus worse. Being under emotional stress and having difficulty concentrating and hearing can also contribute to fatigue. This therapy will help patients to:

- Understand normal sleep patterns.
- Explore the factors that affect their sleep.
- Determine the activities that will promote better sleep.
- Learn relaxation techniques and how to incorporate background sound.

Often, learning about normal sleep cycles and the various stages of sleep is informative for patients with sleep difficulties. We review recommendations for number of hours of sleep for adults (6.5–9 h), and how this may change as we age. Regarding the factors that affect sleep, we specifically emphasize how our thoughts and emotions, such as depression and anxiety influence sleep, and review ways that the environment (i.e., noise, light, temperature) affects sleep. There are both daytime (get regular exercise, avoid napping) and nighttime (go to bed only when you are tired enough to sleep) activities to promote better sleep. We discuss the importance of creating a curfew to separate the day and night, typically about 1½ hours before bedtime. After that time, patients are encouraged to avoid stress, exercise, eating, alcohol, and caffeine. We also discuss how patients arrange the bedroom (▶ Fig. 4.12), specifically that they should eliminate or reduce any distractions and nonsleep-related items, including a TV, cellphone, laptop, food or drink, etc. We also demonstrate relaxation techniques, including progressive muscle relaxation and visual imagery to patients. Finally, we recommend low-level background sound be used to reduce the prominence of tinnitus in the quiet bedroom. There are many ways that low-level background sound can be achieved (e.g., radio, fan, and

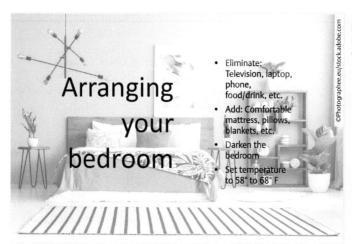

Fig. 4.12 Activities for arranging the bedroom to facilitate sleep. (Source: ©Photographee.eu/stock.adobe.com)

Arranging your bedroom

- Eliminate: Television, laptop, phone, food/drink, etc.
- Add: Comfortable mattress, pillows, blankets, etc.
- Darken the bedroom
- Set temperature to 58° to 68° F

humidifier), and many patients will have already tried something on their own. It is less known by patients that they can control the level of sound to promote better sleep, such as setting a timer to shut off after you will be asleep. For patients who continue to have sleep problems even after we implement these day and nighttime activities, relaxation, and background sounds, we encourage use of a sleep diary to determine which foods, activities, etc., may be contributing to sleep difficulties. See Appendix 4.5 for a guide on good sleep for tinnitus patients. Appendix 4.6 also outlines additional strategies for improving sleep that can be provided to patients.

4.2.4 Concentration

Tinnitus affects one's concentration or the ability to focus the mind on a particular problem or activity. An inability to concentrate can be frustrating or stressful. Here, we address three ways to improve concentration: providing information about the factors that affect concentration, discussing how tinnitus affects concentration, and increasing attention to the task at hand.

Provide Information about Concentration Difficulties

Everyone can be distracted by visual and auditory stimuli. ▶ Fig. 4.13 displays factors that contribute to our ability to concentrate. Some distracting stimuli are:
- Annoying.
- Fearful.
- Competing with the desired target.

- Loud.
- Unpredictable.
- Uncontrollable.

We begin by discussing the differences in concentration skills. We ask patients what problems they have with concentration and discuss how they feel when they have difficulty focusing. Some people cannot study or read in a noisy coffee shop, whereas others can do so easily. Yet, people can learn to focus their attention. An example of this is that some individuals with chronic pain can successfully train themselves to focus their attention away from their discomfort and onto other activities.

Decreasing the Intrusiveness of Tinnitus

Not all people are distracted by tinnitus. However, if it is distracting, focusing attention on tinnitus will make it more difficult to concentrate on other problems or particular tasks. When we focus attention to our tinnitus, it is harder to concentrate on other things. We encourage patients to observe the effects of their tinnitus on concentration for simple (e.g., filing) versus complex (e.g., learning a new computer game) tasks. Simple tasks may not be stimulating enough because tinnitus fills in the "gaps," but tinnitus may be less noticeable while completing complex tasks that are more demanding. We try to figure out what it is about these situations that leads them to be less distracted by their tinnitus, and determine whether or not these characteristics can be transposed to other situations.

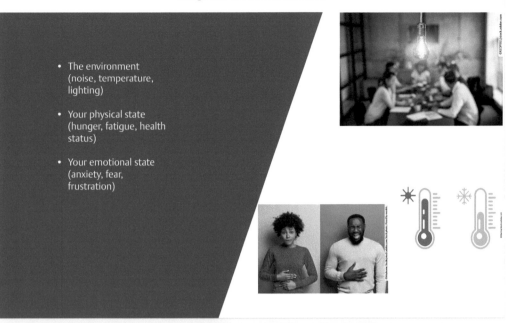

Things that affect concentration

- The environment (noise, temperature, lighting)

- Your physical state (hunger, fatigue, health status)

- Your emotional state (anxiety, fear, frustration)

Fig. 4.13 Things that can affect concentration, including factors in the environment, and one's physical and emotional state. (Source: *Top:* ©REDPIXEL/stock.adobe.com; *bottom left*; ©Wayhome Studio/stock.adobe.com. Stock photo. Posed by models; *bottom right:* ©Marina/stock.adobe.com)

Strategies to improve concentration

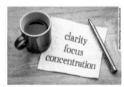

1. Interpret tinnitus as not important

2. Eliminate distractions

3. Stay focused

4. Adjust work habits

5. Decrease prominence of tinnitus

6. Take control of your attention

Fig. 4.14 Strategies to stay focused when concentration is challenged. (Source: ©MarekPhotoDesign.com/stock.adobe.com.)

We discuss the fears that patients have about their tinnitus, and try to dispel fears with a thorough discussion about the mechanisms of tinnitus, and its causes. With the appropriate information, we help patients to realize that they do not need to feel threatened by tinnitus or attend to it.

Strategies to Improve Concentration (▶ Fig. 4.14)

Henry and Wilson[9] describe an "attention diversion" approach to help tinnitus patients learn to control their attention. Patients practice changing the focus of their attention from one stimulus to another (▶ Fig. 4.15). We begin using physical sensations that might be tactile or visual, such as clothing on the skin or an object in a nearby visual field. Practice can then be done by being aware of external sounds, such as a fan noise in the room, and later, directing attention to and from tinnitus. Patients are taught that the focus of our attention is largely under volitional control and that they can divert their attention away from their tinnitus.

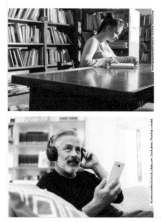

Attention control exercises

- Learn to switch attention from one stimulus to another (e.g., object, sensation, thought, activity) at will

- Allows you to refocus your attention from your tinnitus onto other stimuli

Fig. 4.15 Illustration introducing attention control exercises. (Source: *Top*: ©deyan georgiev/EyeEm/stock. adobe.com. Stock photo. Posed by a model; *bottom*: ©contrastwerkstatt/ stock.adobe.com. Stock photo. Posed by a model.)

Other strategies we recommend are staying focused and adjusting work habits. We encourage patients who are challenged by their tinnitus to actively participate in conversation or problem solving, to take notes on the topic, and to ask questions and stay engaged. Patients can also modify how they approach tasks in which they have difficulty concentrating. For example, a complex task requiring focused and prolonged concentration could be reduced to smaller tasks than can be done in shorter periods of time (20–40 min), taking breaks when needed. Reading is one task that can be easily segmented into shorter intervals. Finally, decreasing the prominence of tinnitus through the use of sound therapy can help to reduce its distracting nature. We recommend partial masking, with either wearable or nonwearable devices as described earlier in the chapter. Refer to Appendix 4.7 for a handout on strategies to improve concentration.

4.3 Conclusion

For some patients, a 5- to 15-minute counseling session that provides a brief overview of the general principles outlined in this chapter will be sufficient.[21,22] During the initial consultation with a patient, we determine if a more thorough counseling session is warranted.

Other patients will require more extensive counseling on several areas that are included in TAT. The content in the counseling sessions includes picture-based materials to be discussed by the patient and clinician, activities to better understand the patient's problems, interests, and motivations, and homework to allow the patients to practice the strategies introduced in each session. Most patients can complete the counseling in three to four sessions, each lasting about 1 hour and separated by 1 or 2 weeks. Presenting the information over several sessions allows for repetition of key concepts and avoids overloading patients with too much information at any given time.

We have recently updated the picture-based materials for activities treatment. Also, we now include notes for the audiologist to guide the discussion with the patient in the counseling sessions. To summarize, our patient-centered approach to tinnitus management uses four areas that are associated with functional impairments: thoughts and emotions, hearing and communication, sleep, and concentration. We include sound therapy to decrease the prominence of tinnitus and recommend administration of the TPFQ to determine the specific areas of difficulty for your tinnitus patient. Finally, we developed a summary session to be covered in a single 30-minute session that highlights the important concepts in activities treatment. TAT is available from Thieme Publishers via this book's companion website.

There are three videos available on the companion website that accompany this chapter. We provide a demonstration of the introduction counseling session of TAT with a patient who has tinnitus, a narration of summary session slides of TAT intended for audiologists who counsel patients with tinnitus, and a demonstration of a tinnitus diary to help tinnitus patients.

References

[1] Tyler RS, Babin RW. Tinnitus. In: Cummings CW, Frederickson J-M, Harker L, Krause CJ, Schuller DE, eds. Otolaryngology: Head and Neck Surgery. St Louis, MO: Mosby; 1986:3201–3217

[2] Tyler RS, Baker LJ. Difficulties experienced by tinnitus sufferers. J Speech Hear Disord. 1983; 48(2):150–154

[3] Stouffer JL, Tyler RS. Characterization of tinnitus by tinnitus patients. J Speech Hear Disord. 1990; 55(3):439–453

[4] Tyler RS, Stouffer JL, Schum R. Audiological rehabilitation of the tinnitus client. J Acad Rehabilitative Audiol. 1989; 22:30–42

[5] Tyler RS, Bentler RA. Tinnitus maskers and hearing aids for tinnitus. Semin Hear. 1987; 8(1):49–61

[6] Coles RRA. Tinnitus and its management. In: Stephens SDG, Kerr AG, eds. Scott-Brown's otolaryngology. Guildford, UK: Butterworth; 1987:368–414

[7] Hallam RS. Tinnitus: living with the ringing in your ears. New York: HarperCollins; 1989

[8] Hallam R, Rachman S, Hinchcliffe R. Psychological aspects of tinnitus. In: Rachman S, ed. 3rd ed. Contributions to medical psychology. Oxford: Pergamon Press; 1984:31–53

[9] Henry JL, Wilson PH. The psychological management of chronic tinnitus: a cognitive-behavioral approach. Boston, MA: Allyn & Bacon; 2001

[10] Henry JL, Wilson PH. Tinnitus: a self-management guide for the ringing in your ears. Boston, MA: Allyn & Bacon; 2002

[11] Sweetow RW. Cognitive-behavioral modification in tinnitus management. Hearing Instruments. 1984; 35:14–52

[12] Wilson PH, Henry JL, Andersson G, Hallam RS, Lindberg P. A critical analysis of directive counselling as a component of tinnitus retraining therapy. Br J Audiol. 1998; 32(5):273–286

[13] Tyler RS, Gogel SA, Gehringer AK. Tinnitus activities treatment. In: Langguth B, Hajak G, Kleinjung T, Cacace A, Moller AR, eds. Tinnitus: pathophysiology and treatment. Progress in Brain Research 2007;166:425–434

[14] Tyler RS, Noble W, Coelho C, Roncanci ER, Jun HJ. In: Katz J, Chasin M, English K, Hood LJ, Tillery KL, eds. Handbook of clinical audiology. New York: Wolters Kluwer; 2014:647–658

[15] Tyler RS, Haskell G, Preece J, Bergan C. Nurturing patient expectations to enhance the treatment of tinnitus. Semin Hear. 2001; 22:15–21

[16] Tyler RS, Bergan C. Tinnitus retraining therapy: a modified approach. Hear J. 2001; 54(11):36–42

[17] Surr RK, Montgomery AA, Mueller HG. Effect of amplification on tinnitus among new hearing aid users. Ear Hear. 1985; 6(2):71–75

[18] Dillon H. Hearing aids. Turramurra, Australia: Boomerang Press;2001

[19] Tye-Murray N. Foundations of aural rehabilitation: children, adults, and their family members. San Diego, CA: Singular;1998

[20] McKenna L. Tinnitus and insomnia. In: Tyler RS, ed. Tinnitus handbook. San Diego, CA: Singular; 2000:59–84

[21] Preece JP, Tyler RS, Noble W. The management of tinnitus. Geriatr Aging. 2003; 6(6):22–28

[22] Tyler RS, Erlandsson S. Management of the tinnitus patient. In: Luxon LM, Furman JM, Martini A, Stephens D, eds. Textbook of audiological medicine. Oxford: Isis Publications; 2000:571–578

Appendix 4.1 Tinnitus Primary Functions Questionnaire (12-Item Version)

Patient name: _____

Date: _____

Instructions: Please indicate your agreement with each statement on a scale from 0 (completely disagree) to 100 (completely agree).

Item	Statement	Your Rating (0–100)
1	I feel like my tinnitus makes it difficult for me to concentrate on some tasks.	
2	I have difficulty focusing my attention on some important tasks because of tinnitus.	
3	My inability to think about something undisturbed is one of the worst effects of my tinnitus.	
4	My emotional peace is one of the worst effects of my tinnitus.	
5	I am depressed because of my tinnitus.	
6	I am anxious because of my tinnitus.	
7	My tinnitus masks some speech sounds.	
8	In addition to my hearing loss, my tinnitus interferes with my understanding of speech.	
9	One of the worst things about my tinnitus is its effect on my speech understanding, over and above any effect of my hearing loss.	
10	I am tired during the day because my tinnitus has disrupted my sleep.	
11	I lie awake at night because of my tinnitus.	
12	When I wake up in the night, my tinnitus makes it difficult to get back to sleep.	

Appendix 4.2 Things You Can Do for Your Tinnitus

Richard S. Tyler

Learn the Situations Where Your Tinnitus Is Worse and the Situations Where Your Tinnitus Is Better. Modify What You Can to Improve Your Situation

Tinnitus is often not bothersome all day long. Some activities seem to reduce its magnitude. Other activities seem to make it worse. By knowing what these activities are, and by making some changes in your daily schedule, you can increase the time that tinnitus is less noticeable and decrease the time it is more noticeable.

	Task	Examples
1	Keep a diary for 2 weeks	List the things you did during the day and whether they reduced your tinnitus or made it worse
2	Make a list of things that reduce or intensify your tinnitus	Activities; situations; environments; food and beverages; time of day; emotions
3	Modify your lifestyle	Use the list and diary above to make changes in you daily life so you are doing more activities where your tinnitus is better and fewer activities where your tinnitus is worse
4	Alternative ways of thinking about your tinnitus	Write down your thoughts and worries about your tinnitus. Check and see if these worries actually happen. List alternative ways of thinking about your tinnitus

Refocus Your Attention Away from Your Tinnitus and on to Activities that You Enjoy

Many patients focus their attention on their tinnitus. They think about their tinnitus much of the day. The more they think about their tinnitus, the worse it gets. The worse it gets, the more they think about it. Refocus Therapy helps you to focus on other activities. It is important to keep yourself busy. Focus your attention on things in life that you enjoy.

	Task	Examples
1	Make a list of activities you enjoy	Hobbies; social activities; individual activities; relaxing activities
2	Create and implement alternative activities when you find tinnitus bothersome	• Make a list of specific activities that you will start doing when your tinnitus is bothersome • Try these activities when you find your tinnitus bothersome and state whether it helped take your mind off the tinnitus
3	Put your tinnitus in the background	• Stop logging in your tinnitus diary after 2 weeks • Stop talking about your tinnitus • Stop reading about tinnitus

Create an Environment so You Are Surrounded by Low Levels of Background Sound

Most patients report that the presence of soft background noise or music is helpful. These sounds can cover up the tinnitus, reduce its loudness, and/or distract your attention from the tinnitus.

The types of sounds that you might find helpful are:

- Broadband noise (heard as "sssshhhh"—an example of this noise is a radio set between stations) or motor noises such as a fan.
- Music—usually soft, light, background music (e.g., classical baroque, simple piano music, music with oboes, flutes, and violins).
- Sound produced particularly for relaxation or distraction (e.g., recorded sounds of rain drops, waves, and waterfalls).

There are several different devices that produce these sounds:

- Wearable devices with earphones or insert earphones (e.g., IPOD, MP3 players).
- Non-wearable devices including radios, CD players, IPAD, televisions, or sound generators specifically produced for relaxation or tinnitus.

Some of these devices can be used at bedside with or without timers to assist with sleep.

	Task
1	Make a list of sounds you enjoy
2	Play these desirable background sounds at low levels when possible
3	Avoid silence

Appendix 4.3a Tinnitus Diary

Richard S. Tyler

NAME: _____

DATE: _____

What are your thoughts & worries about your tinnitus?
e.g., My tinnitus will ....

1

2

3

Do these thoughts & worries actually happen?

1

2

3

Alternative ways of thinking about your tinnitus that will be helpful
e.g., I have tinnitus, but it is really a small part of my life.

1

2

3

4

Week # ___	Activity	Effect on Tinnitus
Day 1		
Day 2		
Day 3		
Day 4		
Day 5		
Day 6		
Day 7		

- Make changes in your daily life so you are doing more activities where your tinnitus is better and fewer activities where your tinnitus is worse.
- Describe modifications you make to your daily living and the effect they have on your tinnitus.

- List new activities you try and how your tinnitus was affected.
- List any low level, background sounds you tried using and their effect on your tinnitus.
- List any "alternative activities" and whether they took your mind off your tinnitus.
- Avoid silence.

Make a list of things that reduce your tinnitus.

These Things Seem to Make My Tinnitus Better
1
2
3
4
5
6
7
8
9
10
11
12

Make a list of things that worsen your tinnitus.

These Things Seem to Make My Tinnitus Worse
1
2
3
4
5
6
7
8
9
10
11
12

Week # ___	Activity	Effect on Tinnitus
Day 1		
Day 2		
Day 3		
Day 4		
Day 5		
Day 6		
Day 7		

- Make changes in your daily life so you are doing more activities where your tinnitus is better and fewer activities where your tinnitus is worse.
- Describe modifications you make to your daily living and the effect they have on your tinnitus.

- List new activities you try and how your tinnitus was affected.
- List any low level, background sounds you tried using and their effect on your tinnitus.
- List any "alternative activities" and whether they took your mind off your tinnitus.
- Avoid silence.

Make a list of sounds you enjoy.

1
2
3
4
5
6
7
8
9
10

Make a list of activities you enjoy.

1
2
3
4
5
6
7
8
9
10
11
12

Create a list of alternative activities to engage in when you find tinnitus bothersome.

1
2
3
4
5
6
7
8

Appendix 4.3b Tinnitus Diary Example Case

Richard S. Tyler

NAME: _____

DATE: _____

What are your thoughts & worries about your tinnitus?
e.g., My tinnitus will ....

1   *My tinnitus will get worse over time.*

2   *Why me? What did I do to cause my tinnitus?*

3   *My tinnitus will interfere with being able to go out with friends.*

Do these thoughts & worries actually happen?

1   *Though some days can be worse, my tinnitus is about the same.*

2   *Tinnitus affects many people. It is not threatening my life to have tinnitus.*

3   *My tinnitus actually does not interfere with socializing with others if I don't focus on it.*

Alternative ways of thinking about your tinnitus that will be helpful
e.g., I have tinnitus, but it is really a small part of my life.

1   *I have tinnitus, but it is really a small part of my life.*

2   *I am seeking help with a professional and they will help me to cope and improve my tinnitus.*

3   *I can learn to ignore my tinnitus.*

4

Week # 1	Activity	Effects on Tinnitus
Day 1	*Walking*	*Heard birds chirping, did not notice tinnitus.*
Day 2	*Dining out at restaurant*	*There was lots of background noise, but I could hear my friend over the noise and my tinnitus.*
Day 3		
Day 4		
Day 5		
Day 6		
Day 7		

- Make changes in your daily life so you are doing more activities where your tinnitus is better and fewer activities where your tinnitus is worse.
- Describe modifications you make to your daily living and the effect they have on your tinnitus.
- List new activities you try and how your tinnitus was affected.
- List any low level, background sounds you tried using and their effect on your tinnitus.
- List any "alternative activities" and whether they took your mind off your tinnitus.
- Avoid silence.

Make a list of things that reduce your tinnitus.

These Things Seem to Make My Tinnitus Better	
1	*Using a fan in the background at night.*
2	*Listening to music during the day.*
3	
4	
5	
6	
7	
8	
9	
10	
11	
12	

Make a list of things that worsen your tinnitus.

These Things Seem to Make My Tinnitus Worse	
1	*Loud and unexpected sounds*
2	*Being in a quiet room*
3	*Being in a loud and crowded room*
4	
5	
6	
7	
8	
9	
10	
11	
12	

Week # 2	Activity	Effect on Tinnitus
Day 1	*Gardening*	*Focused on yard work, tinnitus was less noticeable.*
Day 2	*Working at computer*	*When focused on work project, tinnitus was not bothersome. Took breaks frequently to not be fatigued.*
Day 3		
Day 4		
Day 5		
Day 6		
Day 7		

- Make changes in your daily life so you are doing more activities where your tinnitus is better and fewer activities where your tinnitus is worse.
- Describe modifications you make to your daily living and the effect they have on your tinnitus.

- List new activities you try and how your tinnitus was affected.
- List any low level, background sounds you tried using and their effect on your tinnitus.
- List any "alternative activities" and whether they took your mind off your tinnitus.
- Avoid silence.

Make a list of sounds you enjoy.

1. *Classical music*
2. *Ocean background sound*
3.
4.
5.
6.
7.
8.

Make a list of activities you enjoy.

1. *Running*
2. *Playing in community band*
3. *Reading*
4.
5
6
7
8
9
10
11
12

Create a list of alternative activities to engage in when you find tinnitus bothersome.

1. *Meditation with relaxing music in the background*
2. *Yoga once a week to reduce stress.*
3
4
5
6
7
8

Appendix 4.4 Strategies to Improve Hearing and Communication

Richard S. Tyler

There are many factors that affect our ability to communicate:

1. Hearing loss—sensorineural, conductive, mixed.
2. Background noise—noise covers up speech.
3. Ability to see the talker—need lip reading, facial cues, body language.
4. Familiarity with topic of discussion and talker.
5. Stress level.

Many people with hearing loss and/or tinnitus experience difficulty in certain listening situations. The following strategies can help improve hearing and communication:

1. Amplification:
   - Hearing aids—worn in or behind the ear to make sounds louder.
   - Assistive listening devices—devices that minimize specific listening problems caused by hearing impairment.
   - Cochlear implants—for individuals who have severe to profound hearing loss.
2. Reducing background noise:
   - Position yourself so that the background noise is behind you:
     - Stand or sit close to the person speaking.
     - Go to another room if background noise too loud.
3. Watching faces:
   - Good lighting.
   - Positioning:
     - Face the talker.
     - Minimize noise and visual distractions.
     - Position yourself close to the talker.
4. Anticipatory strategies:
   - Know the topic and key vocabulary words of the discussion.
   - Practice a dialogue of what might be said.
   - Use relaxation techniques.
5. Lip-reading strategies:
   - Consider:
     - Topic of conversation.
     - The expressions and gestures of the person speaking.
   - Ask communication partners to:
     - Slow down.
     - Use clear speech but don't shout.
     - Face you.
     - Avoid chewing and random gestures while speaking.
6. Repair strategies for when communication breaks down:
   - Ask communication partners to:
     - Repeat—say it again the same way.
     - Rephrase—say it again in a different way.
     - Reduce—eliminate unnecessary information and only say the important points.
     - Elaborate—expand on what was said by providing an explanation or description of key points.
7. Positively influencing the communication situation:
   - Communication styles:
     - Assertive—guides communication partner, takes responsibility for communication difficulties.
     - Passive—avoids social situation; bluffs, nods, and pretends to understand.
     - Aggressive—dominates conversation, unwilling to take responsibility for communication difficulties.

Appendix 4.5 A Guide to a Good Night's Sleep for Tinnitus Patients

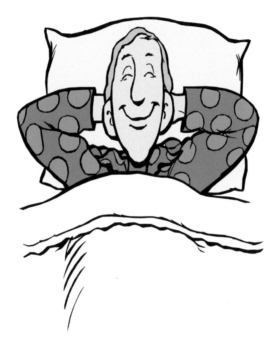

Many people with tinnitus report that their tinnitus interferes with their ability to get a good night's sleep. This guide will give you some options to try to help you get a good night's sleep.

How Tinnitus Affects Sleep

Tinnitus can interfere with the ability to fall asleep initially and/or to return to sleep after waking up. In addition, tinnitus can cause your sleeping problem to be made worse by the "vicious circle." The "vicious circle" occurs when, after having problems falling asleep, you become afraid you will not be able to sleep at all. You feel anxious about not getting enough sleep and this anxiety then keeps you awake.

Things You Can Do to Help with Sleep

1. **Bedroom Environment**
   The first step towards a good night sleep is to ensure that your bedroom is set-up to induce sleep. Changes to your bedroom might include:

- Remove the TV, computer, food, or anything that could distract you from sleep.
- Make sure that your mattress, blankets, pillows, and all other bedding are comfortable.
- Keep the room temperature between 58 and 68 degrees Fahrenheit.
- Play soft background noise or music. These sounds can cover up the tinnitus, reduce its loudness, and/or distract your attention from the tinnitus. Examples of sounds that you might find helpful are:
  - Broadband noise (heard as 'sssshhhh'): An example of this noise is a radio set between stations or motor noises such as a fan.
  - Music: Usually soft, light, background music (e.g., classical baroque, simple piano music, music with oboes, flutes, and violins).
  - Sound produced particularly for relaxation or distraction (e.g., recorded sounds of raindrops, waves, and waterfalls).

2. **Sleep Disrupters**
   The next step is to change aspects of your lifestyle that may be disrupting your sleep pattern:
   - Don't go to bed again until you feel very drowsy.

- Avoid any drink with caffeine (coffee, tea, soft drinks) for 3–4 hours before bedtime.
- Avoid alcoholic beverages for 4–5 hours before bedtime.
- Avoid smoking before bedtime.
- Avoid napping in the middle of the day.
- Avoid taking over-the-counter sleep medicine.
- Don't read, watch TV, or eat in bed.
- Don't go to bed starved or stuffed.

3. **Sleep Inducers**

Try some or all of the following suggestions to assist you in developing good sleep habits:

- Before going to bed try to do something relaxing.
- Only go to bed when you're really tired.
- Get up and go to bed at the same time every day, even on weekends and vacations.
- Get up at the same time every morning, no matter how much sleep you had the night before.
- If you're feeling tired in the middle of the day, do something to keep yourself awake: Drink a cup of coffee, go for a walk.
- Exercise every day – however, refrain from exercise at least 4 hours before bedtime.
- Have a light snack before bed. Warm or hot dairy products and certain proteins like eggs, and turkey contain tryptophan, which acts as a natural sleep inducer. This option may not be appropriate if your sleep is disturbed by the need to urinate.
- Take a hot bath 90 minutes before bedtime. A hot bath will raise your body temperature, but then your body temperature begins dropping rapidly, which may help leave you feeling drowsy.
- Develop a bedtime sleep ritual, this gives your body cues that it is time to slow down and sleep.
- Once in bed, engage in "boring" mind activities by playing an alphabet game, reciting poems, or "counting sheep."
- Play low-level noise to help distract your brain from listening to the tinnitus. Some examples are a motor noise, such as a fan, soothing music or environmental sounds (rain, ocean waves, etc.) found on tapes, CDs or sound therapy machines.
- Do not think about getting to sleep or worry about the day's activities. Instead try to relax your muscles and think pleasant thoughts: Launch yourself into a pleasant daydream.
- It takes time to develop new habits. Try the suggestions listed for at least 21 days.

What to Do When You Can't Sleep

1. If you haven't fallen asleep after 15–20 minutes, go to a different room and read or do a quiet activity using dim lighting until you are sleepy again. Don't expose yourself to bright light while you are up. The bright light gives cues to your brain that it is time to wake up.

Appendix 4.6 Strategies to Improve Your Sleep

Richard S. Tyler

Some people with tinnitus report that their tinnitus interferes with their ability to get a good night's sleep. The following strategies may help you get a better night's sleep.

1. Daytime activities to facilitate sleep:
   - Get regular exercise, at least 3–4 hours prior to sleep.
   - Avoid napping.
2. Evening activities to facilitate sleep:
   - Create a curfew between day and night (at least 1.5 h before bedtime).
   - Avoid stressful activities and exercise before bedtime.
   - Avoid caffeine and alcohol for several hours before going to bed.
   - Avoid eating and drinking close to bedtime.
   - Only go to bed when you are tired enough to sleep.
3. Find ways to relax and reduce your worrying at bedtime:
   - Set aside a time about 1.5 hours before bedtime to write down your worries and then deal with them in the morning.
   - Keep pen and paper by your bed to write down additional concerns at night.
   - Consider using relaxation techniques:
     ○ Progressive muscle relaxation.
     ○ Imagery training.
4. Consider the arrangement of your bedroom:
   - Eliminate the computer, television, food/drink, etc.
   - Be sure you have a comfortable mattress, pillows, and blankets.
   - Darken the bedroom.
   - Set the temperature to 58° to 68 °F.
5. Prepare for sleep using sound:
   - Choose soft, relaxing sounds.
   - Try using nature sounds, music, broadband noise (static or white noise), or motor noise (fan, humidifier, etc.).
   - Consider a pillow speaker if you are concerned that sound will disturb your spouse/partner or use a timer to shut off after a set period of time.
   - Turn sound on during the night if wake up and tinnitus is a problem.
6. Waking up at night:
   - If you are unable to fall back asleep, find something relaxing to do and return to bed when you feel sleepy.
   - Use background sound to reduce the prominence of your tinnitus.
7. Waking up in the morning:
   - Get up at the same time every day.
   - Sunlight will help you wake up.

Appendix 4.7 Strategies to Improve Concentration

Richard S. Tyler

Concentration problems can occur when you are focused on your tinnitus and are not able to attend to other activities or tasks. Remember that we perform best when we focus on one thing at a time. The following strategies can be used to help you improve your concentration.

1. Eliminate distractions:
   - Choose a comfortable environment.
   - Eliminate unwanted noise.
   - Avoid being hungry or tired.
   - Set aside a time to worry or daydream before you need to work.
2. Adjust your work habits:
   - Work in short time spans (e.g., 20–40 minutes).
   - Set a realistic pace.
   - Take breaks as needed.
   - Reward yourself when your task is complete.
3. Stay focused:
   - Actively participate—take notes, ask questions, etc.
   - Repeat information.
   - Organize and categorize important points.
4. Consider task difficulty:
   - Observe the effects of tinnitus on your concentration for simple (e.g., filing) and complex (learning a new computer game) tasks.
   - Vary the amount of time and build up the amount of time spent on each task.
   - Simple tasks may not be stimulating enough to focus away from tinnitus.
   - Try more challenging tasks.
5. Take control of your attention: Don't focus or attend to your tinnitus:
   - The focus of your attention is largely under voluntary control.
   - Practice controlling the focus of your attention under various conditions:
     - Switch your attention from one visual object to another.
     - Switch your attention from one sound to another.
     - Switch your attention from your tinnitus to another sound.
     - Practice reading with various sounds in the room and switch your attention from those sounds to your book.
6. Decrease the prominence of your tinnitus with background sound:
   - Choose a soft, pleasant sound you enjoy.
   - Examples: Broadband noise, such as static or the sound of fans, humidifiers, air purifiers, etc., nature sounds, and/or music.
   - If you have difficulty concentrating, try playing background sound or music.

Appendix 4.8 Daily Listening Diary

Daily Listening Diary for _____

Day of Week	Date	First Daytime Session	Second Daytime Session	Bedtime Session	Additional Times	Music Used
Sunday Example	1/1/04	Yes	Yes	Yes	2 hours after dinner	-Soft rock in day -Sleep relaxation cd at bedtime

Comments
The listening session after dinner helped me relax after a long day at work

Monday

Comments

Tuesday

Comments

Wednesday

Comments

Thursday

Comments

Friday

Comments

Saturday

Comments

Daily Listening Diary for _____

Day of Week	Date	First Daytime Session	Second Daytime Session	Bedtime Session	Additional Times	Music Used
Sunday						

Comments

Monday

Comments

Tuesday

Comments

Wednesday

Comments

Thursday

Comments

Friday

Comments

Saturday

Comments

5 Three-Track Tinnitus Protocol: Counseling Emphasizing the Patient, the Clinician, and the Alliance

Anne-Mette Mohr

"If I want to succeed in guiding a person from one place to another I first and foremost must take care to find him where he is, to understand what he understands and start there.
If I do not do that, then my greater understanding will not help him at all."

Søren Kierkegaard, 1859

Abstract

The Three-Track Tinnitus Protocol provides a method for helping patients to decrease the impact of their tinnitus. The protocol emphasizes the importance of not only addressing tinnitus itself but also to pay attention to how patients are navigating in the existential dimensions of their life and how this can impact their ability to come to terms with tinnitus. Furthermore, the importance of clinicians' way of interacting with patients as well as the importance of clinicians' ability to create and maintain the alliance is being emphasized as important means for successful outcome. The willingness of clinicians to exert self-doubt and to risk surfacing of challenging or painful aspects of their own life also is described. The protocol most importantly encourages the clinicians continuously to be unknowing, open, and curious in order to find the patient "where he is, to understand what he understands and start there."

Keywords: unknowing, self-doubt, existential dimensions, life-world, curiosity, openness, alliance

5.1 Introduction

Through my many years of psychological work with tinnitus patients, I have encountered numerous patients for whom "coming to terms" with a troublesome tinnitus involved more than simply counseling on how to make tinnitus less intrusive. For purposes of this chapter, the phrase "coming to terms with tinnitus" implies that patients are able to lead a satisfactory life which is not dominated by tinnitus, although it sometimes might be experienced as loud and annoying.

When working with this patient population, it is necessary to clarify whether tinnitus affects the existential dimensions of patients' life-world (the physical, the social, the psychological/personal, and the spiritual dimensions of our existence[1]) and also whether stressful challenges in the patients' lives are present alongside tinnitus, preventing patients from coming to terms with tinnitus.

Examples of stressful challenges include anxiety disorder, depression, grief, as well as life-changing events such as serious illness, divorce, stressful challenges at work, or suffering from unfortunate occurrences (traumas) as a child, a teenager, or as an adult.

Some patients do not realize that their difficulty in coming to terms with the annoying tinnitus is connected to the aforementioned challenges. These patients keep looking for the cure for their tinnitus and, as a result, get increasingly frustrated, desperate, and even more focused on tinnitus. In seeking a cure for their tinnitus, they are barking up the wrong tree. Unfortunately, some clinicians do the same, that is, focus on tinnitus rather than on what other issues might be at stake.

Helping these patients realize that there is more to tinnitus than just tinnitus, and devoting some of the counseling sessions to working through different life challenges often provides patients with relief that transforms into energy. This makes patients shift their focus away from the tinnitus, which will make it seem less intrusive. It is important, therefore, that we, as clinicians, do not miss important facts about patients which, when dealt with in a professional manner, could make coming to terms with tinnitus easier.

Consequently, clinicians must remain open to the possibility that other factors beyond tinnitus might need to be attended to during the counseling process. To follow the words of the Danish philosopher, Søren Kierkegaard, clinicians need to endeavor "to find the patient where he is, to understand what he understands and start there." Furthermore, research has shown that the clinician is nine to ten times more important to the outcome of treatment than the method.[2] Therefore, clinicians need to pay careful attention to how they attend to their patients. They need to work actively to build an atmosphere of trust and confidence—the alliance—as well as making sure that they have the full picture of the patients and their problems before initiating the counseling process.

This chapter introduces the three-track tinnitus therapy: the patient–tinnitus track, the patient–life-world track, and the clinician–patient track, a method that takes the abovementioned into account. The method emphasizes that helping the tinnitus patients requires equal and continuous attention to these three tracks during the counseling process. It enables clinicians to let patients stand out as clearly as possible in their life-world before counseling begins, in order to help patients on their own terms. It emphasizes the importance of having clinicians continuously be in "self-doubt" with respect to how they are working and relating to their patients[3] so that they can continue to focus on what patients need and thus ensure a mutually beneficial outcome.

Psychologists, audiologists, and other health care professionals who work with tinnitus patients can use the three-track tinnitus therapy. Depending on the nature of the patients' challenges and the educational background of the clinicians, the clinicians can talk through any issue with their patients or encourage them to seek psychological counseling or encourage them to seek audiological counseling while alongside continuing the psychological counseling.

The three-track tinnitus therapy is based on the existential-phenomenological framework following the thoughts and writings of several existential philosophers as presented by Spinelli.[4,5]

5.2 Protocol

In the three-track tinnitus therapy, we go through these steps.
1. Making initial contact, clarifying:
   - Needs and expectations.
   - Previous treatments.
   - What challenges might surface in the existential dimensions.
2. The first session: The contract.
3. Working in the tracks:
   - "The patient–tinnitus track."
   - "The patient–life-world track."
   - "The clinician–patient track."

5.2.1 Making the Initial Contact

It is important to make sure that clinicians are able to meet the needs of patients prior to beginning the first session. During the initial contact, which can be completed by telephone, the following needs to be clarified.

What Do Patients Need and Expect?

Do the expectations include getting rid of tinnitus? Do patients have unrealistic expectations of the clinician? These examples can disturb the process of counseling by putting increased pressure on the clinician. Patients might end up feeling disappointed and not meeting their expectations. It is important to set appropriate expectations.

What Treatment Have Patients Received Previously?

Have patients sought help from an ENT? Audiologist? Psychiatrist? Psychologist? Have patients tried alternative treatments like acupuncture, chiropractic care, etc.? What was the outcome of these treatments? What medication have patients used? Do patients have problems with alcohol or drugs?

Regarding previous treatment, patients might not have understood what other clinicians have tried to tell them; for instance, why hearing aids can be helpful for tinnitus management. Patients might have previously been diagnosed with depression. Perhaps, patients are having another depressive episode with tinnitus as one of its symptoms. Depression is likely to influence the treatment process. Therefore, depression needs attention.

Do Patients Face Existential Challenges such as Loss and Grief? Are Patients Having Trouble in One or More of the Existential Dimensions? Are Patients in an Existential Crisis Having Lost Meaning and Direction in Life?

During the initial contact with patients, clinicians can seek clarification on the patients' reactions to tinnitus itself (e.g., grief due to loss of silence). Clinicians can ask the patients if they have experienced other stressors in life such as problems at work, at home, or earlier in their life. Clinicians need to store such information at the back of their mind in order for them to address it when appropriate.

When clinicians pose questions around tinnitus, this can make way for patients to consider that there might be more to tinnitus than the ailment itself. This often makes patients realize—even at this early state—how other issues in their lives, for instance, stress or grief, influence their perception of tinnitus. Due to the clinicians' questions, patients gain valuable insight on what tinnitus perhaps is trying to tell them. Clinicians' interest in their patients will help initiate the development of the all-important alliance. As a result, later on patients will be more willing to adopt suggestions provided by clinicians. During the initial contact, patients may feel relieved, even sensing hope. The counseling process has already begun.

If the initial contact leads to a follow-up appointment, it is recommended that the following information is given to patients: (a) duration and fee per session, (b) policy of cancellation, (c) strategies when a change of date is needed, and (d) duration of scheduled session. As patients may be in a crisis and, consequently, not able to take in all the information, it is recommended that this information is given to patients in written form, that is, in a clinic brochure. Misunderstandings on the policy of changing date or time, for example, can cause irritation on behalf of both clinicians and patients, and disturb the alliance. Precise information of the duration of the sessions can help patients prioritize which themes to address during each session.

5.2.2 The First Session: The Contract

"Clients of effective therapists feel understood, trust the therapist, and believe that the therapist can help." "It is the clinician who creates these conditions within the very first moments of interaction. This is done through both verbal and nonverbal communication." During the initial contact, patients "are very sensitive to cues of acceptance, understanding and expertise."[6]

Consequently, from the very start of the counseling process, patients need to be received in a welcoming atmosphere that embodies investment, openness, and compassion on behalf of the clinicians. Typically, informal talk will hopefully break the ice, for example, whether it was difficult to find the clinic or a parking space. Repeating information gained during the initial contact, followed by asking patients: "Did I get it all or is there something that I've misunderstood or forgotten" gives patients the opportunity to add more information. Perhaps new aspects connected to tinnitus have occurred or new questions need to be answered. It gives clinicians the opportunity of checking whether they understand their patients the way as they understand themselves. This will contribute to patients feeling that they have come across a clinician who is actually interested in listening to them. The alliance is developing and the first session can begin.

In order to make sure that clinicians meets patients' needs, the first session should be started out by asking: "Which issues are important for you that we address today?" This way, clinicians are encouraging patients to share responsibility for the outcome of the session. This question emphasizes that the process is not something that is "being done to" patients, but underlines that clinicians and patients are in the situation together, sharing the responsibility of what to address during each session. Therefore, patients should be involved in deciding which step to take from the very start. This will help patients achieve a feeling of strength and of being in control of their circumstances, rather than being helpless victims of tinnitus.

The first session normally targets the patient–tinnitus track, but shifting between the tracks can occur even during the first session. Clinicians should continuously be aware of what is going on in the clinician–patient track to make sure that they help in the ways that are needed, as well as communicate hope and optimism, conveying a firm belief that patients and clinicians are "in it" together and can work through the counseling process successfully.[6]

At the end of the first session, clinicians review with patients in an accepting way what has been understood with respect to their patients' situations, asking patients to confirm or to add things that might have been forgotten. Again, patients will realize that clinicians are truly listening, wanting to hear and understand their patients as they understand themselves. Thus, the alliance is strengthened.

At this point, clinicians will also provide an acceptable and adaptive explanation for the patients' problems with tinnitus, suggesting to the patients what should be addressed during the counseling process.[6] Here, it is important that clinicians invite patients to comment on the treatment plan. Tentatively, clinicians can suggest how many sessions should be included in the process as well as make an agreement with patients on the interval of the sessions. This together with the information of the practical issues (fee, policies of payment, etc.) constitutes the contract between clinicians and patients. It is important that the content of the contract has been heard and understood by both parties in order to avoid annoying misunderstandings.

5.2.3 Working in the Tracks

The following describes how to work on an overall basis in the patient–tinnitus track and the patient–life-world track. The work undertaken in the clinician–patient track aims to support clinicians when working in the patient–tinnitus track and the patient–life-world track.

At the beginning of each session, clinicians need to clarify patients' present needs. Clinicians, as mentioned earlier, also must make it clear to their patients that they share the responsibility of deciding what to focus on during the session. The initial question, "Where would you like to start?" typically indicates this, as well as providing a hint to which track to choose.

During each session, clinicians must repeatedly ask these questions: "Are we on the right track?", "Are we missing anything important?" The patients' replies to these questions will indicate whether to continue in the same track or to change tracks. Monitoring "where we are right now" and "where we are going next" ensures that patients are continuously involved as active partners in the counseling. Involving patients ensures that the sessions address their needs and provide a level of competency to patients, rather than a feeling of helplessness.

This method places a good deal of responsibility on the shoulders of patients. They need to be quite clear about what they actually need. In the beginning, patients may be unsure of their needs, even if they are bothered by their tinnitus.

Patients might start the session by saying, "I don't really know where to start today." Here, clinicians can support by helping patients find out where to start, perhaps by making them describe what has happened since the last session. With time, patients will often be clearer about their needs. It is critical that patients are encouraged to consider topics that need attention at this present session, and then use the time wisely to allow for adequate time on those topics. Otherwise, the unfortunate mistake of failing to address the important concerns will inevitably be brought up in the last minutes of the counseling session. Having an actual clock visible in the clinic, and asking patients to assist in keeping time will make them more aware of which topics to discuss and about using the sessions more efficiently.

During the counseling process, each and every session runs through four different phases where clinicians—metaphorically speaking—position themselves behind their patients (phase one), side-by-side with patients (phase two), face-to-face with patients (phase three), and finally side-by-side with patients again (phase four). The aim is to make patients and their entire situation stand out as clearly as possible before undertaking counseling, to make patients feel heard as well as to make sure that the recommendations from clinicians are feasible to patients. At all times, clinicians must take care to be authentic, warm, and accepting, in control of their emotional reactions toward their patients and prepared to affirm them (see also the clinician–patient track).

Phase one: Unknowing.[4,5] Metaphorically speaking, clinicians stand behind their patients, being the apprentice, and as such, are learning about their situation with tinnitus the way the patients experience it. Therefore, in this phase, clinicians must continually strive to remain open and curious while bracketing their knowledge and assumptions of what might be helpful to patients. They also need to make sure that they have heard and understood not only patients' questions, but also what might lie behind them—be it assumptions, fears, misinformation, trauma, life experience, etc.

Consequently, in phase one, clinicians will attempt to answer patients' questions, but also pose more questions around the patients' questions. Clinicians are not only listening with the aim of understanding, but also are striving to throw light on what might be hidden behind the questions from the patients.

Phase two: Checking. Clinicians stand side-by-side with patients, looking at their life-world with tinnitus, and checking that they both see and understand the same things. This is done by repeating what clinicians have learned from patients, inviting them to correct misunderstandings, and if needed elaborating on a given topic.

Phase three: Counseling. Metaphorically speaking, clinicians are now face-to-face with patients. In phase one and two, clinicians gained knowledge about patients' needs. Bearing this in mind, clinicians are now able to use their professional knowledge and understanding, and offer advice, strategies/tools, opinions, etc. Clinicians continue to make sure that patients have understood the rationale behind the various suggestions (for instance, why it makes sense to use hearing aids).

Most importantly, clinicians will offer advice, tools, and suggestions to patients in the same way as when clinicians at home would offer food to their guests. Alas, clinicians should avoid persuading patients to take what is being offered. Instead, clinicians will let patients decide what to take, and what to be left for now. At the same time, clinicians will try to understand, with a genuine and accepting interest, how it can be that patients choose one thing over another. It might be that patients are not ready for suggestions from clinicians. Perhaps they do not fit into their life-world as it is enfolding presently (see phase four). Whatever the reason, clinicians again have the opportunity to learn and understand more about patients in their life-world.

Phase four: Reflecting upon consequences. Clinicians are again positioned side-by-side with their patients, looking at patients' life-world with tinnitus. Together they reflect on how the information, the new strategies, etc., might influence patients' daily lives as well as patients' relationships with their surroundings. Also, it will be examined how the surroundings might react to a given strategy. For example, if a patient, John, is in need of rest before dinner, John needs to discuss with his wife whether this can be implemented. Perhaps, it is not realistic. Perhaps, John's wife needs help with the kids while she is preparing dinner. Rather than letting John discover this for himself and give rise to a sense of failure (which might affect John's trust in the clinician), it is much better during the session to proactively consider obstacles that might prevent the strategy from becoming a success.

Phase four is often neglected. This might explain why some patients stop using a new strategy or even terminate their counseling.[5] We, as clinicians, have to keep in mind that all patients are part of a bigger "system"—and that their surroundings will typically react to their new strategies, especially if the strategy will make the surroundings exert indulgence and acceptance. Not taking this into consideration during counseling risks letting both patients and their families down. Also, the alliance between clinicians and patients might be influenced in a negative way.

Every session runs through these four phases. As a matter of fact, each and every time patients bring up something new, clinicians should start being un-knowing, checking, counseling, and together with patients end up by reflecting on the consequences of these strategies.

The reader may wonder whether this is not a troublesome and time-consuming way of working. As a matter of fact, it is, at least initially. However, the time spent thoroughly in these phases enables clinicians to help patients in a very precise way. As the counseling process evolves, most of the time will be spent counseling (phase three) because

clinicians very early in the process have achieved a thorough understanding of the total situation of patients. Clinicians, however, should never be tempted to believe that they now know the full truth, but must keep checking their perception of patients and their situation as described in phase two.

Before terminating a counseling session, clinicians will invite patients to reflect on whether the issues they wanted to discuss during the session have been dealt with. As it sometimes takes several sessions to develop a trustful alliance, clinicians must bear in mind that patients might not initially feel like telling the truth. If patients reply that something was not dealt with in this session, it is in fact rather a good thing: it shows that patients feel safe enough to bring out their personal needs without fear of rejection. Some clinicians offer their patients to fill out an evaluation form (mentioned later) but bear in mind that these days many people are fed up with being asked to evaluate every single little thing, and might therefore resent having to do this.

The Patient–Tinnitus Track

Often, tinnitus patients seeking psychological or individual counseling are in urgent need of help for their tinnitus. Therefore, the first sessions are typically spent in the tinnitus–patient track, where issues are addressed such as how to make tinnitus less annoying.

Alongside meeting patients' needs by answering questions, clinicians will also aim to be "unknowing" (phase one). This might take the form of seeking clarification on how patients understands and experiences the tinnitus before giving advice or suggestions. Is tinnitus an illness, a symptom, or a chronic condition? What does tinnitus sound like? Where is it heard and when is it most annoying? Is tinnitus always annoying? Do patients have a physical response to tinnitus like sweating, shaking, palpitations, etc.? When and how did tinnitus start? Out of the blue or in connection with a traumatic event? Do patients have assumptions on what tinnitus is/what have patients read or heard about tinnitus? If so, what did they learn? Have "confidence-inspiring tinnitus-sufferers" in a credible way convinced patients that tinnitus is indeed very difficult to tackle and that tinnitus can ruin their lives?

It is important to be aware that many patients have been so intimidated by scary and wrongful information that initially they may not be able to take in or accept any strategy and advice provided by their clinician, thus making them virtually "deaf" to anything clinicians may offer. This can seriously obstruct and prolong the counseling process. Here, clinicians need to correct misinformation about tinnitus before providing patients with additional strategies.

Listening to patients' worries and needs provides clinicians with important information on what to address early in the process, what may wait for later, and what may need to be addressed in the patient–life-world track (i.e., a concurrent situation with an anxiety disorder or a traumatic event that made tinnitus troublesome). Tinnitus Activities Treatment (TAT; Chapter 4) helps clinicians clarify what to address and when, as well as how to make their patients understand the ideas behind the suggested strategies.

Having made sure that clinicians have heard the present needs of the patients (phases one and two), counseling can be initiated (phase three), providing patients with knowledge and strategies. The range of strategies includes hearing aids, masking, and sound therapy devices (Chapter 8) to progressive muscular relaxation techniques (Chapter 10) as well as exercises that help tinnitus slide into the background. Clinicians proficient in German can find many examples on helpful exercises in "Manual der Hörtherapie" by Dr. Gerhard Hesse et al.[7]

Caveat: Hearing loss is often a very stigmatizing experience. Some patients resent talking about their hearing loss and resent starting to use hearing aids even if they have been told of the positive effects. Therefore, it is important to clarify how patients emotionally feel about hearing loss *before* recommending that they use hearing aids; and it is vital to give patients the time to digest the rationale behind this strategy, and equally vital to respect their decision if they maintain their unwillingness to embrace this strategy.

While working in this track, clinicians should keep in mind that the outcome of the counseling is determined primarily by clinicians' contribution, not by the patients' contribution.[6] Consequently, clinicians need to keep in mind whether the suggested actions or strategies actually match patients' needs as well as whether clinicians are too engaged in talking patients into accepting their model or strategies on what to do (phases three and four). Also, clinicians need to keep an eye on whether they maintain empathy, authenticity, and control of any personal emotional reaction to the patients, thus paying attention to what might go on in the clinician–patient track. Clinicians might even ask patients: "Am I pushing you too much?" Allowing patients to comment on what is going on, as well as respecting patients' comments, will indeed contribute to the development of the alliance and eventually on a positive outcome.

Shifting to the Patient–Life-World Track

After thorough counseling in the patient–tinnitus track, many patients will be able to manage their life with tinnitus in a good way. However, some patients, while working in the patient–tinnitus track, may introduce themes belonging to their life-world which, at some point, might need further attention in the patient–life-world track. Expressions like "I feel stuck in the grip of tinnitus," "I worry all the time and I am never at ease; will tinnitus ever disappear?", "Tinnitus makes me feel sad and lost," all are examples of these subtle indications.

Sometimes the patient, the clinician, or both have a feeling of being "stuck." In spite of all well-intentioned efforts, the counseling process is leading nowhere. This feeling of being stuck may indicate that something needs to be processed in the patient–life-world track (or paid attention to in the clinician–patient track).

Whether it is the narrative of the patients or the feeling of being stuck that makes clinicians consider changing to the patient–life-world track, clinicians should make sure that patients are prepared to shift track. The following are examples of questions that give patients the opportunity to decide whether to shift to the patient–life-world track: "Would you like us to talk more about your sadness or do you prefer to stay with how to use the masking device?" or "If you want, I can teach you a technique that will make your muscles feel less tense?"

Psychologists will normally continue the process with the patients in the patient–life-world track. Depending on the themes that require attention, clinicians without a psychological background may prefer referring patients to a psychologist. If so, clinicians should be aware that sometimes it can be much more helpful simply to let it all out to the clinicians, than to be referred elsewhere. For some patients, feeling heard and understood is sufficient help. Sometimes, however, letting it all out on the clinicians provides many patients with sufficient time to reach their own conclusion that psychological therapy should be the next step. This is a much more caring way of helping patients into a new regime than just referring them to a psychologist. Some patients continue their sessions with the audiologist while at the same time seeing a psychologist.

Of course, flexing back and forth between the tracks is always an option.

The Patient–Life-World Track

In this track, clinicians and patients explore how tinnitus influences the patients' life-world as well as whether stressful themes in the present or unresolved unfortunate occurrences belonging to the past prevent patients from coming to terms with tinnitus. If so, working through reactions to tinnitus and/or the unresolved issues can be an important step toward decreasing the impact of tinnitus.

At this point it can be very informative to let patients fill out the questionnaire presented in "Tinnitus Treatment, Clinical Protocols."[8] The questionnaire addresses all aspects of the life-world of patients, and can bring forth important information that patients might even have forgotten to mention. For instance, early childhood trauma, which in a subtle way influences how patients come to terms with tinnitus, would be reported on the questionnaire, and might not otherwise have been mentioned by patients.

In order to make sure that clinicians and patients achieve a complete picture of how patients live with tinnitus, clinicians can use the existential dimensions, which together constitute our life-world, as a kind of "map."

The existential dimensions are as follows[1]:
- The physical dimension.
- The psychological dimension.
- The social dimension.
- The spiritual dimension.

As an example many tinnitus patients have placed huge demands on themselves and as a result they become increasingly worn out and stressed. Often, these patients initially have experienced sleep disorders, muscular tension and pain, headaches, alertness, hyperacusis followed by the onset of tinnitus (the physical dimension). Due to tinnitus, patients then react by becoming irritable, sad, grieving, depressive, and/or anxious. They might worry about the future: can I continue working this hard with tinnitus in the picture? Who or what am I turning into? (the psychological dimension). Due to tinnitus, patients withdraw from social events like dinners, parties, etc. (the social dimension). Patients might experience uncertainty, hopelessness, and meaninglessness (the spiritual dimension).

Exploring the influence of tinnitus on the four existential dimensions of the lives of patients, clinicians are now able to see the full picture of their entire situation. Clinicians and patients can then explore why patients demand so much of themselves. Sometimes the present situation is simply tough. Patients may be in a situation where home life, workload, and not enough time off constitute a reality that is hard to change. Putting a difficult situation into words may in itself decrease tinnitus. Sometimes a situation with low self-esteem may be the reason why patients place huge burdens on their own shoulders. Patients may constantly work overtime trying to find out what others might want from them in order for them to be liked and loved. Perhaps, patients in early childhood only experienced being loved if they did what their parents wanted them to do. Such patients have learned that they are only worth loving if they work hard. They have not experienced being loved unconditionally by their parents. Together with clinicians, these patients need to find new ways of existing that will allow them to experience being loved, even if they do not work hard to attain that love. Alas, for those patients who normally do everything to please others, it can be a turning point when they experience that they are accepted and respected by clinicians, even when they choose not to follow their suggestions. Furthermore, this principle is illustrated when clinicians are willing to continue working with patients in the way that they need to feel supported. This experience may very well support patients in trying new and less arduous ways of interacting with others. This, too, may very well result in a less intrusive tinnitus.

Quite a few patients will express that their situation with tinnitus has led to an overall feeling of loss of direction and meaning (the spiritual dimension). Patients might say: "Why me?" When patients find an answer as to why, it becomes easier for them to find out how; that is how to recreate meaning in the seemingly meaningless situation with tinnitus. The philosopher Nietzsche expresses it like this: "He who can find a WHY can bear almost any HOW."[9] Viktor E. Frankl, an Austrian psychiatrist and psychotherapist, describes how he created meaning while in a concentration camp during World War II.[9] Interestingly, Frankl observed that the prisoners who were able to create meaning from their challenging situation were the ones who survived the longest.

An example of having recreated meaning is seen when patients say, "On one hand, I wish I had never contracted tinnitus. On the other hand, I wouldn't want to miss all the things that I have learned because of tinnitus."

Undertaking a thorough investigation in the patient–life-world track often provides patients with several answers to the "why me?". Furthermore it provides patients with options of what to do. In other words, the process in this track also provides patients with the "how." In addition, the process sometimes provides patients with important insight and knowledge that they would not have received, had it not been for tinnitus. This insight on how to live their life in a better way, and how to come to terms with difficult challenges like tinnitus can be used both presently and in the future, when most likely new challenges will appear. They also realize that personal development often happens in the wake of crisis and challenge. Even though tinnitus initially was an almost devastating experience and from time to time still may be annoying, some patients realize that it has also given them valuable insight and new options that they would not want to do without. Some patients decide that tinnitus is a kind of friend that signals when they are not navigating their life in agreement with who they are and what they can give to others; or it signals when they are trying to guess the needs of others. In this process, patients have regained meaning. Consequently, they often experience that their tinnitus is less intrusive.

The reaction to tinnitus, and the way in which the existential dimensions influence how the patients come to terms with tinnitus, is different from patient to patient. Bearing this in mind is very important. Not every patient has unfortunate experiences stemming from early life that influence their ability to come to terms with tinnitus in the present. All patients have their own individual version of tinnitus.

Many patients do not even need sessions in the patient–life-world track. Having received sufficient counseling in the patient–tinnitus track has enabled them to come to terms with tinnitus. In this case unresolved issues in their life-world do not impact their tinnitus. My aim has only been to describe what might be going on alongside with tinnitus, influencing patients' ability to come to terms with tinnitus, hopefully encouraging clinicians to work in the patient–life-world track when necessary.

The Clinician–Patient Track

Wampold[6] (and other researchers) has shown that the role of clinicians is immensely important to the outcome of the treatment. The study shows that it is the ability of the therapist to form a working alliance with the patient that is most critical. This working alliance should be "collaborative, purposeful work on the part of the client and the therapist."[6] Establishment of the alliance takes place initially in the treatment process and presupposes that patients from the very start experience clinicians as trustworthy and competent. According to researchers within the field of psychotherapy, the most effective factors in treatment include the ability of clinicians to be (a) authentic and genuine, (b) warm and accepting, (c) open and willing to share their own experiences, (d) in control of their emotional reaction toward patients, and (e) willing and ready to affirm patients.[10,11] According to Nissen-Lie et al,[3] the willingness of clinicians to be self-aware (to exert self-doubt) is a good predictor of outcome.

Consequently, when it comes to helping tinnitus patients the best way possible, the following things should be kept in mind: clinicians, their way of interacting with patients, building and maintaining the alliance, their willingness to exert self-doubt, and their ability to form the alliance needs just as much attention as do the tinnitus patients and their life-world. Therefore, this protocol includes a separate section devoted to clinicians and their interactions with their patients, which aims to support them to work the best way possible in the two other tracks.

Overall, when working in the patient–tinnitus or the patient–life-world track, clinicians should continuously pay attention to what is going on in the clinician–patient track. This attention supports clinicians in being constantly aware of meeting patients in their needs before starting counseling or providing strategies. It also supports clinicians in being constantly aware of themselves—exerting self-doubt—thus paying attention to how they interact with their patients. Are they warm and accepting? Do they remain unknowing, curious, and open, putting assumptions and knowledge aside, with the intention of hearing the patients in their needs? Or are they perhaps allowing themselves to be provoked by patients, or are they actually unable to control their emotional reaction toward patients? In other words, constantly paying attention to what is going on in the clinician–patient track increases the chances of a successful counseling process.

When being unknowing and open, clinicians are able to compartmentalize their professional knowledge, personal attitudes, and assumptions.[4,5]

However, when working with patients it is very easy to forget the openness and curiosity necessary, given the knowledge that clinicians usually have when dealing with tinnitus patients. Clinicians might feel tempted to think something like, "I've been here before—let's go this way. This is normally helpful to tinnitus patients," hereby forgetting the position of un-knowing, the openness, and curiosity. Clinicians must always doubt their own presuppositions because how can the clinician be sure that this particular patient is similar to all other tinnitus patients?

A patient might, for example, say, "Being the father of three children and having a wife working full time is very stressful. Just thinking of it makes my tinnitus feel more intrusive." The clinician might be tempted to answer, "Surely you must feel like this, and as a consequence, it is to be expected that tinnitus may seem louder."

Here, however, this clinician is presupposing what the patient's life at home is like, thus turning off openness and curiosity which might otherwise cause a thorough and open investigation of what is going on in the patient's life at home, and how this might contribute to the tinnitus. Though it is an empathetic response, an open and curious attitude would entail clarifying questions like, "In what way is tinnitus stressful? And is it always stressful?", "Do you sometimes experience other stressful situations where tinnitus either becomes or doesn't become intrusive?", "What is the difference between the situation at home and these other situations?", "What characterizes such situations?", "Does your wife know that you feel stressed?", etc. It might be that patients feel stressed with the chaos in their daily household, for example, the kids are lazy; never getting to talk on a more private level with their spouse; dinner being served too late or too early; iPads and iPhones preventing family members from having a good talk; acoustics in the home perhaps being terrible. The reasons for the increased tinnitus of patients may be manifold. Clarifying the reasons behind what is experienced as stressful might lead to interventions, which target the reasons in a nuanced and fruitful way. Patients will feel that their clinician is paying attention and this will make patients trust the clinician even more. This again will deepen out the alliance.

Sometimes patients present themes or act in a way that might activate challenging or painful themes stemming from the personal life-world of clinicians. This can make it difficult for clinicians to control their emotional reactions toward themselves or toward patients. Clinicians in this situation may be tempted to leave their position of being unknowing, and are unable to bracket their assumptions. They forget to exert "self-doubt," causing the counseling process to become difficult.

Some clinicians, for instance, may experience patients whose personality and behavior resemble the erratic behavior of a difficult parent. In this case, clinicians may feel unable to help patients, and sometimes, clinicians might develop negative assumptions on what kind of person this patient is, for example, difficult, negative, and not willing to comply. If clinicians feel stuck and perhaps even at a loss, they might resort to presenting some new strategies to patients without checking whether these fit into their life-world. This gives clinicians a provisional good feeling of "doing something." For instance, clinicians might try very hard to persuade patients to start using hearing aids without acknowledging and working with the stigma connected to hearing loss. If patients do not want hearing aids, clinicians might presume that patients are showing resistance to improvement. Clinicians might even find that patients are annoying, irritating, and impossible to help (just like the clinician's difficult parent!), whereas patients might feel wrong and misunderstood and start resenting clinicians, thus engaging in a vicious circle that might very well lead patients to terminate counseling without having received adequate help.

Before jumping to these perhaps erroneous conclusions, self-doubt needs to be exerted by asking, "Am I correct in my assumptions? Am I ignoring what patients' ways of being emotional evokes in me?" These questions might very well lead clinicians to realize that something unfortunate from their own personal life-world has been activated.

One way of tackling this feeling of being stuck is to ask patients: "I get the sense of being in a kind of a deadlock. Do you share this experience?" This question invites patients to take an active part in the clinician–patient track, so that clinicians and patients can start exploring what could be done differently. Often simply to addressing the situation makes way for a change and movement.

From time to time clinicians might feel so overwhelmed by their frustration toward patients that it becomes difficult for them to involve patients in how to proceed. Even though some patients can in fact be difficult to deal with, elements from clinicians' own life-world often interact and interfere with the counseling process. Some choose to bring the counseling to an end, others seek supervision to find the root of the problem.

In other cases, patients might for instance share feelings of grief and sadness that resonate with a former or present painful situation in the clinicians' private lives, making them turn off their position of unknowing and their curious and open attitude. In order to alleviate their personal discomfort, clinicians might be tempted to offer interventions that do not match the needs of the patients. Here, too, patients might end up feeling wrong and not good enough; and likewise, clinicians will also feel wrong and not very clever, because their interventions failed. Both are stuck—and this may lead to a premature termination of the counseling.

In emotionally challenging situations like these, clinicians must first of all acknowledge that patients' pain resonates with their own, and that while this may be difficult, clinicians must nevertheless maintain their position of being un-knowing, open, and curious. Clinicians, needless to say, must respect their own boundaries but can express empathy by ensuring patients that they understand how difficult this is.

Secondly, supervision by their peers will help clinicians become more clear about what patients trigger, and how to deal with emotional reactions toward themselves and their patients. This often makes continued work with patients possible.

Paying attention to what goes on between patients and clinicians in the clinician–patient track presupposes that clinicians are prepared to exert self-doubt as well as facing and exploring themes that are not only challenging or painful to patients, but also to clinicians. Coming to terms with how personal emotions are affecting the counseling can be helpful and a source of personal development for clinicians. And in the future, clinicians might experience that working with these kind of patients is less difficult.

As a means of ensuring that patients feel that they are heard and met in their needs, some clinicians administer a rating scale at the end of every patient session. For example, Miller et al[12] developed a scale that gathers feedback from patients on how well they felt themselves heard, understood, and respected. The scale assesses if the clinicians' approach is a good fit for the patients as well as whether the session is meeting their needs. It is recommended that patients fill out the scale 10 minutes before the end of the session to give ample time to discuss the results. Though we should acknowledge that feedback may need to be taken with a pinch of salt, especially in the beginning of the counseling process, feedback will provide an indication of whether an alliance has developed positively and whether patients' needs have been met. Use of such scales is another example of how the clinician can pay attention to what is going on in the clinician–patient track.

5.3 Conclusion

This protocol provides a method for helping patients decrease the negative impact of tinnitus (the patient–tinnitus track). The method also addresses how the patients are navigating in the existential dimensions of their life-world (the patient–life-world track) and how this might have an influence on tinnitus and vice versa. As a consequence, the impact of tinnitus on the existential dimensions is addressed, as well as how different aspects of these dimensions might influence the patients' journey toward coming to terms with tinnitus. Furthermore, the critical role of clinicians has been described. This role has been incorporated into the protocol as the clinician–patient track, thus emphasizing the importance of clinicians' way of interacting with patients as well as the importance of clinicians' ability to create and maintain the alliance as an important means for a successful outcome. Furthermore, the importance of clinicians' willingness to exert self-doubt and to risk surfacing of challenging or painful aspects of their own life has been presented.

Most importantly: During the whole counseling process, clinicians must be un-knowing, open, curious, and consequently willing to find the patient "where he is, to understand what he understands and start there."[13]

To illustrate the Three-Track Tinnitus Protocol, there are three interviews of tinnitus patients discussing their experiences with tinnitus in a psychology counseling session available on the companion website.

References

[1] Deurzen EV. Everyday mysteries. Existential dimensions of psychotherapy. London: Routledge; 2006
[2] Bertolini M, Miller SD. What works in therapy: a primer. In: Miller SD, Bertolini M, eds. The ICCE manuals on feedback-informed treatment (FIT). International Center for Clinical Excellence; 2012

[3] Nissen-Lie HA, Rønnested MH, Høglend PA. Love yourself as a person, doubt yourself as a therapist? Clinical Psychology and Psychotherapy. Wiley Online Library; 2015. doi:10.1002/cpp.1977

[4] Spinelli E. Tales of un-knowing: therapeutic encounters from an existential perspective. London: Duckworth; 1997

[5] Spinelli E. Practising existential therapy: the relational world. London: Sage; 2015

[6] Wampold BE. The contribution of the therapist to psychotherapy: characteristics and actions of effective therapists. In: Von der Lippe A, Niessen-Lie HA, Oddli HW, eds. Psykoterapeuten: En antologi om terapeutens rolle i psykoterapi. Oslo: Gyldendal Akademisk; 2014:51–67

[7] Hesse G, Schaaf H. Manual der Hörtherapie. Schwerhörigkeit, Tinnitus und Hyperacusis. Stuttgart: Georg Thieme Verlag; 2012

[8] Mohr A-M, Hedelund U. Tinnitus person-centered therapy. In: Tyler R, ed. Tinnitus treatment: clinical protocols. New York: Thieme Medical Publishers, Inc.; 2006:198–216

[9] Viktor E. Frankl: man's search for meaning—the classic tribute to hope from the Holocaust. Boston, MA: Beacon Press; 1959

[10] Jørgensen CR. Den Psykoterapeutisk Holdning. København: Hans Reitzels Forlag; 2018

[11] Norcross JC. Psychotherapy: relationships that work. 2nd ed. New York: Oxford University Press; 2011

[12] Miller SD, Duncan BL, Brown J, Sorrell R, Chalk MB. Using formal client feedback to improve retention and outcome: making ongoing, real-time assessment feasible. Columbus J Brief Ther. 2006; 5(1)

[13] Kierkegaard S. Synspunkter for min Forfatter-Virksomhed. København: C.A. Reitzels Forlag; 1859

Suggested Readings

Cohn HW. Existential thought and therapeutic practice. An introduction to existential therapy. London: Sage; 1992

Hesse G. Tinnitus. 2. Überarbeitete und erweitere Auflage. Stuttgart: Georg Thieme Verlag KG; 2016

Madsen, PL. Doktor Zukarovs Testamente. København: Gyldendal, Epub, 2019, version 2.0

May R. The art of counseling. A true classic in the literature of the helping professions. New York: Gardner Press, Inc.; 1989

Mohr A-M. Reflections on tinnitus by an existential psychologist. Audiol Med. 2008; 6:73–77

Mohr A-M. Your life and tinnitus. In: Tyler R, ed. The consumer handbook on tinnitus. 2nd ed. Sedona: Auricle Ink Publishers; 2016:91–110

Spinelli E. The interpreted world. An introduction to phenomenological psychology. London: Sage; 1989

Spinelli E. Demystifying therapy. London: Constable; 1994

Spinelli E. The mirror and the hammer. Challenges to therapeutic orthodoxy. London: Continuum; 2001

Strasser F. Emotions. Experiences in existential psychotherapy and life. London: Duckworth; 1999

Thielst P. Man bør tvivle om alt - og tro på meget. Filosofiens historie fra Thales til Habermas. Frederiksberg: Det Lille Forlag; 2002

Yalom ID. Terapiens essens. København: Gyldendal; 2002

6 The Psychological Management of Tinnitus-Related Insomnia

Laurence McKenna and Elizabeth Marks

Abstract

Many tinnitus patients report sleep disturbances or insomnia that can significantly impact overall function. This chapter overviews our approach to addressing sleep disturbances using cognitive behavioral therapy that includes information on group and individual therapy sessions. We also discuss sleep titration, sleep hygiene, and relaxation techniques for improved sleep.

Keywords: insomnia, tinnitus, sleep, cognitive behavioral therapy, sleep management

6.1 Introduction

Insomnia is a sleep–wake disorder that can involve a range of problems. These include difficulty in getting to sleep, staying asleep, waking too early; insufficient duration of sleep, or feeling that sleep is nonrestorative or otherwise of poor quality. These problems occur despite an adequate opportunity to sleep. Insomnia has daytime effects that can include impaired functioning, tiredness, and distress. Like tinnitus, insomnia is very prevalent in the general population,[1] affecting up to 30% of adults.[2] Sleep disturbance is one of the most important aspects of tinnitus complaint among adults[3,4] and children,[5,6] with most studies indicating at least 40% of tinnitus patients report insomnia.[7] Tinnitus tends to be more distressing when it is associated with difficulties sleeping.[8,9,10,11,12,13] There is an obvious need to address the issue of tinnitus-related insomnia and its management, and recent research suggests that a cognitive behavioral (CB) approach is likely to be effective.

6.2 The Cognitive Behavioral Model

A case can be made for the use of pharmacological treatment of insomnia in the short term, that is, up to 2 weeks (National Institute for Health and Care Excellence [NICE] guidelines)[14] to break an unhelpful cycle of sleeplessness and worry. There are strong arguments against pharmacological treatment of insomnia beyond the short term.[15]

Psychological management with Cognitive Behavioral Therapy for insomnia (CBTi) is the treatment of choice for primary insomnia, as it has been proven effective.[16,17] The authors have recently published an evaluation of a CBTi group for patients reporting distressing tinnitus and insomnia based on the standard CB model,[18] indicating that this approach also seems effective in cases where insomnia is occurring secondary to tinnitus.

CBTi is based on the CB theory that suggests that an individual's distress arises out of an interaction between their environment, thoughts (cognitions), behavior, and physiological experiences.[19] The cognitive component of the CB model emphasizes that it is the way we *interpret* and *think* about a situation rather than the situation per se that influences our emotions. The behavioral component of the CB model suggests that the way a person behaves also influences well-being. A person may engage in behaviors that end up making the problem and the distress worse, or they may stop doing things (behaviors) that could help reduce the problem.

Cognitive therapy was first introduced by Beck[20] as a treatment for depression. The CB approach has since been developed and evaluated for use with many other problems such as anxiety disorders,[21] specific phobias, and, more recently, personality disorders[22] and psychosis.[23] As argued by some researchers, CB "can be applied to the assessment and treatment of almost every chronic medical problem."[24] The intervention emphasizes self-management to help people cope with the medical problem and to reduce the level of distress accompanying the condition.

When applied to tinnitus, the CB model would suggest that it is the thoughts that people have about their tinnitus, and their related behaviors that determine how distressed they are, rather than the tinnitus alone. If a person is able to think about tinnitus as "just another noise," and to continue with life as normal, then they will not likely experience significant emotional or physical changes, and it is unlikely that they will feel distressed. Conversely, if someone interprets tinnitus as threatening, unmanageable, or potentially catastrophic, they will understandably begin to feel emotions such as anxiety, fear, sadness, or frustration. Such strong negative emotions often have a physical impact and usually lead people to change their behavior in some way, for example, they may start to avoid certain activities, or spend more time checking and monitoring tinnitus and their hearing. This can become a vicious cycle, whereby a person's thinking becomes increasingly negative, their emotional and physical state becomes more distressing and aroused, behavior alters even more, and attention becomes increasingly focused on tinnitus.

Thus, the CB model suggests that tinnitus-related difficulties continue because changes in thinking, behavior, attention, emotion, and physiological arousal affect one another. For example, a woman who believes that tinnitus will spoil her enjoyment of social events checks the state of her tinnitus, and feels physically tense and emotionally anxious, before meeting friends. As a consequence, she cancels her arrangement to go out with friends, resulting in more time to attend to her tinnitus. Initially, she may feel a sense of relief; however, the process confirms her belief that tinnitus spoils her social life, maintains her vigilance for the perceived threat, and leaves her feeling depressed.

Hallam et al[25] and Scott et al[26] were among the first to formulate a CB approach to tinnitus, and since then many studies support the benefits of this approach as indicated by recent systematic reviews and meta-analyses.[27,28] More recently, McKenna et al[29] proposed a CB model of tinnitus distress that places a conceptual framework on the earlier therapeutic studies.

6.2.1 Cognitive Behavioral Therapy and Insomnia

The CB model has been applied to insomnia.[30] People with insomnia are thought to engage in negative thoughts about sleep during the night and the impact of sleeplessness during the day. Insomnia is, therefore, regarded as a 24-hour process or a sleep–wake disorder (and not just a sleep disorder). Most people with insomnia worry about insufficient sleep, such as the impact of loss of sleep during the night and how this lack of sleep will affect their health or functioning during the day. These thoughts and worries fuel anxiety and increase autonomic arousal; this, in turn, interferes with the person's ability to sleep well. As sleep becomes more difficult, people then start to change their behavior around sleep in an attempt to improve things. For example, people tend to

spend increasing amounts of time in bed, begin to rest or nap more in the day, and may try to use stimulants such as caffeine to stay awake. They also become increasingly hypervigilant toward signs of insomnia and sleepiness. These behaviors, in fact, interfere with the natural process of sleep, making insomnia more likely. Again, a vicious cycle of thoughts, emotions, behaviors, attention, and physical sensations becomes established and maintains the problem.

Cognitive and behavioral interventions are helpful in the management of insomnia, and the gold-standard treatment for primary insomnia is CBTi (e.g., Espie et al,[15] Harvey et al,[31] Morin et al,[32] and Morin et al[16]). More recently, studies have found that CBTi can be very effective when treating insomnia that is secondary to other conditions, such as chronic pain or cancer.[33,34,35,36] The present authors are currently running a clinical trial to evaluate the effectiveness of CBTi in patients with insomnia secondary to distressing tinnitus, providing further evidence that CBTi may also benefit patients with tinnitus.

6.2.2 The CB Model, Tinnitus, and Sleep

It is our view that tinnitus is not a specific sleep antagonist. Rather, the CB model of insomnia can be applied to the person who suffers from tinnitus-related insomnia. Our hypothesis is that anxiety associated with tinnitus, and with poor sleep, leads to insomnia. The anxiety is manifested in terms of altered cognitions, altered behavior, elevated levels of arousal, and a distressed emotional state. A vicious cycle of anxiety, tinnitus, and poor sleep is established. It is common for anxiety about either the tinnitus or poor sleep to assume dominance and there may be desynchrony in the extent to which each component of the anxiety is present. Many, but not all, of our patients have some previous history of sleep difficulties. Our suggestion to address sleep difficulties, based on clinical observation is as follows: (1) A person may become aware of tinnitus when trying to sleep, or to go back to sleep, because the presleep period with its few other distractions offers an opportunity to focus on tinnitus, and because of low levels of ambient noise. (2) The greater awareness leads to unhelpful cognitions about tinnitus and changes in behavior (e.g., delaying going to bed where tinnitus is more intrusive, drinking alcohol, checking tinnitus), increased arousal, and distress. (3) This anxiety leads to poor sleep. (4) The sleep difficulties give rise to anxiety again in the form of unhelpful cognitions about sleep, to changed behavior, and increased arousal and distress. (5) This anxiety maintains the insomnia and leads to greater awareness of tinnitus. (6) Poor sleep maintains the environment that fosters continued awareness of tinnitus. We envisage the process as akin to the "five element" CB model of emotional problems described by Greenberger and Padesky[19] and Williams.[37] We recognize that many of our patients suffer from significant levels of depression, but it is our observation that anxiety processes are the key factors in determining our patients' poor sleep; it may be that the anxiety represents an aspect of depression in many cases.

6.3 Group Therapy

In our clinic, we offer both group therapy and individual therapy for insomnia. Most people that we see are offered group therapy and the focus of this chapter is a description of our group therapy approach that involves several weeks of therapy for adults with this problem. The CBT interventions used in individual therapy do not differ fundamentally from those used in the group approach. Individual therapy can, however, permit a greater flexibility for people whose problems are multifactorial or who, for some reason, are not suited to group therapy. We use a "closed group" format, that is, once the group has commenced, there is no opportunity for others to join the sessions. A new member entering after the first few sessions will gain little benefit because the content of the sessions builds upon the knowledge gained in previous sessions. A closed group can enable a sense of cohesion and trust between members. Group therapy allows people to meet others who are in a similar situation; this can normalize a person's experiences and reduce anxiety.

Patients can also serve as role models for each other. A group milieu may also reduce any tendency for patients to dispute the therapist's ability to understand or help because the therapist does not have tinnitus. Such assumed differences can become barriers to the therapeutic process. From a service perspective, group therapy can be cost effective and may result in more patients receiving the required input. Nonetheless, care needs to be taken that the group setting does not lead to disadvantages. It was suggested by Jakes et al[38] that observing other group members improving may elicit helplessness and envy in some people, or

confirm a patient's belief that their problems are unique and, therefore, much harder to address. In addition, the group environment may result in reinforcement of each other's negative opinions. It is our practice to use two therapists in each group to help safeguard against such difficulties.

6.4 Selection and Definitions

The problems of insomnia include difficulty falling asleep (initial or early insomnia), waking in the middle of the night and having difficulty returning to sleep (middle insomnia), and waking too early in the morning (terminal or late insomnia). Problems with the quality of sleep translate into complaints of sleep being light, broken, or restless, and not being restorative or refreshing. Complaints about associated daytime problems such as tiredness or sleepiness, mood disturbance, and poor performance are also common.

By itself, the quantity of sleep that a person gets is not an accurate guide to whether sleep will be regarded as problematic. Some of our patients complain of poor sleep while reporting that they get eight, or more, hours of sleep a night; others manage well on little sleep. Subjective complaint about sleep is, therefore, a key factor in the clinical consideration of sleep problems. To obtain some measure of objectivity, however, we follow guidelines that are set out in the insomnia literature. We regard a delay in getting to sleep or getting back to sleep in the middle of the night, of at least 30 minutes,[39] as a criterion for describing sleep as problematic. This benchmark is based largely on the observation that normal sleep-onset latency is usually less than 30 minutes.[40,41] In the case of several awakenings, a total time awake of 45 minutes or more is regarded as problematic. We accept Morin's[39] suggestions that waking after a total of less than 6½ hours be used to define late insomnia and that these difficulties should occur at least three nights a week for the classification of insomnia. To be regarded as insomnia, problematic sleep should include a complaint about an impact on daytime functioning. While a critical aspect of the definition, the variability inherent in this aspect of the complaint, however, makes this a challenging aspect of the assessment.

Sticking to criteria that are rigidly based on time or frequency of problem alone can be problematic. Considerable variability in sleep patterns is seen in the general population and with variations associated with age.[42] There is also variability among people complaining of insomnia. Good and bad nights are interspersed and a defining feature of the problem for many sufferers is the unpredictability of sleep rather than simply a lack of it. In fact, Chambers and Keller[43] concluded from a review of studies comparing good sleepers with insomniacs that the mean total sleep time (TST) of the latter was only 35 minutes less than good sleepers. The importance of complaints about insomnia is often a matter of clinical judgment. Nonetheless, adherence to the time and frequency criteria results in greater homogeneity in the group and avoids the inclusion of people with problems that others regard as implausible.

Another important criterion in our selection process is the establishment that the insomnia is related to the person's tinnitus. Insomnia, like tinnitus, is a symptom rather than a single disorder and it can occur for a variety of reasons. Dement and Vaughan[44] list disruption of the circadian rhythm and psychological disorder as among the main causes of persistent insomnia. Both these problems are commonly reported by our sleep-disturbed tinnitus patients. Provided the psychological disorder is related to the patient's struggle with tinnitus or the circadian rhythm disturbance is a result of their inappropriate efforts to deal with their insomnia, then such patients are included in our group. People whose problems arise from something like shift work, however, are not included. Dement and Vaughan[44] also suggested that restless legs syndrome, periodic limb movement disorder, gastroesophageal reflux, and fibrositis syndrome or other pain states be considered when investigating possible reasons for persistent insomnia. Breathing disorders are also a common cause of insomnia.[45] It is also possible for some medications to disturb sleep by producing arousal or by disturbing the phases of sleep.[46] Alcohol and illicit drug abuse can also lead to sleep disturbance. Having tinnitus does not give a person immunity from these other possible sources of sleep disturbance. We suggest that therapists be mindful of these causes when assessing people complaining of tinnitus-related insomnia and, if necessary, refer the person to another professional appropriately. Some of these problems are easier to consider and exclude than others. Countries vary in the license that they extend to different professional groups to diagnose or exclude; practitioners must be guided by their local regulations.

Our sleep management program employs psychological rather than pharmacological treatment; however, many of our patients with tinnitus-related insomnia are already taking hypnotics or other psychotropic medication that affects sleep. We request that people do not alter their medication during the program, unless there is a clear indication that they are taking the medicine improperly, or unless a reduction in dose is established as a specific therapeutic goal. In such cases, reference is made to the prescribing physician. We do not include people who are significantly abusing alcohol. Many of our patients, however, use alcohol as a sleeping agent, and inclusion or exclusion from our program is dependent on whether the primary problem is the insomnia or the alcohol use. To obtain some homogeneity, we restrict membership of the group to the "adult" population, that is, 18 to 70 years of age. Older adults are seen on an individual basis.

6.5 Assessment

6.5.1 Questionnaire Measures

A number of questionnaire measures are used in the evaluation of our therapy. They are administered 2 weeks before the start of the therapy, at the start and end of the therapy, and at 1-month follow-up.

Tinnitus

The Tinnitus Questionnaire (TQ)[10] and the Tinnitus Primary Functions Questionnaire[47] include questions directly related to sleep disturbance and tinnitus. We consider these useful instruments that often reveal changes in sleep and other tinnitus complaint factors.

Sleep

We assess clinical insomnia using the Insomnia Severity Index (ISI),[48] an easily completed, seven-item scale that assesses the core features of insomnia. A score of 15 indicates clinically significant insomnia, and a drop of 6 points or more indicates a clinically meaningful change.[49] One of the seven questions refers to daytime functioning.

We also assess sleep quality with the Pittsburgh Sleep Quality Index (PSQI).[50] The PSQI assesses sleep quality during the previous month in terms of seven components: subjective sleep quality, sleep latency, sleep duration, habitual sleep efficiency, sleep disturbances, use of sleeping medications, and daytime functioning. The seven-component scores are then summed to yield a global PSQI score. A disadvantage is that it involves retrospective and somewhat global judgments about sleep that may be subject to reporting biases. An advantage of the PSQI is that it assesses sleep across a range of dimensions, has a high specificity, and is easily administered. This questionnaire is perhaps more helpful for research applications, and it cannot substitute for a detailed nightly sleep diary.

Psychological Distress

We assess psychological distress in three ways. We use the CORE-OM as a pandiagnostic measure of psychological well-being, which has the advantage of indicating levels of distress regardless of whether an individual meets the criteria for psychiatric diagnoses, such as anxiety and depression. The CORE-OM has been validated in a tinnitus sample.[51] We also screen for depression using the PHQ9[52] and the GAD7[53] as these questionnaires are freely available and widely used as screening and outcome tools. These measures allow for comparisons with other interventions conducted elsewhere.

6.5.2 Sleep Diaries

The use of diaries on a nightly basis is the most useful and sensitive self-report instrument for assessing insomnia. The person provides information about their sleep on a nightly basis that supports therapeutic intervention and shows progress. The diary is integral to the CBTi intervention, as the information recorded here is used to develop personalized sleep programs for each member of the group. The individual records the following each night:

- Time they get into bed.
- Time they then first go to sleep.
- The number of times they wake in the night.
- In total, the length of time that they are awake during the night.
- The time they finally wake up.
- The time they get out of bed.

This allows calculation of the key measures: total time in bed (TIB) and the total sleep time (TST). From this, a sleep efficiency (SE) is calculated that represents the percentage of time that the person is asleep while in bed.

The sleep diary also asks people to rate (on a 0–10 Likert scale) the quality of their sleep, how refreshed they felt upon waking, and how intrusive tinnitus was during the night. At the end of the day, the person is also asked to rate their daytime functioning and to record any naps or ingestion of caffeine, alcohol, or sleep medication.

An example of a sleep diary used in tinnitus management is given by McKenna.[3] It is our practice to provide the sleep diary in an Excel spreadsheet, allowing for graphical representation of sleep change over time, particularly of changes in TIB, TST, and sleep quality. Summary data in terms of mean values can be calculated for final evaluations.

6.6 Group Structure

Our group sessions contain 6 to 10 patients and usually are led by 2 clinical psychologists. This number of participants allows time to address individual problems within the group, to prevent the quieter members feeling overwhelmed, and to help the group feel contained. There are six treatment sessions. The first four occur weekly, to provide the necessary support to help patients make changes to sleep. The fifth session occurs 2 weeks after that and the sixth after another 2 weeks; these intervals provide some time for the new sleep programs to develop and stabilize. We also offer a follow-up appointment 1 month later.

6.7 Treatment Protocol: Key Components

6.7.1 Group Support

A key part of the group is the supportive milieu and the opportunity for patients to meet others in a similar situation and to realize that they are not alone. The first session involves introductions, setting of ground rules, and some ice-breaker activities. Some time is allotted for patients to set their goals for the group sessions. All information provided is supported by handouts and the participants are given pen and paper to make notes and, thus, build up a folder to use as an aide memoire. Homework is given each week, and this is reviewed every session.

6.7.2 Psychoeducation

Following this, the clinical psychologists provide comprehensive psychoeducation about tinnitus, sleep, insomnia, and how these conditions interact. The intention is to demystify tinnitus and sleep, and to provide a framework to normalize some of the patients' experiences, for example, frequent awakenings and light sleep in the second half of the night, and within which to set realistic goals.

This educational component is the key as there are many unhelpful myths about sleep and tinnitus that often drive the unhelpful thoughts and behaviors described previously. The first session also introduces the idea of the cognitive model, and how sleep, tinnitus, anxiety, behavioral changes, and physiological arousal cause a vicious cycle that maintains the problem. Thus, the target of treatment is less focused on "silencing" tinnitus, but more about escaping from the vicious cycle and returning to a healthy sleep cycle.

Psychoeducation about Tinnitus

The information provided about tinnitus is based on the habituation model described by Hallam et al[25] and the cognitive model of tinnitus distress proposed by McKenna et al.[29] Emphasis is placed on the observation that most people respond increasingly less to tinnitus with the passage of time, and the majority of people who have tinnitus are not greatly distressed by it. We emphasize that high levels of arousal (or "tension") and negative beliefs about tinnitus impede the process of habituation. Further, the physical parameters of tinnitus (e.g., as identified through matching and masking assessments) are less important in determining distress.

Psychoeducation about Sleep and Insomnia

The sleep education element is derived from psychological writings within the insomnia literature (e.g., Espie[54] and Morin[39]) and particularly, from a CB model of insomnia.[30] Therapists should acquire some basic knowledge about sleep and insomnia before offering a sleep-management program to tinnitus patients. At this stage, the information presented is restricted to a number of points about sleep stages, normal sleep times, and the effects of sleep deprivation.

Information about Normal Sleep Times and Sleep Stages

Most people get 7 to 8 hours of sleep. There is, however, a considerable range in normal sleep times. We illustrate the point that some people manage well on little sleep by reference to a high achieving person such as Margaret Thatcher who famously got only four hours sleep a night. It is a commonly held belief that older people do not need as much sleep as they did when younger.

Although older people do tend to get less sleep at night,[42] they may also nap more in the daytime, so the total amount of sleep achieved remains relatively stable from middle age to later life.[39,55] An attempt is made to normalize the experiences of the group members by reference to the literature.[56]

Sleep stages (rapid eye movement [REM] sleep and non-REM stages 1–4) are described and the cycle of REM and non-REM sleep throughout the night is outlined. Patients are informed that this cycle takes about 90 minutes to complete, but that it can vary from 70 to 120 minutes. This cycle is repeated four or five times a night in healthy young adults. A normal night's sleep also includes several awakenings. These are usually brief, and many people are unaware of them. For most people, the first obvious awakening occurs after 2 or 3 hours of sleep. Awakenings become more common as the hours of sleep increase. The first awakening often represents a watershed after which the periods of REM sleep become longer. Clinically, the experience is often described in terms of little really deep sleep after the first awakening.

Age-related changes in sleep patterns are described. Older people experience less deep sleep and REM sleep[42] and the number of awakenings increases with age. Young adults commonly experience two awakenings in a normal night's sleep; older people may experience as many as nine awakenings a night. For many elderly people, sleep is experienced as light and fragmented. This information is illustrated by using a histogram representation of sleep stages[3] and by reference to the experiences of the group members. Many people find it difficult to clearly distinguish light sleep from wakefulness. This difficulty may be accounted for by the observation that people may continue to think about things even during periods of light sleep; mental activity is mistaken for wakefulness.

Information about the Effects of Insomnia

The exact function of sleep remains unclear,[57] but there is virtually universal agreement that sleep is necessary.[58] It is more helpful to consider some of the commonly reported difficulties associated with lack of sleep rather than to discuss the possible function of sleep. A distinction is made between total sleep deprivation and the less severe sleep loss that is characteristic of clinical insomnia. People with insomnia complain of a range of deficits such as daytime sleepiness, poor concentration and memory, and poor performance on daily tasks.

Such complaints are part of the definition of insomnia and clearly need to be treated with respect. Reviewing the evidence, Walker concludes that sleep loss can have profound detrimental effects.[58] The literature on the effects of insomnia, however, also contains other reports about the objective evidence for such difficulties and it can be questioned whether, when present, they can be attributed to sleep loss per se or to other factors such as stress. Individual people with insomnia vary in their ability to do tasks. However, some research studies have found no difference between insomniacs and people who sleep well on psychological tests.[43,56,59,60,61,62,63]

During the group sessions, we inform participants that the negative effects of insomnia seem to be caused as much by the anxiety surrounding it as by the sleep loss per se, a finding that was published by the American Academy of Sleep Medicine.[64] A discussion of these points is encouraged and an attempt is made to relate patients' experiences to the research evidence. Patients may be skeptical about these ideas and knowledge of the literature may be vital for the therapist's credibility. Notwithstanding this, it is our experience that formulating their problems in terms of the effects of increased arousal is credible to most patients. Nonetheless, a pragmatic approach is needed, and patients are directed to ensure good self-care and safety.

Information about Tinnitus and Sleep

Patients are asked to consider the fact that tinnitus does not lead inevitably to one or another negative consequence. The varying experiences of the group members are drawn upon to illustrate this point. Next, this association is discussed for tinnitus and insomnia. The group members are informed that only about half of people attending a tinnitus clinic complain of sleep problems. Emphasis is placed on the idea that tinnitus does not inevitably lead to insomnia. The factors that give rise to, and more importantly that maintain insomnia, are likely to be psychological in nature and susceptible to psychological treatment. It is our observation that our patients awaken in the night at about the times predicted from a typical sleep cycle and it is our contention that tinnitus does not wake people up. Once awake, tinnitus may be the first thing a person is aware of and they may then remain awake for the reasons set out above. We stress the point that we do not view tinnitus as a specific sleep antagonist.

6.7.3 Individual Goal Setting

Formal research programs commonly use sleep-onset latency (i.e., the time taken to fall asleep) as an outcome measure (see Espie,[54] for definitions). As it applies to the individual patient, greater care is needed when setting treatment outcome goals. Given the subjective nature of insomnia, it is inadequate to set a standard goal for all patients, even to the extent of suggesting that an increase in the amount of sleep obtained should be the goal. Patients' aspirations for treatment are individualistic and imposing standard outcome criteria may lead to a sense of failure for both patients and therapists. Many patients do hope for an increase in the number of hours of sleep obtained, but other, equally valid goals are expressed by patients. These may include sleep without the aid of alcohol or pills, improved sleep efficiency (time asleep as an expression of time in bed), more predictable sleep, better quality sleep, a reduction in daytime deficits, or to feel less anxious or depressed. The therapist must consider the individual goals compared to what is known about normal sleep, what is possible within the clinic setting and the time available, etc. For example, a goal of 8 hours of uninterrupted deep sleep in a 60-year-old patient may be unrealistic.

6.7.4 Creating an Individualized Sleep Program

Developing a new and reliable sleep routine underpins the CBTi program. Every patient will learn to create a sleep pattern that is appropriate for them. The sleep routine is based upon the average numbers that are collected in a sleep diary 2 weeks prior to the first session of CBTi. Every patient will calculate their TST, TIB, and SE based on the preceding 2 weeks.

From these numbers, they will be asked to note the discrepancy between TIB and TST. Most individuals with insomnia will spend much longer in bed than they actually sleep for, and this will be linked to their SE; this is usually between 40 and 80% in people with insomnia. It will be explained that good sleepers have an SE of 90% or more and that the program is designed to help them become good sleepers by improving their SE to 90% or above. The only way in which they can reach this point is to restrict how long they spend in bed.

Each patient will, therefore, be asked to restrict their TIB to the average TST achieved over the last 2 weeks, plus 30 minutes. TIB, however, should never be set below 5½ hours. Thus, if an individual recorded having 5¼ hours of sleep on an average in the last fortnight, they will be permitted 5¾ hours TIB (or "sleep window"). If the person reports having 5 hours or less per night, they will have a 5½-hour sleep window. The individual is asked to choose a regular wake time that he or she can adhere to throughout the week (including weekends), and is asked to count backwards from that *wake time* by the number of hours they are permitted. So, an individual with a sleep window of 5¾ hours may choose to get up at 6 a.m., in which case, they will be asked to go to bed at 12.45 am.

This change can be very challenging; so, time is spent discussing the rationale for this change as it relates to the information given about sleep. It is also important to note that the aim of this change is to restrict time in bed and not to restrict time asleep. In fact, everyone will be given enough time in bed to get at least the same amount of sleep they are already getting. The key aim of this stage of the sleep program is to help people begin to consolidate their sleep and become more efficient. Then, their sleep window can be extended and over time, they will get more and more sleep.

6.7.5 Sleep Titration

Participants keep a sleep diary for the entire duration of CBTi. In each session, the numbers from the previous week are used to continue to develop the individual's sleep program. There are some very simple rules to follow, based on whether or not SE has improved.

1. If SE has increased to, or remained above 90%, the individual may add another 15 minutes to their sleep window. It is recommended that 15 minutes is taken at the start of the night, that is, going to bed 15 minutes earlier. It is best to keep the wake time the same throughout, unless otherwise indicated.

2. If SE lies between 80 and 90%, then the individual is asked to keep their sleep window the same for the following week.

3. If SE lies below 80%, then the individual is asked to remove 15 minutes from their sleep window, that is, going to bed 15 minutes later, as it is best to keep the get up time the same throughout, unless otherwise indicated.

Every week, diaries are checked and sleep windows updated in line with the average sleep over the preceding sleep. The intention is to train the participants to be able to do this independently so

that the person will be able to manage his or her sleep pattern effectively when the sessions move to once every 2 weeks. This self-management can then continue after the end of the program, until the person is sleeping well and no longer need to make changes.

This part of the program can be difficult, and the therapist spends time troubleshooting and managing motivation. Many participants complain of feeling more tired at the start of the program. This is actually helpful as it means they tend to fall asleep more quickly at night and sleep more soundly. It is *critical* that the participant does not nap during this process, or it will not be effective.

A common difficulty is staying awake while being tired late at night. This is managed by planning low-intensity activities such as doing household chores or puzzles in the evening. Another common difficulty is getting up early and this is managed by having an alarm clock that one has to get up to switch off. Another difficulty is feeling sleepy in the day; this is managed by getting more daylight, more physical activity, and avoiding naps.

6.7.6 Stimulus Control

Negative associations with the bed, bedtime, and sleep are common in insomnia. These associations are thought to feed into the anxiety and distress that can occur in the bedroom, or in preparation for bedtime. Stimulus control refers to the part of the intervention that aims to break these associations. Participants are introduced to the idea of associative learning, and how this might relate to insomnia. They are then given clear advice on how to break these unhelpful associations in a number of ways:

1. Bed is for sleep and sex only: Participants are advised that no other activity should take place in bed (i.e., no TV, reading, telephones, radio, etc.).

2. The "20-minute rule": If a person does not fall asleep within 20 minutes, or if they wake up and do not fall back to sleep within 20 minutes they are advised to get up, leave the bedroom, and go and do a quiet activity in a different room. This activity should not involve bright lights or screens or be too stimulating (i.e., no TV, no Internet, no caffeine). The person can return to bed when they feel sleepy. If they do not fall asleep within 20 minutes, then they should get up again. They repeat this until they fall asleep within 20 minutes.

3. Evening routine: People are advised to have a pre-bedtime routine to help them and their

bodies recognize that it is time to slow down, relax, and sleep. The routine can be very individual to each person and some of the sleep hygiene can be incorporated. It is helpful to discuss with people what their plans for a new routine are and to caution against potentially unhelpful behaviors. For example, people often think that exercise pre-bed will help to exhaust them, but it is more likely to "energize" their system. Suggest to the person that exercises earlier in the day are likely to be helpful.

6.7.7 Motivation and Video Modeling

There is evidence that seeing other people cope with a problem can be therapeutic for patients with some psychological problems. The present authors are not aware of any studies that have formally employed coping models in tinnitus management, but Davies et al[65] postulate that improvements in tinnitus patients undergoing group therapy may be due to the modeling seen in group environments. We, therefore, show video-recorded interviews with past patients who had a history of considerable tinnitus-related suffering, including insomnia, but who are now coping well following CBTi. These patients talk about how they managed some of their challenges, and what the benefits were from CBTi therapy.

6.7.8 Relaxation

Patients are given a rationale for relaxation therapy in terms of reducing sympathetic autonomic nervous system arousal. The reduction of muscle tension provokes a similar reduction in other autonomic subsystems such as heart rate, respiration, blood pressure, etc. Elevated levels of arousal decrease the likelihood of initiating sleep and, therefore, relaxation therapy increases the chances of sleep. Muscle relaxation has also been found to be effective in reducing intrusive thoughts.[66,67] It is suggested that the experience of tinnitus is related to heightened levels of sympathetic autonomic arousal[25] and that by reducing the level of this arousal, the distress associated with tinnitus may also be reduced. We believe that the provision of a clear rationale may enhance the face validity, thus promoting these nonspecific effects and encouraging compliance. By distinguishing relaxation therapy from other activities commonly thought to be "relaxing" (e.g., watching television or reading a

novel), the rationale may also reduce these alternative, possibly arousing behaviors.

Participants are taught three types of relaxation: Progressive Muscular Relaxation; Diaphragmatic Breathing; and Relaxing Imagery. These are taught in sessions 2, 3, and 4, with practice done in the session and a CD or downloadable-guided relaxation exercises available for home practice. Regular relaxation is part of weekly homework, and advice is to begin by doing this before going to bed, with the aim of learning how to relax when awake, rather than as a way of falling asleep. A guide for relaxation listening for sleep is provided in Appendix 6.1.

6.7.9 Cognitive Restructuring (Cognitive Therapy)

The cognitive therapy element focuses on the process of "cognitive restructuring." The initial aim of this intervention is to help people understand the relationship between thoughts, emotions, behavior, and bodily sensations. This is achieved by using simple illustrations that demonstrate the link between thoughts and emotions, for example, a friend does not say hello because (a) he is ignoring you—resulting in you being emotionally upset or (b) he does not see you—resulting in a less distressing emotional state. This illustrates that the same physical event can be interpreted differently and, thus, can lead to different emotional states.

Once this basic relationship is understood, the point is reiterated that unhelpful thoughts about tinnitus and poor sleep contribute to a cycle of distress, increased tinnitus perception, and sleep disturbance. Patients are asked to think of ways that their own thoughts contribute to their experience of distress. Initially, the therapist may help by pointing out the thoughts that patients have expressed when relating their history. If need be, they help patients in other ways, such as the use of imagery, to access their thoughts. The process of cognitive distortion wherein thoughts acquire an overly negative bias is also described and illustrated.

The patients are asked to monitor their emotions and thoughts using diaries as a homework task.[19] This adds to the information learned in the session and encourages participants to recognize their unhelpful thoughts. The next step is to help people to reevaluate these unhelpful thoughts. The role of the therapists is to help patients consider alternative, more helpful thoughts about their situation. There are many questions people can ask themselves to consider a different perspective about a situation. For example, "What's the evidence for my thoughts?" (very often, it is scarce) or "Is my thought fact or is there another way to think about this?"[19] Once the conviction in the initial thought is weakened, the person is encouraged to think about another way of viewing the situation. For example, rather than thinking "I'll never get to sleep and won't be able to do *anything* at work tomorrow," it may be more helpful to think "I've never had a night when I haven't slept at all, and I've always been able to do *something* at work even when I've been very tired." It is important that these new thoughts and beliefs are tested, and work done outside the group setting is reviewed within the session. For example, with the above situation, the person may be encouraged to record what they do at work. This will help to provide evidence against the biased, or distorted, belief that they will not be able to do *anything* and will offer evidence in support of the new belief.

6.7.10 Worry Period

Another way to manage repetitive negative thinking is to use a "worry period." Worries are common at nighttime, and yet this is rarely the time of day when we are best equipped to respond to them. We offer a suggestion to some patients (though it is not appropriate for all patients) to set aside 15 minutes per day when they can focus on their worries—a "worry period." This should be during the day or early evening, and at least several hours before bed. During this time, people are encouraged to sit without other distractions and allow their mind to think freely. People should then write down thoughts that are causing them to feel anxious. They can then, if they wish, write down possible first steps (or next steps) for responding to these worries. Should the worry reoccur at night, the person can then recall that he or she has attended to the worry, has done all they possibly can, and that tomorrow is the next time when they will consider the problem.

6.7.11 Sleep Hygiene

As the cognitive model suggests, thoughts and feelings influence people's behavior. When people have difficulty sleeping, they do things that they believe will help them sleep. Such strategies may include taking medication or drinking alcohol, avoiding going to bed, remaining in bed for long periods of time, or watching television in their bedroom. These strategies may offer short-term

benefits, but in the long term, they may perpetuate the insomnia.[68] If the person continues to attribute sleep difficulties to the tinnitus, rather than to these behaviors, then he or she will unwittingly reduce the chances of sleep—and so a cycle is established. Helping the person with insomnia to gain insight into this cycle is an important intervention. Once the group members have begun to question some of their behaviors, the next step is to discuss "sleep hygiene" and the behavioral changes they could begin to make to promote sleep. Sleep hygiene interventions must be considered for all people who have poor sleep because even if poor sleep hygiene is not the primary cause of sleep disturbance it may be a secondary factor that is playing a role in maintaining sleep problems.[68]

Alcohol

Alcohol may help to induce sleep, but it can also cause sleep disruption throughout the night, especially the second half. The result is broken sleep and early morning wakening. Patients are encouraged to avoid using alcohol as a sleep or relaxation aid.

Caffeine

Although it is widely known that caffeine is a stimulant, many people drink tea or coffee before going to bed and/or if they wake in the night. People are advised to slowly reduce their caffeine intake, to avoid it in the evenings, and to be aware that it is present in a range of foods and drinks, for example, chocolate, soda, and energy drinks.

Nicotine

People often have a cigarette before bed or when they wake up in the night. As with alcohol, they may be viewing cigarettes as a means of relaxation. People are advised about the physiological stimulating effect of nicotine and advised to reduce and carefully regulate their intake.

Diet

Hunger can result in difficulty initiating sleep, but so too can a heavy meal near bedtime. It is important to gain a balance between going to bed hungry and on a full stomach. People are advised to not eat while awake in the night. Throughout the day, eating well can reduce feelings of fatigue, and participants are advised that sugary snacks may give a quick energy "high," but that this can exacerbate fatigue later. Eating regular, healthy, complex carbohydrates, and protein-based snacks can help.

Exercise

Regular exercise helps well-being and promotes sleep. During exercise, and for some time following exercise, the body is in an increased level of arousal. It is, therefore, advisable to engage in regular exercise; however, intense exercise should not be taken just before going to bed. Gentle movement, such as slow yoga or a gentle stroll would be fine.

6.7.12 Sound Enrichment

Many patients use sound in the bedroom to alleviate their tinnitus, and this can be helpful, unless it is too stimulating. Using the TV as a source of sound is common, but it is unhelpful because the light from the screen can be bright enough to affect melatonin production, and interfere with natural sleepiness. Radio, although it does not have light, often has variability in noise levels (particularly commercial radio) and can also keep people focused on the time (e.g., with regular news updates and time checks). We encourage people to use alternative sources of sound enrichment at night. If a radio is all that is available, we suggest a nonstimulating station that rarely mentions the time. Even better is the use of a sound-ball or sound-enrichment Apps that offer a range of noises such as white noise, ocean waves, rain, etc. For tinnitus-habituation purposes, it is important that the noise is set to a volume *below* that of tinnitus. The aim here is not to completely mask the tinnitus, but to give the brain an alternative noise to receive and process. Setting the noise above the level of tinnitus can lead to an exacerbation of tinnitus intrusiveness in the longer term. If sound is used, then it is often useful to keep it on for 24 hours a day so that it quickly becomes part of the bedroom environment and any arousing effects are minimized.

6.7.13 Clock Watching

For people who have sleep problems, looking at the clock during the night may serve to increase anxiety or dread, decreasing the chances of sleep. The best strategy is to not have a clock in the bedroom, or if an alarm is needed then turn the clock face so it cannot be seen. We also explain how hypervigilance to something like the time can even distort the perception of the problem and lead the person to overestimate how poor their sleep is.

6.8 Conclusion

Complaints about sleep disturbance are common in patients with medical problems and are a key feature in the presentation of tinnitus patients. It has been argued that improving sleep facilitates healing, well-being, and the ability to cope with illness.[69] Improving the sleep of tinnitus patients may not "heal" tinnitus, but the other points in this argument seem as relevant to people with tinnitus as to those with other medical problems. Overall, however, outcome studies of psychological treatment for tinnitus have not produced encouraging results in the management of insomnia.[70] Reviewing this evidence, McKenna[3] noted that in many outcome studies, no measures or only very crude measures of sleep disturbance were included. Even where some measure of sleep disturbance was included, treatments were rarely directed specifically at insomnia management. There is currently no published controlled outcome study that targets tinnitus-related insomnia as the central variable and that includes the sorts of measures that are commonly reported upon in the insomnia literature. This chapter has described the clinical approach employed by the authors and reported by them in the form of uncontrolled outcome study.[18] The work is informed as much by the insomnia literature as by the tinnitus literature. Our central proposition is that tinnitus is not a sleep antagonist, but that both tinnitus distress and insomnia are provoked by a process akin to anxiety. As yet, our assumptions have not been empirically tested, but our work is being systematically evaluated. It is possible at this stage to report only our most preliminary impressions. The vast majority of our patients report some benefit from the group therapy described here. Most achieve their treatment goals, although such goals vary considerably between individuals and are not restricted simply to increased sleep time.

We have created a video discussing sleep hygiene, sound therapy, and relaxation before bedtime, which is available on the companion website.

References

[1] Shapiro C, Dement W. Impact and epidemiology of sleep disorders. In: Shapiro C, ed. ABC of sleep disorders. London: BMJ Publishing; 1993

[2] Morphy H, Dunn KM, Lewis M, Boardman HF, Croft PR. Epidemiology of insomnia: a longitudinal study in a UK population. Sleep. 2007; 30(3):274–280

[3] McKenna L. Tinnitus and insomnia. In: Tyler RS, ed. Tinnitus handbook. San Diego: Singular; 2000

[4] Tyler RS, Baker LJ. Difficulties experienced by tinnitus sufferers. J Speech Hear Disord. 1983; 48(2):150–154

[5] Gabriels P. Children with tinnitus. In: Vernon JA, Reich GE, eds. Proceedings of the 5th International Tinnitus Seminar. Portland, USA: American Tinnitus Association; 1995:270–274

[6] Kentish RC, Crocker SR, McKenna L. Children's experience of tinnitus: a preliminary survey of children presenting to a psychology department. Br J Audiol. 2000; 34(6):335–340

[7] Asnis GM, Majeed K, Henderson MA, Sylvester C, Thomas M, De, La Garza R. An examination of the relationship between insomnia and tinnitus: a review and recommendations. Clin Med Insights Psychiatry. 2018; 9. DOI: 1179557318781078

[8] Axelsson A, Ringdahl A. Tinnitus: a study of its prevalence and characteristics. Br J Audiol. 1989; 23(1):53–62

[9] Folmer RL, Griest SE. Tinnitus and insomnia. Am J Otolaryngol. 2000; 21(5):287–293

[10] Hallam RS. Correlates of sleep disturbance in chronic distressing tinnitus. Scand Audiol. 1996; 25(4):263–266

[11] Miguel GS, Yaremchuk K, Roth T, Peterson E. The effect of insomnia on tinnitus. Ann Otol Rhinol Laryngol. 2014; 123(10):696–700

[12] Schecklmann M, Pregler M, Kreuzer PM, et al. Psychophysiological associations between chronic tinnitus and sleep: a cross validation of tinnitus and insomnia questionnaires. BioMed Res Int. 2015; 2015:461090

[13] Scott B, Lindberg P, Melin L, Lyttkens L. Predictors of tinnitus discomfort, adaptation and subjective loudness. Br J Audiol. 1990; 24(1):51–62

[14] NICE. National Institute for Health and Care Excellence. 2015. https://cks.nice.org.uk/insomnia

[15] Espie CA, Inglis SJ, Tessier S, Harvey L. The clinical effectiveness of cognitive behaviour therapy for chronic insomnia: implementation and evaluation of a sleep clinic in general medical practice. Behav Res Ther. 2001; 39(1):45–60

[16] Morin CM, Savard J, Bliss FC. Cognitive therapy. In: Lichstein KL, Morin CM, eds. Treatment of late-life insomnia. California: Sage; 2000:207–230

[17] Okajima I, Komada Y, Inoue Y. A meta-analysis on the treatment effectiveness of cognitive behavioral therapy for primary insomnia. Sleep Biol Rhythms. 2011; 9(1):24–34

[18] Marks E, McKenna L, Vogt F. Cognitive behavioural therapy for tinnitus-related insomnia: evaluating a new treatment approach. Int J Audiol. 2019; 58(5):311–316

[19] Greenberger D, Padesky CA. Mind over mood. 2nd ed. New York: Guilford Press; 2015

[20] Beck A. Cognitive therapy and the emotional disorders. New York: Penguin Books; 1976

[21] Clark DM. A cognitive approach to panic. Behav Res Ther. 1986; 24(4):461–470

[22] Persons JB, Bertagnolli A. Cognitive-behavioural treatment of multiple problem patients: application to personality disorders. Clin Psychol Psychother. 1994; 1(5):279–285

[23] Fowler D, Garety P, Kuipers E. Cognitive behaviour therapy for psychosis: theory and practice. Chichester: Wiley; 1995

[24] White C. Cognitive behaviour therapy for chronic medical problems. Chichester: Wiley; 2000

[25] Hallam RS, Rachman S, Hinchcliffe R. Psychological aspects of tinnitus. In: Rachman S, ed. Contributions to medical psychology, Vol. 3. Oxford: Pergamon Press; 1984:31–53

[26] Scott B, Lindberg P, Lyttkens L, Melin L. Psychological treatment of tinnitus. An experimental group study. Scand Audiol. 1985; 14(4):223–230

[27] Hesser H, Weise C, Westin VZ, Andersson G. A systematic review and meta-analysis of randomized controlled trials of cognitive-behavioral therapy for tinnitus distress. Clin Psychol Rev. 2011; 31(4):545–553

[28] Fuller T, Cima R, Langguth B, Mazurek B, Vlaeyen JW, Hoare DJ. Cognitive behavioural therapy for tinnitus. Cochrane Database Syst Rev. 2020 08;1:CD012614

[29] McKenna L, Handscomb L, Hoare DJ, Hall DA. A scientific cognitive-behavioral model of tinnitus: novel conceptualizations of tinnitus distress. Front Neurol. 2014; 5:196

[30] Harvey AG. A cognitive model of insomnia. Behav Res Ther. 2002; 40(8):869–893

[31] Harvey L, Inglis SJ, Espie CA. Insomniacs' reported use of CBT components and relationship to long-term clinical outcome. Behav Res Ther. 2002; 40(1):75–83

[32] Morin CM, Hauri PJ, Espie CA, Spielman AJ, Buysse DJ, Bootzin RR. Nonpharmacologic treatment of chronic insomnia. An American Academy of Sleep Medicine review. Sleep. 1999; 22(8):1134–1156

[33] Jungquist CR, Tra Y, Smith MT, Pigeon WR, Matteson-Rusby S, Xia Y, Perlis ML. The durability of cognitive behavioral therapy for insomnia in patients with chronic pain. Sleep Disord. 2012;2012:679648

[34] Espie CA, Fleming L, Cassidy J, et al. Randomized controlled clinical effectiveness trial of cognitive behavior therapy compared with treatment as usual for persistent insomnia in patients with cancer. J Clin Oncol. 2008; 26(28):4651–4658

[35] Jungquist CR, O'Brien C, Matteson-Rusby S, et al. The efficacy of cognitive-behavioral therapy for insomnia in patients with chronic pain. Sleep Med. 2010; 11(3):302–309

[36] Savard J, Simard S, Ivers H, Morin CM. Randomized study on the efficacy of cognitive-behavioral therapy for insomnia secondary to breast cancer, part II: immunologic effects. J Clin Oncol. 2005; 23(25):6097–6106

[37] Williams C. Overcoming depression: a five areas approach. London: Arnold; 2001

[38] Jakes S, Hallam RS, McKenna L, Hinchcliff R. Group cognitive therapy for medical patients: an application to tinnitus. Cognit Ther Res. 1992; 16(1):67–82

[39] Morin C. Insomnia: psychological assessment and management. New York: Guildford Press; 1993

[40] Budur K, Rodriguez C, Foldvary-Schaefer N. Advances in treating insomnia. Cleve Clin J Med. 2007; 74(4):251–252, 255–258, 261–262 passim

[41] Ringdahl EN, Pereira SL, Delzell JE, Jr. Treatment of primary insomnia. J Am Board Fam Pract. 2004; 17(3):212–219

[42] Ohayon MM, Carskadon MA, Guilleminault C, Vitiello MV. Meta-analysis of quantitative sleep parameters from childhood to old age in healthy individuals: developing normative sleep values across the human lifespan. Sleep. 2004; 27(7):1255–1273

[43] Chambers MJ, Keller B. Alert insomniacs: are they really sleep deprived? Clin Psychol Rev. 1993; 13:649–665

[44] Dement WC, Vaughan C. The promise of sleep. London: MacMillan; 1999

[45] Williams A. Insomnia: doctor I can't sleep. UK: Amberwood Publishing; 1996

[46] Idzikowski C, Shapiro C. Non-psychotropic drugs and sleep. In: Shapiro C, ed. ABC of sleep disorders. London: BMJ Publishing; 1993

[47] Tyler R, Ji H, Perreau A, Witt S, Noble W, Coelho C. Development and validation of the tinnitus primary function questionnaire. Am J Audiol. 2014; 23(3):260–272

[48] Bastien CH, Vallières A, Morin CM. Validation of the Insomnia Severity Index as an outcome measure for insomnia research. Sleep Med. 2001; 2(4):297–307

[49] Yang M, Morin CM, Schaefer K, Wallenstein GV. Interpreting score differences in the Insomnia Severity Index: using health-related outcomes to define the minimally important difference. Curr Med Res Opin. 2009; 25(10):2487–2494

[50] Buysse DJ, Reynolds CF, III, Monk TH, Berman SR, Kupfer DJ. The Pittsburgh Sleep Quality Index: a new instrument for psychiatric practice and research. Psychiatry Res. 1989; 28 (2):193–213

[51] Handscomb L, Hall DA, Hoare DJ, Shorter GW. Confirmatory factor analysis of Clinical Outcomes in Routine Evaluation (CORE-OM) used as a measure of emotional distress in people with tinnitus. Health Qual Life Outcomes. 2016; 14(1):124

[52] Kurt K, Spitzer R. The PHQ-9: A New Depression Diagnostic and Severity Measure. Psychiatr Ann. 2002; 32:9:1–7

[53] Spitzer RL, Kroenke K, Williams JBW, Löwe B. A brief measure for assessing generalized anxiety disorder: the GAD-7. Arch Intern Med. 2006; 166(10):1092–1097

[54] Espie CA. The psychological treatment of insomnia. Chichester: Wiley; 1991

[55] Reynolds CF, III, Kupfer DJ, Hoch CC, Sewitch DE. Sleeping pills for the elderly: are they ever justified? J Clin Psychiatry. 1985; 46(2 Pt 2):9–12

[56] Stepanski E, Zorick F, Roehrs T, Young D, Roth T. Daytime alertness in patients with chronic insomnia compared with asymptomatic control subjects. Sleep. 1988; 11(1): 54–60

[57] Shapiro C, Falnigan M. Function of sleep. In: Shapiro C, ed. ABC of sleep disorders. London: BMJ Publishing; 1993

[58] Walker M. Why we sleep: the new science of sleep and dreams. Penguin; 2018

[59] Mendleson WB. Insomnia: the patient and the pill. In: Bootzin RR, Kihlstrom JF, Schacter DL, eds. Sleep and cognition. Washington: American Psychological Association; 1990:139–147

[60] Mendelson WB, Garnett D, Linnoila M. Do insomniacs have impaired daytime functioning? Biol Psychiatry. 1984; 19(8): 1261–1264

[61] Schneider-Helmert D. Twenty-four-hour sleep-wake function and personality patterns in chronic insomniacs and healthy controls. Sleep. 1987; 10(5):452–462

[62] Seidel WF, Ball S, Cohen S, Patterson N, Yost D, Dement WC. Daytime alertness in relation to mood, performance, and nocturnal sleep in chronic insomniacs and noncomplaining sleepers. Sleep. 1984; 7(3):230–238

[63] Sugerman JL, Stern JA, Walsh JK. Daytime alertness in subjective and objective insomnia: some preliminary findings. Biol Psychiatry. 1985; 20(7):741–750

[64] Sateia MJ, Doghramji K, Hauri PJ, Morin CM. Evaluation of chronic insomnia. An American Academy of Sleep Medicine review. Sleep. 2000; 23(2):243–308

[65] Davies S, McKenna L, Hallam RS. Relaxation and cognitive therapy: a controlled trial in chronic tinnitus. Psychol Health. 1995; 10:129–143

[66] Nicassio PM, Mendlowitz DR, Fussell JJ, Petras L. The phenomenology of the pre-sleep state: the development of the pre-sleep arousal scale. Behav Res Ther. 1985; 23(3): 263–271

[67] Sanavio E. Pre-sleep cognitive intrusions and treatment of onset-insomnia. Behav Res Ther. 1988; 26(6):451–459

[68] Spielman AJ, Anderson MW. The clinical interview and treatment planning as a guide to understanding the nature of insomnia: The CCNY Insomnia Interview. In: Chorkroverty S, ed. Sleep disorders medicine, basic science, technical considerations and clinical aspects. 2nd ed. Woburn: Butterworth-Heinemann; 1999:385–426

[69] Shapiro CM, Devins GM, Hussain MR. Sleep problem inpatients with chronic illness. The ABC of sleep disorders. London: BMJ Publishing; 1993

[70] Andersson G, Lyttkens L. A meta-analytic review of psychological treatments for tinnitus. Br J Audiol. 1999; 33(4): 201–210

[71] Sweetow RW. Adjunctive approaches to tinnitus patient management. Hear J. 1989; 42:38–43

Appendix 6.1 Relaxation Listening for Sleep

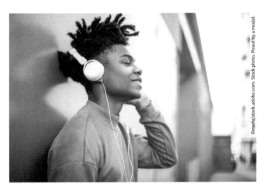

(Source: ©merla/stock.adobe.com. Stock photo. Posed by a model.)

There are many benefits to listening to music or background sound for tinnitus, including increased relaxation, stress reduction, and personal enjoyment. We are asking you to listen to music or a low-level background sound every night as you prepare to fall asleep.

Things to Remember

- Choose a comfortable and distraction-free place in which to listen. Listening in your bedroom is ideal.
- Close your eyes and turn off the lights.
- Set the volume of the music or background sound to a comfortable level.

- Observe your heart rate and breathing rhythm and notice as they slow down with the music or sound.

Listening Guidelines

We would like you to follow this listening routine every night for 30 minutes. Allow yourself to use this time to unwind from the stresses of your day and prepare for sleep. Keep in mind that you cannot be relaxed and anxious at the same time. If while listening you find your mind wanders to thinking about your tinnitus or other worries you have, refocus your thoughts on the music or background sound and the rate of your breathing.

7 Optimizing Hearing Aid Fittings for Tinnitus Management

Grant D. Searchfield and Alice H. Smith

Abstract

Most clinical guidelines support the use of hearing aids in the management of tinnitus accompanied by hearing loss. Hearing aids may improve tinnitus through: improved communication enabling participation in daily activities, attention diversion, masking, and disruption of tinnitus processing neural networks. The effectiveness of hearing aids as a tinnitus management tool may be enhanced by applying the protocol described in this chapter.

Keywords: hearing aids, tinnitus, therapy, clinical protocol

7.1 Introduction

"Nothing is more effective in curing tinnitus than diminishing deafness and nothing so harmful as increasing deafness." (Fowler,[1] p. 36)

This quote from Fowler is 70-years old but it still has currency. We are awaiting pharmacological cures for tinnitus and hearing loss, until then hearing aids are the most effective solution for managing both hearing loss and tinnitus.[2] Current clinical guidelines recommend a hearing aid evaluation for clients with hearing loss and persistent bothersome tinnitus.[3] In the decade since the first edition of this book, there have been significant advances in hearing aid technology and our knowledge of how to apply hearing aids to the task of tinnitus management. The protocol described here is not revolutionary; rather, it is an evolution of the principles established in 2006. The recommendations were originally based on clinical experience. There is now a substantial volume of research exploring hearing aid features and benefits.[4] Hearing aid technology continues to develop with implications for tinnitus as well as hearing loss. This chapter will briefly consider the existing literature on the mechanisms underpinning hearing aid benefit for tinnitus before focusing on the practical aspects of fitting these instruments for treating tinnitus.

7.2 Benefits, Modes, and Mechanisms

Retrospective surveys of tinnitus clinic populations illustrate the benefits of hearing aids. In one study, a third of respondents reported that the primary benefit of attending a tinnitus clinic was the fitting of hearing aids[5]; in another study, 64% of respondents rated hearing aids effective or very effective[6]; and in a third clinic, approximately 90% of tinnitus clients with hearing loss benefitted from hearing aids.[7]

Coles hypothesized five benefits for tinnitus from the fitting of hearing aids[8]:
1. Psychological benefit from assisting hearing.
2. Less attention is paid to hearing and consequently to tinnitus.
3. Understanding that hearing loss is the main cause of communication problems, not tinnitus.
4. Ambient noise and internal circuit noise, making tinnitus less audible.
5. The counseling accompanying hearing aid fitting provides an understanding of tinnitus.

We are beginning to get a clearer picture of how multiple factors contribute to the success of hearing aids. Counseling is a very important component of tinnitus therapy, but it is not the sole benefit of the hearing aid fitting process. The combination of hearing aids with counseling results in better outcomes than counseling alone[9] and hearing aids without any counseling also improve tinnitus.[10,11] Improved quality of life accompanying reduced hearing handicap likely plays a role in tinnitus reduction, but it too is not the only reason for benefits. The degree of masking predicts hearing aid outcome.[12] If total masking was achieved when the hearing aids were turned on at the fitting, long-term reduction in tinnitus handicap was greatest. Partial masking resulted in some reduction in tinnitus handicap. No masking resulted in no long-term reduction in tinnitus handicap. These results imply that masking, not just reduction in hearing handicap, determines the effect of hearing aids on tinnitus. Tinnitus was also more likely to be reduced if its primary pitch was within the frequency range of amplification.[12] It is possible that the greater the complex sounds interrupt tinnitus processing[13] or reduce central auditory gain,[14] the greater the benefit. The use of hearing aids also appears to improve sleep and concentration in persons with tinnitus.[15]

In summary, hearing aids may reduce tinnitus mechanisms in many ways. Our protocol attempts to optimize outcomes by matching individual needs to the multiple benefits of hearing aids.

7.3 Clinic Protocol

The core to our protocol is to correct hearing loss, to connect the individual with their auditory environment, and to provide additional low-level sound stimulation to mask and divert attention from tinnitus. Most tinnitus therapies agree that use of hearing aids should be accompanied by instruction[16] and/or counseling.[17] It is important that clients understand that the aids are part of a therapy, not just prosthetic replacements for lost function. The philosophy underpinning our approach is an ecological framework for tinnitus.[18] Tinnitus perception is governed by the balance of tinnitus and normal sound-related neural activity, individual psychology including personality, and the context in which tinnitus is perceived.[19] The Sound Therapy and Aural Rehabilitation of Tinnitus (START) framework was developed to assist audiologists tailor individualized sound therapy plans.[20] Some elements within the protocol, such as the assessment of tinnitus and counseling, will be discussed only briefly here.

7.3.1 Audiometry and Evaluation

The first step in the evaluation of tinnitus, and then its management, is a comprehensive case history, including questions regarding onset, description, location, possible cause (noise, medications, and stress), context of perception, and severity. The case history questionnaire developed by the Tinnitus Research Initiative is very useful.[21] If the tinnitus is objective, pulsatile, unilateral, or associated with a temporomandibular joint complaint, referral to a physician is made.

Assessments of hearing and tinnitus undertaken: Air and bone conduction pure-tone audiometry, speech and immittance audiometry, and otoacoustic emissions, all assist in determining the focus for rehabilitation and basis for instruction about the physiological basis for the individual's tinnitus.[16] Discretion is needed when measuring acoustic reflex threshold due to the potential for loudness discomfort accompanying tinnitus. Measurements of loudness discomfort levels are valuable for individual setting of the maximum output of hearing aids, but these too must be undertaken with care due to the risk of loudness discomfort. Beginning at a low level and then ascending in small intensity steps is necessary. For persons with severe intolerance to sound, suprathreshold measures may have to be estimated as direct measurement may cause

discomfort and hinder the building of trust between the clinician and client. Psychoacoustical measures such as tinnitus pitch and loudness have little diagnostic value[3]; however, they are useful in counseling[22] (Chapter 8). Device selection is also assisted by knowledge of the degree of low-frequency hearing loss and predominant pitch of tinnitus.[12] If hearing loss is greater than mild in low frequencies, we combine sound therapy with hearing aid use (Chapter 8). If tinnitus pitch is outside the amplification range of hearing aids (practically above 8 kHz), then hearing aids may be less useful[12] and we then trial combination sound therapy or assistive tinnitus devices. Other psychoacoustic tinnitus measures may be useful in selection of sound therapy (Chapter 8).

Self-report questionnaires (e.g., the Tinnitus Functional Index[23] and Tinnitus Primary Function Questionnaire[24]) assist in identifying the most bothersome aspects of the individual's tinnitus. These results are used to identify the different areas of tinnitus to be discussed at counseling sessions and are elaborated upon during needs assessment.

7.3.2 Aural Rehabilitation and Goal Setting

A shared vision for therapy between the clinician, client, and significant others needs to be mapped out in order to focus rehabilitation and to create realistic goals for management. A tinnitus version of the Client Oriented Scale of Improvement (COSI) is used.[26] The original COSI assessed client's communication needs, and outcomes achieved following the fitting of hearing aids. Using the open-ended format of the Client Oriented Scale of Improvement in Tinnitus (COSIT[27]), the clinician and client identify specific situations in which tinnitus is bothersome, for example, "Tinnitus affects my ability to concentrate at work," and negotiate between what the client may want (tinnitus gone completely) and realistic outcomes (diminished awareness of tinnitus). If the client is experiencing strong anxiety or depression, referral to a psychologist is organized and counseling is emphasized. Strong reaction to the nature of the tinnitus sound itself may point toward the use of therapeutic sounds, while high hearing needs suggest hearing aids. Once individual needs are understood we apply one or more of four aural rehabilitation components: (1) Instruction, (2) counseling, (3) sensory management, and (4) perceptual training.[28]

7.3.3 Instruction

Instruction is a directive form of psychoeducation and considers the mechanisms of hearing and neurophysiology of tinnitus.[16] Knowledge about a condition leads to better therapeutic outcomes.[29] Often understanding what tinnitus is (and isn't) is all that is needed to reassure clients to its usually benign nature. We describe how hearing loss, thoughts, and environmental factors all contribute to tinnitus. The level of detail provided is adjusted to the individual's understanding.

Clients are told:

- Most tinnitus appears to be the consequence of the auditory systems' interpretation of altered activity from the inner ear.
- Changes in the spontaneous (background) output of the cochlea accompanying hearing loss are exaggerated by central auditory processing which can eventually lead to a change in the functional organization of the auditory cortex.
- Tinnitus severity is not fully explained by the degree of ear damage as there is poor correlation between hearing threshold and tinnitus distress.
- It is thought that much of the severity of tinnitus relates to enhancement by central auditory processing and the individuals' reaction to the abnormal perception.
- Because tinnitus is a new and unusual auditory perception, the brain struggles to place it in context and it takes on an unusual importance.

With respect to hearing aids they are told:

- Hearing aids should improve communication and divert attention from their tinnitus.
- Hearing aids also amplify background sound, which should decrease the prominence of their tinnitus.
- They should enrich their listening environment with music or other sounds to divert attention away from the tinnitus and to partially mask it.
- Sound therapy using hearing aids and an enriched listening environment along with counseling may assist in adaptation to tinnitus.

7.3.4 Counseling

For chronic bothersome tinnitus, instruction alone may be insufficient. A person-centered counseling approach may be needed that addresses specific emotional and quality-of-life concerns.[17] There are many excellent protocols and guidelines for tinnitus counseling. In our clinic we focus on four primary areas: attend, react, educate, and adapt (AREA). The structure of the counseling is based on Wilson and Gilbert's theories of affective adaptation.[30] We use a slide show presentation and online material (www.tinnitustues.com) to supplement the discussions. It is important that the client's perspectives are sought and they guide the areas addressed. Each session is altered according to individual needs and incorporates instruction along with discussion; topics typically covered include:

Attend:
- Attention grabbing aspects of tinnitus.
- Attention refocusing.

React:
- Tinnitus and stress.
- Perceived threat.

Educate:
- Why understanding tinnitus is important.
- How we hear.
- Adaptation-level theory.
- Reality of tinnitus perception.
- Adaptation-level theory of tinnitus and role of sound.

Adapt:
- Meaning of adaptation.
- Perceptual adaptation.
- Affective adaptation.
- Assistance through sound therapy, visualization, and guided imagery.
- Hearing and active listening and brain/attention training.

7.3.5 Sensory Management: Selection of Hearing Aids and Their Features

We define sensory management as the use of hearing aids and sound therapy.[31] A person's environment and the context in which tinnitus is heard can indicate the need for sensory management.[18] Hearing loss accompanying tinnitus can result in anxiety, social isolation, and a reduction in sound-driven auditory.[32] It makes sense that reducing this "auditory isolation" through the fitting of hearing aids should reverse some of the circumstances leading to bothersome tinnitus. In severe losses, cochlear implants may be needed. In the sections below, we describe our hearing aid selection and fitting method.

We select hearing aids as our sensory management approach when tinnitus pitch is less than 8 kHz (within the amplification range of most aids) and the person has normal hearing to mild hearing loss in the low frequencies. Outside of this range, we recommend the combination of hearing aids and sound therapy (Chapter 8) and for severe to profound hearing loss—cochlear implants (▶ Fig. 7.1).

The principle underpinning hearing aid fitting in our approach is to provide as much gain of low-intensity ambient sound as possible without louder sounds causing discomfort. So, in the selection of hearing aids the ideal devices are those that allow the dual, but potentially antagonistic, goals of improving the audibility of speech and amplifying ambient sound to interfere with tinnitus. Flexibility in programming is very useful so we often select hearing aids where the audiologist has control over as many fitting parameters as possible.

Recommended Features and Settings

Understanding the degree to which a particular hearing aid, or aid setting, results in the amplification of low-intensity sounds is fundamental to knowing how to adjust hearing aids to reduce tinnitus audibility.

Binaural Fitting and Processing

For bilateral hearing loss, we aim to provide more normal auditory balance. If unilateral tinnitus is associated with unilateral hearing loss, then a single device may be an option.[33] This sometimes results in perception of tinnitus moving toward the opposite ear. Binaural processing in which the hearing aids apply processing linked between ears, as opposed to working as two separate units, is a new technology, and merits for tinnitus management have yet to be ascertained.

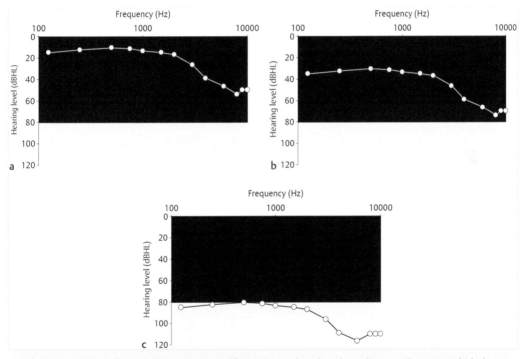

Fig. 7.1 A rough guide for the selection between different devices based on the audiogram. The area in which the audiogram falls suggests the device type. If the audiogram and tinnitus pitch is primarily within the *gray* area, **(a)** hearing aids are likely to be successful; if primarily in the *black* area, **(b)** hearing aids combined with sound therapy may be a better option, and if in the *white* area, **(c)** cochlear implants may be the only option for success of therapy using device. Hearing aids appear most effective when there is little or no low-frequency hearing loss. (Based on Searchfield 2014.[34])

Open Fit When Possible

Reduction in environmental sound, from blocking the ear canal, can result in increased tinnitus awareness. Thin tube receiver over-the-ear and receiver in-the-ear hearing aids have been a great development for clinicians working with tinnitus hearing losses. Both their cosmetic appeal and acoustic benefits in avoiding occlusion have assisted client adoption of hearing aids as tinnitus therapeutic devices. Open fittings avoid occlusion from the user's own voice while providing targeted amplification to high-frequency hearing loss. There are also occasions in which less venting is appropriate such as low-frequency hearing losses.[36] With low-frequency hearing loss, custom earmolds may be necessary to allow low frequencies to be heard; with severe high-frequency hearing loss, they may be needed to prevent feedback.

We do not recommend custom in the ear devices for tinnitus, but as long as they are appropriately fit they also can meet the goals of a tinnitus fitting. In the ear long-wear devices (the Phonak Lyric) have been trialed successfully but despite their ability to provide long duration doses of sound through continuous use, they do not appear to provide clinically significant benefits over other aid types.[37] It is possible that intermittent sound exposure is more likely to lead to helpful neuroplastic changes than constant sound exposure.[35]

Flexible Compression Settings

Low-compression kneepoints enable the amplification of low-intensity environmental sounds to audible levels without causing discomfort to louder sounds. Low-compression kneepoints and wide dynamic range compression allow more amplification of quiet ambient sounds than linear strategies. A low-compression kneepoint with higher than normal compression ratio also limits the amount of high intensity sound being amplified. If the amount of gain to moderate inputs is maintained and the kneepoint is lowered, the level of ambient noise perceived should increase. Wide dynamic range compression with low-compression kneepoints (20- to 45-dB SPL) is recommended. The circuit noise generated by the hearing aid has been useful in tinnitus management in the past[36] but is often inaudible due to expansion or "soft squelch" in digital hearing aids. Expansion results in a more rapid reduction in gain below the kneepoint than in conventional compression. The goal of expansion is exactly the opposite of what is desirable for reducing tinnitus audibility in quiet: the reduction of ambient sound and circuit noise. In cases were circuit noise or amplification of environmental noise is insufficient or annoying to the hearing aid user, therapeutic sounds may be substituted (Chapter 8).

Omnidirectional Microphone Setting in Quiet Environments

In quiet environments an omnidirectional setting facilitates hearing sounds from around the user, not just from in front. Conveniently, manufacturer's automatic acoustic classifiers switch to omnidirectional modes in the absence of background noise.

Noise Reduction Algorithms Switched Off

Noise reduction digital signal processing algorithms monitor temporal and spectral characteristics of sound and attempt to reduce amplification in channels in which speech-like stimuli are not present.[38] While useful for providing comfort in noise, these are counterproductive when the tinnitus user is in quiet. They effectively reduce the ambient sounds used to partially mask tinnitus. Our preference is for hearing aids in which noise reduction features can be tuned by the dispensing clinician.

Frequency Lowering

There is contradictory evidence as to the value of frequency lowering as a digital signal processing strategy for tinnitus. One study[39] reported linear frequency transposition as being very beneficial, while another study found frequency compression to be less helpful than standard amplification.[40] Further investigation is required before frequency lowering is adopted as a tinnitus amplification strategy.

Manual Volume Controls

We believe that in most cases automatic volume controls are advantageous for tinnitus management. When appropriately set, automatic volume adjustment may result in less attention being paid to the aids, ears, and consequently tinnitus. Constant volume control manipulation may focus attention to the ears, which will hamper attempts to ignore tinnitus. However, volume controls can be useful to increase amplification in quiet environments, or reducing sound for persons experiencing loudness intolerance. Volume controls may also be needed for control sound therapy provided in combination with the amplification.

Multiple Programs

In the previous edition of this chapter, we recommended a separate amplification program for tinnitus, which placed a strong emphasis on amplification of very quiet environmental sounds. This was advocated due to the absence of modern combinations of hearing aid processing with therapy sounds at the time. This option is less of a necessity now because advanced amplification processing is available with programmable sound therapy options. Rather than programming "noisy" hearing aid settings, we now favor using onboard tinnitus therapy sounds (also called "noisers") if normal amplification isn't sufficient in reducing tinnitus audibility (Chapter 8). Much lower gain along with low maximum outputs and high-compression ratios are needed when tinnitus is accompanied by hyperacusis. These settings can be increased gradually over time as the person becomes used to hearing more in their environment and physically managing the devices. Manufacturer listening programs labeled as "comfort" or "loudness" may be selected on a more regular basis to manage the intolerance to sound.

Automatic Acoustic Classifiers

Most hearing aid manufacturers have developed acoustic sound classifiers that select settings on the basis of the sound environment sampled. Sensing of different environments (e.g., quiet, speech, and speech in noise) results in a selection of signal processing settings believed to be most suited to those environments. These automatic sound classifiers appear useful when the goal is optimizing speech recognition.[41] Benefits for tinnitus do not appear to have been ascertained; however, if the classifier correctly identifies loud noisy environments and the aids adjust by reducing amplification, we would predict benefits for persons with decreased tolerance for sound. If the aids select no noise reduction and omnidirectional settings in quiet, this may benefit in tinnitus masking. Some manufacturers allow for the sensitivity of settings to be tuned. This should allow the clinician some flexibility to manipulate the automatic processes to the tinnitus sufferers' needs.

Streaming

Wireless communication between hearing aids and smartphones, tablets, or computers enables access to a wide range of therapy sounds from manufacturer apps or downloaded from the Internet. This added flexibility in sound choice can be useful when the internal therapy sounds aren't tolerated (Chapter 8). The ability to select from a wide range of treatment sounds also provides the user with a sense of control. Control is often a high-priority treatment goal. Music which evokes positive emotions for the individual may be used. Music which diverts attention and is vigorous is recommended for short-term relief from their tinnitus at its worst, while slower pieces of music that enable a progression to a relaxed state may be more helpful in the longer term.[42] On occasions, a separate amplification program optimized for music listening may be necessary.

Datalogging

Datalogging (onboard recording of hearing aid use) is not a feature that results in a direct impact on tinnitus. The information obtained, including hours of use, programs used, volume settings, and the environments users experience, can be helpful to the clinician. The information can be used at follow-up appointments to compare compliance with recommended use and reports of problems encountered. The clinician can then use this information to discuss impact on the therapy plan and the negotiated outcomes determined with the COSIT.

Remote Programming

Remote programming of hearing aids potentially can address client concerns with fewer face-to-face consultations. This may be valuable for anxious clients who request frequent consultations. However, the demand on clinicians for immediate action needs to be carefully managed, and time allocated in clinic schedules for this programming.

Artificial Intelligence, Sensors, and the Internet

Advances in Internet connectivity, miniaturized sensor technology, and artificial intelligence offer exciting opportunities for tinnitus treatment. Although yet to be directly applied to tinnitus, biometric information may enable hearing aid and sound therapy tuning in real time, for example, in response to heart rate.

Over-the-Counter Devices

Over-the-counter hearing aids may provide some of the benefits described in this chapter. However, in clinical practice we value the flexibility offered in the programming of hearing aids. The counseling accompanying the device fitting is also very important and would be difficult to replicate in self-fitting aids.

Fitting

Prescriptive procedures for hearing aid amplification have been developed to determine the most appropriate amount of amplification for an individual based on their hearing loss. The amount of amplification that best assists hearing speech and that which is optimized to reduce tinnitus audibility in quiet environments is different. Also, the amount of amplification normally prescribed by these formulas for high-intensity sounds may exceed the usually low loudness tolerance of tinnitus sufferers. In the 2006 edition of this book, we recommended two listening programs: one optimized for hearing speech and the other for masking tinnitus. Now that most hearing aid technology incorporates tinnitus therapy sounds (Chapter 8), the need for a dedicated tinnitus amplification program is reduced. Instead, our recommended selection of first-fit prescription varies according to an individual's priorities. We had suggested the Desired Sensation Level series of targets be used as a starting point for the tinnitus because evidence indicated that tinnitus was less audible with hearing aids set to DSL(I/O) than NAL-NL1.[4,43] The most likely reason for reduced tinnitus audibility using the DSL prescription was that it prescribed greater low-intensity low-frequency amplification than other prescriptions and this is the frequency

region for most background noise.[44] The relative merits of the newer prescription versions DSL v 5.0 and NAL-NL2 on tinnitus have yet to be determined. An alternative approach to hearing aid amplification has tried using notched amplification to achieve lateral inhibition.[45] It is too early to draw any conclusions as to the merits of notched amplification relative to conventional approaches. If necessary, multiple prescriptions, including manufacturer's proprietary prescriptions, can be trialed to determine the best responses for the individual.

All fittings need to be able to be verified against prescribed amplification using real-ear measurements (▶ Fig. 7.2). When undertaking the real-ear measures, the response to a moderate intensity (65-dB SPL) stimulus is matched to the chosen target. A quiet background sound (of approximately 30-dB SPL) is amplified to meet or exceed auditory threshold across as wide a frequency range as possible. The level of sound used is lower than that produced by real-ear measurement equipment; hence, this requires that the real-ear equipment signal is switched off and replaced by a signal external to the equipment. The ambient sound within the clinic room or just audible sound from a recording of environmental sound can be used as the stimulus to be measured. The amount of amplification finally chosen is usually that which results in the tinnitus being less easily detected without discomfort to the listener. For some clients, total masking can be achieved with little

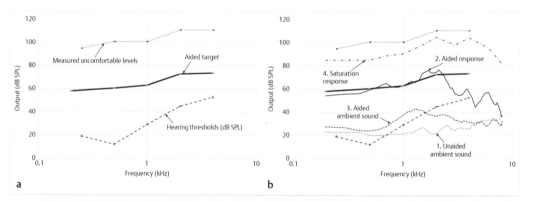

Fig. 7.2 Hearing aid fitting process using real ear measures and amplification of ambient sound to exceed threshold. **(a)** Real ear targets for a high-frequency hearing loss. **(b)** Step-by-step process: (1) Measurement of ambient sound with probe microphone in ear, no aid in, sound stimulus from equipment turned off. (2) Aid in place and measurement of moderate-level stimulus (65-dB sound pressure level [SPL]) through hearing aid, adjusted as necessary to match to prescription target. (3) Measurement of ambient sound through hearing aid (real-ear equipment sound off—or at lowest level) to determine audible spectrum based on exceeding hearing threshold. (4) Measurement of maximum output (saturation response) of hearing aid to high-level sound (depending on tolerance 80- to 90-dB SPL) to ensure levels do not exceed measured discomfort levels. (Based on Searchfield 2006.[47])

amplification of sound. If the degree of ambient sound amplification is unpleasant for the client, the amount of gain for low-level inputs is reduced. When clients have a history of sound intolerance, it is recommended that uncomfortable loudness levels are measured[46] rather than being predicted from the audiogram. The hearing aid output to high-intensity sound is measured (80- to 90-dB SPL, swept tones) using the probe microphone system and the maximum output of the aid is altered where necessary to be below uncomfortable loudness levels.

Physical Comfort and Occlusion Measures

We do not want our clients to focus unduly on the ears as this simply reminds them of their tinnitus. The physical comfort of the devices is evaluated by placing the aids switched off in the ear. Alterations should be made to avoid any physical discomfort. The extent to which the chosen hearing aid prevents transmission of sound by occluding the ear canal can be determined using real ear measurements.[48] A comparison between the real-ear unaided and occluded (aid in but switched off) responses indicates the extent to which the device attenuates sound. If the hearing aid significantly blocks quiet sounds, steps can be taken to overcome this by increasing vent size or changing earmold style. Some occlusion of the ear with the aid switched off is acceptable only if the aid switched on can amplify sounds to overcome any insertion loss of ambient sound.

7.3.6 Perceptual Training

We use both informal and guided attention-based listening tasks.[49] Here we will discuss a self-directed approach.[50] The guided training approach is discussed in the accompanying chapter on sound therapy (Chapter 8). Rather than just passive use of the hearing aids, clients are counseled to actively train their ears. They are coached to try and reduce their focus on tinnitus by improving attention to external sounds. The hope is that by increasing the cognitive load used for real-world listening, fewer resources are available for tinnitus processing. We teach the client wearing hearing aids to first try and identify their tinnitus and how it sounds, accept this and then direct attention to the real-world soundscape. The intention is the sufferer understands the perceptual reality of tinnitus and through this learns to place it in context.[25] They then allocate resources to the useful role of evaluating their soundscape. They are told to "scan the environment, listen, detect and localize, sounds around you, focus on these real sounds. Notice how focus on other sounds reduces focus on tinnitus. Now practice this every day, especially when tinnitus is on your mind. As you become better at listening to other sounds the tinnitus will reduce."

7.3.7 Appointment Scheduling and Follow-Up

The time allocated to each task will need to vary according to the clinic structure. Our customer service team screen direct client enquiries in an attempt to identify those persons who are just curious about their tinnitus (booked for a hearing evaluation) from those with tinnitus likely needing management (booked for both a tinnitus evaluation and needs assessment and instruction). We originally undertook assessment and first management appointments as a continuous appointment; however, this is demanding on both the client and the clinician. Now assessment takes place in one session and the clients return for needs assessment, and first instruction and counseling session in the afternoon of the same day or on a separate day. A break helps improve concentration and it enables formulation of questions by the client and a preliminary management plan by the clinician. At the end of the session a membership to our online tinnitus resource is provided. We have found that the 24/7 adjunct support provided by the online material reduces the frequency of enquiries from anxious clients, lightening the administrative burden of frequent enquiries to the clinic. It is also reassuring to clients that instruction and counseling support is available even when the clinician is not. Typically, 2 weeks following needs assessment, those receiving devices will return for fitting, and then these are trialed for 3 weeks followed by a follow-up appointment and, typically, a further 3 weeks of trial and follow-up. We encourage 6- and 12-month follow-up consultations, and frequently evaluate outcomes through client surveys. Adaptation to tinnitus is likely to be demonstrated by a progressive decrease in tinnitus effects across time. Hearing aids appear to reach maximum benefit by 9 to 12 weeks with benefit plateauing 12 to 24 weeks following fitting.[2] Additional benefits and maintenance of effect may be dependent on further counseling and client's adherence to sensory management and perceptual training recommendations.

The clients most likely to require on-going assistance are those who report little or no change in tinnitus audibility when the hearing aids are first switched on. The initial prescription of amplification is not going to suit every client. Fine-tuning should be undertaken to address self-reported difficulties with the aids. If hearing aids are not reducing the audibility of tinnitus then a change to settings, such as increasing low-level gain or introduction of alternative therapeutic sound, should be implemented. At stages throughout the tinnitus rehabilitation process, the problems identified using the COSIT are re-examined and improvement in tinnitus in each situation is determined. If improvement is not shown, appropriate steps are undertaken to address the problem until realistic goals are achieved. The focus of intervention should move from high-priority COSIT goals to the next priorities with progression in therapy. Any adverse response to the hearing aids needs to be managed so as to prevent the client from being forced to focus on their hearing and consequently the tinnitus. Clients need to be reminded that treating tinnitus is a journey of many steps.

Occasionally, intolerance to sounds can be a barrier to hearing aid success. When clients complain that hearing aids exacerbate their tinnitus, it is often found that the maximum output of the hearing aids had been set above the client's loudness tolerance levels. In order to accommodate reduced loudness tolerance, extra caution must be applied in the amount of amplification recommended. Optimal amplification of speech sounds may have to be sacrificed and preference instead given to comfort and amplification of soft sounds. Amplification can gradually increase as sound tolerance permits. As long as the sound intolerance is not severe, management of the tinnitus can occur concurrently. When a client cannot tolerate any amplification, onboard sound therapy is used and amplification is gradually introduced as progress permits. Real-ear measures can be used to illustrate what the ideal target for amplification is, and where the individual's preferred setting currently sits. It is important that an explanation be provided of why ideal amplification cannot be achieved until there has been some improvement in sound tolerance.

7.4 Conclusion

The basic premise in hearing aid fitting for tinnitus is to do your best to improve your clients' hearing and stimulate the auditory system with low-level sounds.

- Hearing aids are useful in managing tinnitus when combined with counseling.
- Amplification of speech serves to divert attention away from tinnitus.
- Amplification of ambient noise serves to partially mask tinnitus.
- The most effective hearing aid settings for communication are not necessarily the best for reducing tinnitus audibility.
- Clinicians need to be flexible in their device selection and fitting strategy.

There is still a need for strong randomized controlled trials of the role of hearing aids in tinnitus therapy; however, the volume of research supporting hearing aid effectiveness has increased significantly over the past decade.[2]

To demonstrate hearing aid fitting for a tinnitus patient, there is a video available on the companion website. The video developed by the editors describes fitting and verification of sound therapy devices using real ear measures and psychoacoustic measures of tinnitus.

References

[1] Fowler EP. Nonvibratory tinnitus; factors underlying subaudible and audible irritations. Arch Otolaryngol. 1948; 47(1):29–36

[2] Shekhawat GS, Searchfield GD, Stinear CM. Role of hearing AIDS in tinnitus intervention: a scoping review. J Am Acad Audiol. 2013; 24(8):747–762

[3] Tunkel DE, Bauer CA, Sun GH, et al. Clinical practice guideline: tinnitus. Otolaryngol Head Neck Surg. 2014; 151 (2) Suppl:S1–S40

[4] Shekhawat GS, Searchfield GD, Kobayashi K, Stinear CM. Prescription of hearing-aid output for tinnitus relief. Int J Audiol. 2013; 52(9):617–625

[5] Sanchez L, Stephens D. Survey of the perceived benefits and shortcomings of a specialist tinnitus clinic. Audiology. 2000; 39(6):333–339

[6] Aazh H, Moore BC, Lammaing K, Cropley M. Tinnitus and hyperacusis therapy in a UK National Health Service audiology department: patients' evaluations of the effectiveness of treatments. Int J Audiol. 2016; 55(9):514–522

[7] Liang F, Han F, Li L. (2017). Study on treatment effect of hearing aids on bilateral prolonged tinnitus in Chinese patients. Paper presented at the BIO Web of Conferences

[8] Coles RRA. Tinnitus and its management. In: Kerr AG, ed. Scott-Brown's otolaryngology. London: Butterworths; 1985:368–414

[9] Searchfield GD, Kaur M, Martin WH. Hearing aids as an adjunct to counseling: tinnitus patients who choose amplification do better than those that don't. Int J Audiol. 2010; 49(8):574–579

[10] Shekhawat GS, Searchfield GD, Stinear CM. Randomized trial of transcranial direct current stimulation and hearing aids for tinnitus management. Neurorehabil Neural Repair. 2014; 28(5):410–419

[11] Sheldrake JB, Coles RRA, Foster JR. Noise generators ("maskers") for tinnitus. In: Reich GE, Vernon JA, eds. Proceedings of the Fifth International Tinnitus Seminar. Portland: American Tinnitus Association; 1996:351–352

[12] McNeill C, Távora-Vieira D, Alnafjan F, Searchfield GD, Welch D. Tinnitus pitch, masking, and the effectiveness of hearing aids for tinnitus therapy. Int J Audiol. 2012; 51(12):914–919

[13] Andersson G. A cognitive-affective theory for tinnitus: experiments and theoretical implications. Paper presented at the Proceedings of the seventh international tinnitus seminar, Perth; 2002

[14] Pienkowski M. Rationale and efficacy of sound therapies for tinnitus and hyperacusis. Neuroscience. 2019; 407:120–134

[15] Zarenoe R, Hällgren M, Andersson G, Ledin T. Working memory, sleep, and hearing problems in patients with tinnitus and hearing loss fitted with hearing aids. J Am Acad Audiol. 2017; 28(2):141–151

[16] Jastreboff PJ, Hazell JW. Tinnitus retraining therapy: implementing the neurophysiological model. Cambridge: Cambridge University Press; 2008

[17] Tyler RS, Gogel SA, Gehringer AK. Tinnitus activities treatment. Prog Brain Res. 2007; 166:425–434

[18] Searchfield GD. Tinnitus what and where: an ecological framework. Front Neurol. 2014; 5(271):271

[19] Searchfield GD, Kobayashi K, Sanders M. An adaptation level theory of tinnitus audibility. Front Syst Neurosci. 2012; 6:46

[20] Searchfield GD, Linford T, Durai M. Sound therapy and aural rehabilitation for tinnitus: a person centred therapy framework based on an ecological model of tinnitus. Disabil Rehabil. 2019; 41(16):1966–1973

[21] Langguth B, Goodey R, Azevedo A, et al. Consensus for tinnitus patient assessment and treatment outcome measurement: Tinnitus Research Initiative meeting, Regensburg, July 2006. Prog Brain Res. 2007; 166:525–536

[22] Tyler R. The psychoacoustical measurement of tinnitus. Tinnitus handbook, 2000:149–179

[23] Chandra N, Chang K, Lee A, Shekhawat GS, Searchfield GD. Psychometric validity, reliability, and responsiveness of the tinnitus functional index. J Am Acad Audiol. 2018; 29(7):609–625

[24] Tyler R, Ji H, Perreau A, Witt S, Noble W, Coelho C. Development and validation of the tinnitus primary function questionnaire. Am J Audiol. 2014; 23(3):260–272

[25] Feldmann H. Tinnitus: reality or phantom. In: Aran JM, Dauman R, eds. Tinnitus 91: Proceedings of the Fourth International Tinnitus Seminar. Amsterdam: Kugler Publications; 1992

[26] Dillon H, James A, Ginis J. Client Oriented Scale of Improvement (COSI) and its relationship to several other measures of benefit and satisfaction provided by hearing aids. J Am Acad Audiol. 1997; 8(1):27–43

[27] Searchfield GD. A client oriented scale of improvement in tinnitus for therapy goal planning and assessing outcomes. J Am Acad Audiol. 2019; 30(4):327–337

[28] Boothroyd A. Adult aural rehabilitation: what is it and does it work? Trends Amplif. 2007; 11(2):63–71

[29] Lucksted A, McFarlane W, Downing D, Dixon L. Recent developments in family psychoeducation as an evidence-based practice. J Marital Fam Ther. 2012; 38(1):101–121

[30] Wilson TD, Gilbert DT. Explaining away: a model of affective adaptation. Perspect Psychol Sci. 2008; 3(5):370–386

[31] Hoare DJ, Searchfield GD, El Refaie A, Henry JA. Sound therapy for tinnitus management: practicable options. J Am Acad Audiol. 2014; 25(1):62–75

[32] Zaugg T, Schechter MA, Fausti SA, Henry JA. Difficulties caused by patient's misconceptions that hearing problems are due to tinnitus. In: Patuzzi R, ed. Proceedings of the Seventh International Tinnitus Seminar (pp. 226–228). Perth: University of Western Australia; 2002

[33] Tsai BS, Sweetow RW, Cheung SW. Audiometric asymmetry and tinnitus laterality. Laryngoscope. 2012; 122(5):1148–1153

[34] Searchfield GD. Selecting and optimising hearing aids for tinnitus benefit: a rough guide. ENT and Audiology News. 2014; 22(6)

[35] Sheppard A, Liu X, Ding D, Salvi R. Auditory central gain compensates for changes in cochlear output after prolonged low-level noise exposure. Neurosci Lett. 2018; 687:183–188

[36] Tyler RS, Bentler RA. Tinnitus maskers and hearing aids for tinnitus. Semin Hear. 1987; 8(01):49–60

[37] Henry JA, McMillan G, Dann S, et al. Tinnitus management: randomized controlled trial comparing extended-wear hearing aids, conventional hearing aids, and combination instruments. J Am Acad Audiol. 2017; 28(6):546–561

[38] Schweitzer C. Development of digital hearing AIDS. Trends Amplif. 1997; 2(2):41–77

[39] Peltier E, Peltier C, Tahar S, Alliot-Lugaz E, Cazals Y. Long-term tinnitus suppression with linear octave frequency transposition hearing AIDS. PLoS One. 2012; 7(12):e51915

[40] Hodgson SA, Herdering R, Singh Shekhawat G, Searchfield GD. A crossover trial comparing wide dynamic range compression and frequency compression in hearing aids for tinnitus therapy. Disabil Rehabil Assist Technol. 2017; 12(1):97–103

[41] Searchfield GD, Linford T, Kobayashi K, Crowhen D, Latzel M. The performance of an automatic acoustic-based program classifier compared to hearing aid users' manual selection of listening programs. Int J Audiol. 2018; 57(3):201–212

[42] Hann D, Searchfield GD, Sanders M, Wise K. Strategies for the selection of music in the short-term management of mild tinnitus. Aust N Z J Audiol. 2008; 30(2):129–140

[43] Wise K. Amplification of sound for tinnitus management: a comparison of DSL[i/o] and NAL-NL1 prescriptive procedures and the influence of compression threshold on tinnitus audibility. Master of Audiology, The University of Auckland, Auckland; 2003

[44] Moreland JB. Ambient noise measurements in open-plan offices. J Acoust Soc Am. 1988; 83(4):1683–1685

[45] Strauss DJ, Corona-Strauss FI, Seidler H, Haab L, Hannemann R. Notched environmental sounds: a new hearing aid-supported tinnitus treatment evaluated in 20 patients. Clin Otolaryngol. 2017; 42(1):172–175

[46] Hawkins DB, Ball TL, Beasley HE, Cooper WA. Comparison of SSPL90 selection procedures. J Am Acad Audiol. 1992; 3(1):46–50

[47] Searchfield GD. Hearing aids and tinnitus. In: Tyler RS, ed. Tinnitus treatment. New York: Thieme; 2006

[48] Mueller H, Hawkins D, Northern J. Probe microphone measurements—hearing aid selection and assessment. San Diego, CA: Singular; 1992

[49] Searchfield GD, Morrison-Low J, Wise K. Object identification and attention training for treating tinnitus. Prog Brain Res. 2007; 166:441–460

[50] Henry J, Wilson PH. The psychological management of chronic tinnitus: a cognitive-behavioural approach. Massachusetts: Allyn & Bacon; 2001

8 Combining Sound Therapy with Amplification

Grant D. Searchfield, Mithila Durai, and Tania Linford

Abstract

Hearing aid amplification alone may not always be sufficient as a sound therapy. The use of therapeutic sounds in combination with hearing aids increases their versatility as devices for tinnitus management. The heterogeneity in tinnitus and individual preferences for different sounds are challenges for clinicians, but they can be overcome by careful consideration of client goals. This chapter describes a clinical protocol for incorporating sound therapy with amplification.

Keywords: sound therapy, hearing aids, tinnitus, clinical protocol

8.1 Introduction

Sound therapy and aural rehabilitation form the basis of audiological approaches to tinnitus.[1] Sound therapy is the use of any sound to manage or treat tinnitus. All management methods using sound, irrespective of type, level, and duration are encompassed by this definition.[2] Sound therapy is a common approach to tinnitus, but its effectiveness is often questioned.[3] Some individuals show strong benefits from sound therapy while others do not benefit.[4] This chapter is concerned with the process of providing sound therapy generated by, or in connection with, a hearing aid. These aids were once called combination aids and were only available from a few manufacturers. Now almost all hearing aids have tinnitus treatment sounds as selectable options. Although the evidence supporting hearing aids for tinnitus has reached a level of general acceptance for their benefit (Chapter 7), evidence for additional benefit by combining with therapeutic sound is not as strong.[5]

Therapeutic sounds generated by hearing aids are usually variations of broadband noise (BBN),[6] although fractal tones are also used.[7] Many hearing aids can also be used in combination with sound players (e.g., wireless streaming via Bluetooth connectivity with Smartphones), and recorded sounds (e.g., sounds from nature), or customized sounds can also be used as sound therapy. Numerous tinnitus apps (software applications for mobile devices) are also now available, providing a greater range of treatment sounds. There is limited evidence that combination aids are superior to hearing aids.[8,9]

Most studies have been unable to separate the benefits for tinnitus suppression of combined amplification with sound therapy from amplification alone,[5] and other studies have suggested that use of different therapy sounds do not affect outcomes greatly.[10,11] There is a great deal of variability in response to sound, with approximately one-third of patients responding well to partial masking.[4] Another contributing factor to the limited evidence for efficacy of sound therapy is its diversity and plural modes of action.[12] We do not believe that "sound therapy" is a single strategy; rather, it consists of many different sound stimulation approaches, targeting many different mechanisms. Compelling arguments in favor of sound therapy could be made if it was viewed in a similar light to cognitive behavioral therapy (CBT), which is as an omnibus therapy using a combination of strategies tailored to an individual's needs.[13] The efficacy of CBT is judged on its effect as a combination of approaches rather than its constituent components. Like CBT, sound therapy consists of many components that can, for any given individual, be more useful than another component.[14] In this chapter, we first briefly describe this approach to organizing sound therapy before focusing on the practical aspects of providing sound therapy in combination with hearing aids.

8.2 Sound Therapy Framework

We use a unifying "omnibus" framework for tinnitus sound therapy.[2] On the basis of a review, we categorized the modes of action of different approaches to sound therapy into three nonexclusive organizing themes of: (1) the presence of sound, (2) the context of sound, and (3) the reaction to sound, with a fourth global theme of adaptation (▶ Fig. 8.1[12]). Sounds can have an effect through one or more of these pathways. We briefly describe these organizing principles of sound therapy below.

8.2.1 The Presence of Sound Effect

The simplest argument in favor of sound as a tinnitus therapy is that tinnitus is often at its most annoying when the person experiences it in a quiet environment, and is less noticeable when sound is present. This presence of external sound can mask the tinnitus, reduce its audibility, or

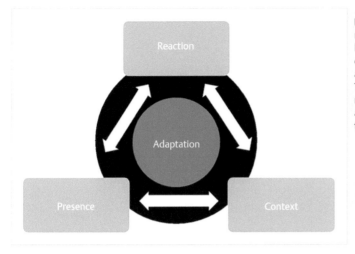

Fig. 8.1 Sound therapy and aural rehabilitation themes. Sound therapy has three organizing themes (presence, context, and reaction to sound) and a global theme of adaptation.[12] The categories are nonexclusive and need to be balanced against positive and negative effects across each theme.

change its perceived magnitude.[12] Whatever the stated theoretical goal of a sound therapy is, some of its effect will be elicited by its presence interfering with tinnitus perception. This is a bottom-up process and is less dependent on the meaning of sound as its ability to change activity in the auditory pathways. Even if the tinnitus is not totally masked, some people find comfort from having the presence of another sound; often they report it "just takes the edge off the tinnitus" and helps them to feel a little more in control. Variations of BBN (e.g., white or pink noise) are typically used within this theme.

8.2.2 The Context of Sound Effect

The goal of this approach is to change the perception of tinnitus by placing it in a context of real sound.[14] Attention to real-world sounds (e.g., speech and environmental sounds) reduces the resources available to attend to tinnitus. Reducing the emphasis on tinnitus and refocusing of attention to normal sounds may facilitate both perceptual and affective adaptation to the tinnitus. Amplification may be the best means to achieve this goal; however, use of guided imagery and perceptual training (see Chapter 9) that encourages an outward focus on listening, rather than a focus on the tinnitus, may aid rehabilitation.[2]

8.2.3 Reaction to Sound Effect

Sound may elicit positive psychological benefits to reduce tinnitus distress.[15,11] Individuals vary in their reaction to sound therapy based not only on how the sound affects tinnitus but also on

how they react emotionally to the sound. This emotional response will also guide the best level and type of sound for therapy. Music (e.g., classical, piano), fractal sounds (i.e., computer-generated chime), and nature sounds (e.g., ocean waves, rain) have been used for this purpose.[12]

8.2.4 Adaptation to Sound

Adaptation is a two-way process allowing both an increase and a decrease in response; it includes both sensory and psychological changes.[16] An overarching goal of many sound therapies is to elicit a long-term reduction in tinnitus. It is clear that the majority of persons with tinnitus do not experience a complete elimination of their tinnitus with sound therapy. However, studies that have examined the effects of sound over time have shown a progressive reduction in tinnitus can occur over months of therapy.[17] The mechanisms for lasting changes are uncertain, but may be due to affective and sensory adaptation,[16] habituation, or a combination of mechanisms broadly classified as auditory plasticity.[18] Experience with tinnitus clients tells us that long-term reductions in tinnitus are possible, as long as psychosocial and individual psychological factors do not counteract the gains achieved with sound.

8.2.5 WHO International Classification of Functioning, Disability, and Health

An ecological view of sound therapy[19] can be described with respect to the WHO International

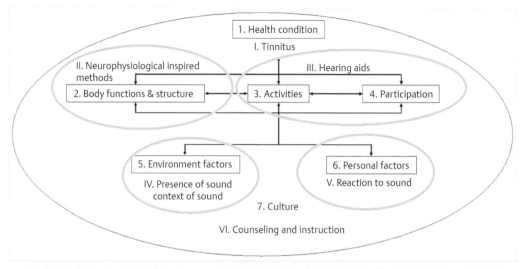

Fig. 8.2 Tinnitus sound therapy (*gray* text) in context of WHO International Classification of Functioning, Disability and Health.[20] (1) The health condition is tinnitus. (2) Sound therapy methods that act via specific neurophysiological mechanisms (e.g., synchrony of neural ensembles),[21] central gain,[22] inhibition[23] (see also Chapter 1), or address hearing loss[24] act on body systems. Hearing aids also play an important role in: (3) increasing activities and (4) participation by reducing social isolation. (5) Environmental factors are the physical, social, and attitudinal environment in which people live and conduct their lives. Sound therapy and awareness of the external sound environment can facilitate better functioning. (6) Personal factors include identifiers such as gender, age, race, lifestyles, and profession. Some of the reaction to sound therapy is governed by who we are. (7) Culture is added as beliefs, including non-western perspectives of health, should be considered in counseling and sound therapy selection.[19]

Classification of Functioning, Disability, and Health (ICF,[20] ▶ Fig. 8.2). Sound therapy and counseling for tinnitus address many aspects of the ICF framework.

8.3 Protocol

This protocol is similar in structure to the protocol we use when fitting hearing aids (Chapter 7). It is based on four aspects of aural rehabilitation including instruction, counseling, sensory management, and perceptual training. Here, we focus on those components of our strategy that relate to use of sound therapy in addition to amplification. The basic foundation principles of our approach are: (1) most sound is good for tinnitus relief; silence is generally not; (2) hearing aid amplification is usually needed for most patients due to the high incidence of hearing loss among tinnitus patients, but is sometimes not enough; (3) sound alone is not a complete therapy, but needs to be accompanied by instruction and counseling; and (4) the effect of sound on tinnitus annoyance needs to be balanced against the annoyance of the therapy sound.

8.3.1 Audiometry and Evaluation

Our evaluation protocol is described in Chapter 7. As well as the audiogram and assessment of the tinnitus pitch, we find the measurement of minimum masking levels (MMLs) is often helpful (see Chapter 12 for a general overview of tinnitus measurement). Narrow band masking sounds centered at 0.5, 1, 2, 4, and 6 kHz are used for identifying MMLs. The sounds are presented in an ascending manner from hearing threshold in 1- to 2-dB steps until the listener reports not hearing their tinnitus, and this is repeated for three total trials to achieve a consistent result. If the tinnitus cannot be masked or the level of sound becomes uncomfortable for the patient, this is noted and the testing is discontinued. MMLs for sounds 0.5 to 6 kHz assist in identifying frequencies most susceptible to masking through hearing aids. If the tinnitus pitch is outside of this range, and 0.5- to 6-kHz MMLs are high, the effectiveness of hearing aids, and the aids as a sound therapy device, may be limited. If the MML at tinnitus pitch is low, and not within the specified frequency range of hearing aids, headphones, or other transducers with broader frequency range, may need to be used for therapy. The MMLs are considered alongside self-report measures to guide the nature of sound to be used, and the likelihood that some degree of masking will be practical. MMLs help identify whether the focus of sound therapy can be on the presence of sound (low MMLs) or the focus should be on less direct methods such as modifying the context or reaction to tinnitus perception (when MMLs are high or not able to be obtained, e.g., due to discomfort).

8.3.2 Aural Rehabilitation and Goal Setting

Research has not shown clear evidence for the superiority of one sound type or strategy over any other[25,5]; however, individuals can have clear preferences for certain sounds. The selection of sounds for an individual can be based on these preferences alongside individual goals and priorities.[26] Personal preferences for sounds can play an important role in sound selection, but the selection should not solely be determined by what sound the person finds most pleasant. The most pleasant sound may not meet the client's needs and goals to reduce their tinnitus.[25] A trial investigating the merits of nature sounds and BBN found natural sounds more pleasant to listen to but BBN more effective in reducing tinnitus effects.[11] The establishment of needs using the Client Oriented Scale of Improvement in Tinnitus (COSIT, a goal-setting and outcome tool)[26] facilitates conversation between clinician and client on the goals for tinnitus therapy, and can be used to select the best sounds for trial to meet these different goals. A trial of various sounds is often required before choosing one or two best options.

8.3.3 Instruction

A clear understanding of the effects of sound therapy on tinnitus and how it should be used has to be communicated clearly to the client. Descriptions of the basis of tinnitus and the effects of sounds being used are often helpful and can be reinforced through the use of diagrams and posters of the ear and brain.[27] Instructions are provided to tinnitus patients on how to undertake relaxation, incorporate positive imagery, and use perceptual training strategies as part of the overall treatment.[27] Our instructions are combined with the patient's treatment goals. For example, this might mean that we instruct on masking for

a patient seeking some control of their tinnitus, we would instruct on use of relaxation and relaxing sounds for a person who has difficulty relaxing, and we may instruct on use of perceptual training for another patient who is continually focusing on their tinnitus. As individuals progress through their treatment goals, instructions are revisited to ensure best use of sound for our patients' circumstances. We also recommend clients subscribe to our online clinic (www.tinnitustunes.com) so that instructions can be accessed any day and time.

8.3.4 Counseling

The use of sound is just one part of a solution that should include counseling.[28] The ecological model of tinnitus predicts that positive adaptation to tinnitus can occur if tinnitus audibility is reduced, if it is placed in context, and if emotional associations and drivers are controlled or removed.[14] Factors that may exacerbate tinnitus need to be managed, including negative associations or memories of tinnitus,[29] anxiety,[30] and excessive attention or poor coping strategies.[31] In the majority of patients we see, informational counseling provided by the audiologist is sufficient. When there are concerns of unmanaged depression and anxiety, or mention of self-harm, referrals made to psychologists and the client's physicians are advised.

8.3.5 Sensory Management: Selection and Use of Different Sounds

Our clients usually do well with amplification alone if they have normal low-frequency hearing and mild high-frequency sensorineural hearing loss (see Chapter 7). If patients have greater than a mild low-frequency hearing loss, we recommend hearing aid amplification with additional sounds. With moderate and greater hearing losses, the large amount of gain required to make quiet sounds sufficiently loud to partially mask tinnitus may not be possible, or result in acoustic feedback. For severe-profound hearing losses, sound therapy with hearing aids is difficult. The sound level may exceed safety recommendations for intensity and duration of exposure.[32] With severe-profound hearing loss, cochlear implants are more likely to provide benefit and similar principles to the use of sound can be applied to the use of implants.[33] Used in a conventional way cochlear implants benefit people with severe-profound hearing loss and severe tinnitus, but the reduction in tinnitus usually disappears when the implant is switched off.[34,35] It is possible that sustained benefits might be achieved by use of sound therapy in combination with the normal implant processing. As an example, the use of an app to stream sounds to the cochlear implant has been shown to be beneficial.[33]

In our practice, almost all our clients try one or more of the sounds available onboard their hearing aids. Many clients do not like these sounds and prefer other sounds streamed to their aids from an external device. Some clients, predominantly older, struggle pairing their aids with external devices and prefer the simple option of using their aids to amplify sounds, such as music, played via their home stereo system. In these cases, participants are provided with a selectable music program.

The client's goals and preferences form the priorities for sound therapy. Individuals respond to sound in different ways based on their memories and personality, but generally, some sounds are more likely to act with different therapeutic modes than others (▶ Table 8.1).

When possible, we address the client's highest priorities first; however, if we feel a particular approach is going to provide benefit toward multiple therapy goals, we may encourage its selection. For example, our first approach is often to try and normalize peripherally driven auditory activity as much as possible by amplification.[24] Hearing aids may achieve this, but when amplification of low-intensity sounds is ineffective, sound customized to the client's hearing loss (Threshold Adjusted Noise) may be necessary.[36] Comfort and acceptance are further important considerations in the selection of sound therapy.

Onboard Sounds

We define onboard sounds as those playable from the hearing aids themselves without the need for a transmitting device (e.g., sounds streamed from smartphone, music played over a stereo system).

Broadband Noise

BBN has energy across a wide range of frequencies (e.g., white noise, pink noise). It has been used historically as it was easier to generate than the more complex sounds available now.[10] BBN has been shown to provide the most improvement in tinnitus compared to NBN alone or BBN and NBN combined.[6] When BBN and recorded nature sounds were compared in an 8-week clinical trial, BBN had a superior effect.[11] Long-term usage of BBN may facilitate adaption toward external sounds because of its neutral nature. However, BBN may have lower spontaneous acceptance compared to nature sounds, so a trial over several weeks may be necessary to determine if it will be accepted.

Threshold Adjusted Noise

Threshold adjusted noise is BBN that has been filtered to mirror the audiogram.[36] Greater sound energy is provided in regions of hearing loss,

Table 8.1 Suggested sound therapy approach based on individuals' goals (based on Searchfield 2018,[26] p. 5)

Goal	Theme	Suggested sound therapy
Cover tinnitus Control tinnitus Reduce tinnitus volume Make tinnitus less obvious	Presence of sound	Amplification Broadband noise Threshold adjusted noise
Improved hearing Socialize more Reduce focus on tinnitus Want to ignore tinnitus Hear speech better Better sound localization Want to hear real sounds Sleep better	Context of sound	Amplification Environmental sounds Modulated noise Sleep aids Perceptual training
Want to relax Sounds to be comfortable Don't want to stress Need to be calmer	Reaction to sound	Nature sounds Music Fractal sounds
I don't want to hear tinnitus so often Not having it...not aware	Adaptation to sound	Sum of all above along with instruction and counseling

rather than a flat spectrum of noise. This filtered noise attempts to provide a more even stimulation across the frequency range, when otherwise sounds in the region of hearing loss would not be heard. This also has the advantage of providing sound energy in the tonotopic region associated with tinnitus pitch, reducing the level of sound needed for some people with tinnitus.[36] This type of BBN noise has been widely adopted by hearing aid manufacturers.

Simulated Water Sounds

Amplitude-modulated sounds resembling ocean surf have been implemented by many hearing aid manufacturers, but there is only limited evidence for their benefit.[37] Amplitude-modulated ocean wave/surf-like sounds have been shown to reduce tinnitus loudness and distress following 30-minute exposures, with random amplitude-modulated surf reducing tinnitus audibility more than constant surf sound.[38] Clinical experience suggests amplitude-modulated sounds are more beneficial than static sounds in managing pulsatile tinnitus.

Streaming Sounds

Many hearing aids can now receive and play sounds streamed from smartphones using Bluetooth connections. Most hearing aid manufacturers have also developed apps for this purpose, and there are various websites where sounds for tinnitus treatment can be accessed and downloaded to the client's music library. The sounds used most often in this way are recordings from nature, or music, less often people may find audio books or podcasts effective sound therapies. The ability to stream sounds selected from a variety of sources provides the opportunity for the clinician to work with clients for whom standard sounds are ineffective or unpleasant. Providing more options for masking helps the client feel they have greater control that assists in the emotional response to tinnitus. However, endless searching by the client for the perfect sound is unhelpful, as tinnitus remains at the forefront of thoughts. Unrealistic expectations for a perfect treatment need to be managed with counseling.

Recorded Nature Sounds

Nature sounds are generally well tolerated by users and often evoke more positive emotional responses than BBN. A multisite trial with clinics in Italy and our clinic in New Zealand tested this idea.[10] A group using amplification and BBN (17 participants) was compared to a group using hearing aids with nature sounds streamed from the user's phone (19 participants). The participants selected their preferred sound from a wide range of recordings of naturally occurring sounds. The preferred nature sounds were some form of running water.[10] Significant improvements were achieved at 3 and 6 months compared to baseline, but there was no distinct advantage of one sound type over another. The allocation to the nature group or BBN group was not made on the basis of needs assessment or preference; some individuals may have benefitted more from one sound than another. A final recommendation of therapy sound for long-term use should be on the basis of user preferences, intent of the sound, and trial.

Music

Music has been used in various forms as a therapeutic tool for tinnitus. Most people prefer music that had a calming effect and complexity that can redirect attention from tinnitus to the music, and has positive memory associations.[39] Most clients are already aware of music that they find helps their tinnitus. The audiologist's role is most often ensuring that the quality of the music played through hearing aids is adequate; this may involve the programming of specific music programs.

Fractals

A fractal is a random, harmonic tone or chime, based on a fractal mathematical algorithm so that the music is similar to itself without being repetitive. One hearing aid manufacturer has adapted fractal sound "zen tones" as the basis of their tinnitus platform that offers a useful alternative approach to variations of BBN.[40,41,7]

Apps

The common catch phrase "there's an app for that" also applies to tinnitus. There are many hearing aid manufacturers and third-party developers who have created apps for tinnitus. They commonly include sounds or activities for relaxation and distraction. The benefit provided by apps and other smart technology for tinnitus relief is only now being evaluated.[42] As the technology develops, they may serve a useful role bridging the gap between clinicians and clients, and improving accessibility to services.

8.3.6 Device Selection and Fitting

It is important to ensure physical comfort of any device so that users are able to comply with the expected duration of use. Although smartphones and other audio-players are an inexpensive alternative to hearing aids, their headphones are often occluding, meaning that the user hears their voice as boomy when talking while wearing, and they tend to block external sounds. New generation "Hearables" may soon assist hearing as part of their headphone function. In our research, we have found low compliance (e.g., low hours used) to therapy with MP3 players and headphones.[38,11] Users report extended wear with current MP3 players and headphones is difficult. Consequently, we find that open-fit solutions produce higher satisfaction for clients.

We prefer hearing aids that provide flexibility in fitting and enable modification of many sound parameters. Ease of pairing with Bluetooth devices is also important, given that many of our clients stream therapy sounds from their smartphones. The quality of the support material (marketing and instructional material for clients) provided by device manufacturers varies a great deal. This support material is particularly helpful when beginning in tinnitus practice.

Level

There has been a lot of debate about the best level of sound to use for sound therapy. There is mixed evidence as to whether the level of the background sound changes the overall sound therapy effectiveness.[43,25, 44] We believe that the level used should be selected on the basis of the underlying goals of the therapy (i.e., control, masking, and habituation) and individual emotional response to the sound selected. An ideal sound has a strong effect on tinnitus while not being annoying, and can be assessed using rating scales as a function of level, from threshold to MML (▶ Fig. 8.3). Although there is variation between listeners, a rain-like sound results in a similar reduction to constant BBN as a function of MML, but is less annoying.[11]

Real-Ear Measures

Real-ear measures can be helpful in objectively evaluating the amount and spectrum of sound the user will receive with different settings. The real-ear equipment sound is turned off and instead the sound generated by the device can be used as a stimulus, and compared to threshold. Although there are no targets to match the sound to, the therapeutic sound can be considered relative to auditory threshold and the degree of overlap between the sound and tinnitus pitch can be observed.

Duration of Use

Sound therapy can be used intermittently, on an as-need basis, or be used fairly constantly. We

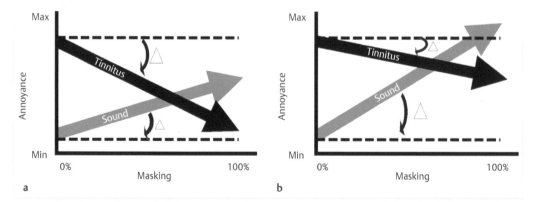

Fig. 8.3 The interaction between therapy sound and the tinnitus perception is complex. As a general rule, an increase in the level of sound will affect tinnitus by decreasing its annoyance; however, simultaneously the annoyance of the sound will increase. **(a)** An ideal sound: Tinnitus annoyance reduces rapidly with small increases in level, while the annoyance of the sound itself only increases a small degree. **(b)** Less than ideal sound: The tinnitus annoyance reduces only a small amount, while the therapy sound becomes annoying with small increases in level. The selection of sound level must be based on a combination of both the effect on tinnitus and the annoyance of the therapy sound. This relationship will differ between sounds and individuals.[11]

strongly encourage regular and consistent use of hearing aids during awake hours. As the hearing aids alone may be effective in many environments, users are empowered to select additional therapeutic sounds when and where they may be most useful, often in quiet environments. BBN can often be used for long periods of time with limited disruption to the listener as its constant and uninteresting nature lends itself to habituation.[11] Music, on the other hand, can be used (1) as an example of sound suitable for short-term use or (2) as a facilitator of relaxation or distraction, due to its complex and repetitive nature.[39] Some researchers have recommended two[45] or three[46] stages of sound use, progressing from total masking to partial masking. An alternative recommendation is to alternate between masking and sounds targeting emotional response.[11] For pragmatic reasons, most research on tinnitus therapy follows participants up to 12 to 18 months. The treatment period for sound therapy will depend on when clients reach their therapy goals, this may be much earlier, or later, than 12 months. In some cases, the sound therapy may be used as a temporary intervention while an underlying pathology is treated, or during times of high stress.

8.3.7 Negative Effects

Although sound generally has a positive effect, some individuals do have negative reactions to sound that can exacerbate their tinnitus. If this is the case, there needs to be an emphasis in rehabilitation of the client's reaction to sound. Any goals of treating tinnitus may need to lag behind managing the hyperacusis.[47,48] Some clients find constant sounds cause the tinnitus to be perceived as louder. If so, we try music, modulated noise, or ask the client to record sounds they find helpful and use those. Streaming of sounds to hearing aids from manufacturer apps or online sound libraries might be the solution. We ask the client to list, or record, five sounds that do not exacerbate their tinnitus and use them, or similar sounds, for therapy. If hyperacusis, not tinnitus, is the primary concern, various desensitization approaches can be used.[47]

Early in the development of sound therapy, concerns were raised as to the possibility of sound overexposure causing hearing loss[32] and recently there has been speculation that central plasticity in response to BBN may have negative consequences.[49] There is little or no evidence of long-term negative effects of BBN used for tinnitus sound therapy on humans.[50,51] Most manufacturers limit the output of their onboard sound generators to reduce the possibility of noise-induced hearing loss, and persons with tinnitus are not deprived of other sound stimulation. Hearing aids reduce auditory deprivation, and hearing is increasingly being seen as a contributor to healthy aging and to improve quality of life.[52] There is the possibility that over-the-counter hearing devices and sounds streamed to hearing aids and then amplified might be damaging. When an audiologist is dispensing the devices, they should check outputs using real-ear measures or test-box measures to ensure safe output levels.

8.3.8 Perceptual Training

Most sound therapy is passive. Perceptual training is an active process involving listening and then responding. Perceptual training is usually undertaken over a short period of time on a daily basis, and may help clients who are struggling to adapt, not suited to, or are unwilling to wear ear-level devices regularly. Attention-based training methods have shown promise.[53,54] We use a structured approach based on auditory object identification and localization described by Searchfield et al[55] and available online (www.tinnitustunes.com). The training consists of MP3 files that are downloaded and played over several weeks for 20 to 30 minutes per day. The training can be employed by streaming through the user's hearing aids, facilitating acclimatization to hearing aids as well as reducing one's focus on tinnitus. The training provides benefit, in reducing masking levels, for most who have tried it, and it appears to improve the acceptance of sound among persons with "normal" hearing.[56] A combination of passive and active sound therapy may ultimately be the best solution for tinnitus as it combines the relatively quick improvements possible with training with the sustaining effects of longer-term passive sound exposure.

8.3.9 Follow-Up

Further instruction and counseling are often needed on follow-up. Clients may need to be encouraged to persevere if their immediate expectations are not initially met. We schedule clients to be seen two to three times over the first 2 months of therapy, and then 6 months and 12 months following. We make supplementary appointments when needed. At these appointments, we consider progress toward the client's goals identified through the COSIT, and whether new goals are needed. If issues have arisen during the trial of devices, we address these and provide further instructions on use. Further counseling is undertaken to work through ongoing or new concerns raised.

Common issues and their solutions with sound therapy at follow-up are:
- Not liking the on-board maskers—trial streaming of sounds.
- Intolerant to feel of devices—change form factor, for example, move to open fitting with domes.
- Streaming unreliable, causing frustration—consider benefits of streaming versus use of an onboard sound.
- Those with limited cognitive ability struggle to use the devices—look to simplify use (simple on/off rather than user selection of sounds); involve family and friends in the rehabilitation.
- High battery drain if streaming often—consider rechargeable aids or the cost-benefit of streaming compared to the onboard sounds.
- Dislike of high-frequency sound despite this having the greatest effect on their tinnitus—place a priority on comfort, as they adapt to the sound, increase high-frequency content.

Due to the high comorbidity of anxiety with tinnitus, requests for urgent appointments and frequent phone calls or emails to the clinic can be expected from clients. However, we have found that with the development of the tinnitustunes.com clinic website, the number of out-of-schedule requests have reduced. Our clinic's customer service team directs enquiries to the website where clients can access many of our clinic resources online. Subscribers also receive automated emails for 12 weeks, providing tinnitus management tips consistent with the messages provided by the clinician.

8.3.10 New and Emerging Concepts

Many innovative concepts are being developed for sound therapy and trialed with hearing aids. Head-related transfer functions have been used to customize masking sounds to localize and then mask the tinnitus perception in 3D sound space,[57] and tonal stimuli have been used to alter the synchrony of neural ensembles potentially responsible for tinnitus.[58] Ultra-high-frequency sounds have been explored.[59] There are likely to be many innovations in this area over the next few years. However, many existing sound therapy concepts still lack adequate evidence to support their use.[5] Audiologists should be critical consumers of tinnitus technology and be mindful of not putting technology solutions ahead of the needs of their clients.

8.4 Conclusion

Sound is a useful tool for tinnitus management but should be considered as part of an omnibus approach that consists of not just one type of sound or the use of sound devoid of counseling. Appropriate application and then evaluation of clinical methods should recognize this diversity. Sound therapy can be applied to reduce the audibility of tinnitus, reduce focus on tinnitus, and provide relaxation. Long-term sound therapy may aid adaptation to tinnitus. To be successful, clinicians are encouraged to consider their clients as individuals and use unique combinations of sound, instruction, counseling, and training to address their needs and goals. At this point in time, the recommendations made in this chapter should be considered in light of the limited evidence at hand. Clinical judgment and understanding of your individual clients' needs are essential for success.

The editors have created a slide deck on hearing aids and wearable tinnitus devices that can be used to help you guide sound therapy for tinnitus patients. The materials are available on the companion website.

References

[1] Tyler RS, Bentler RA. Tinnitus maskers and hearing aids for tinnitus. Semin Hear. 1987; 8(1):49–62

[2] Searchfield GD, Linford T, Durai M. Sound therapy and aural rehabilitation for tinnitus: a person centred therapy framework based on an ecological model of tinnitus. Disabil Rehabil. 2019; 41(16):1966–1973

[3] Mckenna L, Irwin R. Sound therapy for tinnitus—sacred cow or idol worship?: An investigation of the evidence. Audiol Med. 2008; 6(1):16–24

[4] Tyler RS, Perreau A, Powers T, et al. Tinnitus sound therapy trial shows effectiveness for those with tinnitus. J Am Acad Audiol. 2020; 31(1):6–16

[5] Tutaj L, Hoare DJ, Sereda M. Combined amplification and sound generation for tinnitus: a scoping review. Ear Hear. 2018; 39(3):412–422

[6] Kim BJ, Chung SW, Jung JY, Suh MW. Effect of different sounds on the treatment outcome of tinnitus retraining therapy. Clin Exp Otorhinolaryngol. 2014; 7(2):87–93

[7] Sweetow RW, Sabes JH. Effects of acoustical stimuli delivered through hearing aids on tinnitus. J Am Acad Audiol. 2010; 21 (7):461–473

[8] Bauer CA, Berry JL, Brozoski TJ. The effect of tinnitus retraining therapy on chronic tinnitus: a controlled trial. Laryngoscope Investig Otolaryngol. 2017; 2(4):166–177

[9] Henry JA, Frederick M, Sell S, Griest S, Abrams H. Validation of a novel combination hearing aid and tinnitus therapy device. Ear Hear. 2015; 36(1):42–52

[10] Barozzi S, Del Bo L, Crocetti A, et al. A comparison of nature and technical sounds for tinnitus therapy. Acta Acust United Acust. 2016; 102(3):540–546

[11] Durai M, Searchfield GD. A mixed-methods trial of broad band noise and nature sounds for tinnitus therapy: group and individual responses modeled under the adaptation level theory of tinnitus. Front Aging Neurosci. 2017; 9:44

[12] Searchfield GD, Durai M, Linford T. A state-of-the-art review: personalization of tinnitus sound therapy. Front Psychol. 2017; 8:1599

[13] Andersson G. Psychological aspects of tinnitus and the application of cognitive-behavioral therapy. Clin Psychol Rev. 2002; 22(7):977–990

[14] Feldmann H. Tinnitus: reality or phantom. In: Aran JM, Dauman R, eds. Tinnitus 91: Proceedings of the Fourth International Tinnitus Seminar. Amsterdam: Kugler Publications; 1992

[15] Durai M, O'Keeffe MG, Searchfield GD. Examining the short term effects of emotion under an Adaptation Level Theory model of tinnitus perception. Hear Res. 2017; 345: 23–29

[16] Searchfield GD, Kobayashi K, Sanders M. An adaptation level theory of tinnitus audibility. Front Syst Neurosci. 2012; 6:46

[17] Jastreboff PJ. 25 years of tinnitus retraining therapy. HNO. 2015; 63(4):307–311

[18] Hoare DJ, Adjamian P, Sereda M, Hall DA. Recent technological advances in sound-based approaches to tinnitus treatment: a review of efficacy considered against putative physiological mechanisms. Noise Health. 2013; 15(63):107–116

[19] Searchfield GD. Tinnitus what and where: an ecological framework. Front Neurol. 2014; 5(271):271

[20] WHO. International classification of functioning, disability and health. Geneva: ICF, World Health Organization; 2001

[21] Tass PA, Adamchic I, Freund H-J, von Stackelberg T, Hauptmann C. Counteracting tinnitus by acoustic coordinated reset neuromodulation. Restor Neurol Neurosci. 2012; 30(2):137–159

[22] Noreña AJ. An integrative model of tinnitus based on a central gain controlling neural sensitivity. Neurosci Biobehav Rev. 2011; 35(5):1089–1109

[23] Stein A, Wunderlich R, Lau P, et al. Clinical trial on tonal tinnitus with tailor-made notched music training. BMC Neurol. 2016; 16(1):38

[24] Shekhawat GS, Searchfield GD, Stinear CM. Role of hearing AIDS in tinnitus intervention: a scoping review. J Am Acad Audiol. 2013; 24(8):747–762

[25] Pienkowski M. Rationale and efficacy of sound therapies for tinnitus and hyperacusis. Neuroscience. 2019; 407:120–134

[26] Searchfield GD. A client oriented scale of improvement in tinnitus for therapy goal planning and assessing outcomes. J Am Acad Audiol. 2019; 30(4):327–337

[27] Searchfield GD, Magnusson JE, Shakes G, Eberhard B. Counselling and psycho-education for tinnitus management. In: Moller A, Langguth B, Ridder DD, Kleinjung T, eds. Textbook of tinnitus. New York: Springer; 2010:535–556

[28] Tyler RS, Gogel SA, Gehringer AK. Tinnitus activities treatment. Prog Brain Res. 2007; 166:425–434

[29] De Ridder D, Elgoyhen AB, Romo R, Langguth B. Phantom percepts: tinnitus and pain as persisting aversive memory networks. Proc Natl Acad Sci U S A. 2011; 108(20):8075–8080

[30] Fagelson MA. The association between tinnitus and post-traumatic stress disorder. Am J Audiol. 2007; 16(2):107–117

[31] Andersson G, Kaldo V, Stromgren T, Strom L. Are coping strategies really useful for the tinnitus patient? An investigation conducted via the Internet. Audiol Med. 2004; 2(1):54–59

[32] McFadden D. Tinnitus: facts, theories, and treatments. Washington, DC: National Academies Press; 1982

[33] Tyler RS, Owen RL, Bridges J, Gander PE, Perreau A, Mancini PC. Tinnitus suppression in cochlear implant patients using a sound therapy app. Am J Audiol. 2018; 27(3):316–323

[34] Cabral Junior F, Pinna MH, Alves RD, Malerbi AF, Bento RF. Cochlear implantation and single-sided deafness: a systematic review of the literature. Int Arch Otorhinolaryngol. 2016; 20(1): 69–75

[35] Ramakers GG, van Zon A, Stegeman I, Grolman W. The effect of cochlear implantation on tinnitus in patients with bilateral hearing loss: a systematic review. Laryngoscope. 2015; 125 (11):2584–2592

[36] Searchfield G, Warr A, Kuklinski J, Purdy S. Digital instruments for tinnitus: mixing point identification and threshold-adjusted noise. Paper presented at the Proceedings of the Seventh International Tinnitus Seminar; 2002

[37] Sereda M, Davies J, Hall DA. Pre-market version of a commercially available hearing instrument with a tinnitus sound generator: feasibility of evaluation in a clinical trial. Int J Audiol. 2017; 56(4):286–294

[38] Durai M, Kobayashi K, Searchfield GD. A feasibility study of predictable and unpredictable surf-like sounds for tinnitus therapy using personal music players. Int J Audiol. 2018; 57(9): 707–713

[39] Hann D, Searchfield G, Sanders M, Wise K. Strategies for the selection of music in the short-term management of mild tinnitus. Aust N Z J Audiol. 2008; 30(2):129–140

[40] Herzfeld M, Enza C, Sweetow R. Clinical trial on the effectiveness of widex zen therapy for tinnitus. Hear. Rev. 2014; 21:24–29

[41] Sweetow R, Jeppesen A. A new integrated program for tinnitus patient management: Widex Zen Therapy. Hearing Review. 2012; 19(7):20–27

[42] Kalle S, Schlee W, Pryss RC, et al. Review of smart services for tinnitus self-help, diagnostics and treatments. Front Neurosci. 2018; 12:541

[43] Henry JA, Schechter MA, Zaugg TL, et al. Clinical trial to compare tinnitus masking and tinnitus retraining therapy. Acta Otolaryngol Suppl. 2006(556):64–69

[44] Tyler RS, Noble W, Coelho CB, Ji H. Tinnitus retraining therapy: mixing point and total masking are equally effective. Ear Hear. 2012; 33(5):588–594

[45] Davis PB, Paki B, Hanley PJ. Neuromonics tinnitus treatment: third clinical trial. Ear Hear. 2007; 28(2):242–259

[46] López-González MA, López-Fernández R. Sequential sound therapy in tinnitus. Int Tinnitus J. 2004; 10(2):150–155

[47] Pienkowski M, Tyler RS, Roncancio ER, et al. A review of hyperacusis and future directions: part II. Measurement, mechanisms, and treatment. Am J Audiol. 2014; 23(4):420–436

[48] Searchfield GD. Hearing aids and tinnitus. In: Tyler R, ed. Tinnitus protocols. New York: Thieme; 2006

[49] Attarha M, Bigelow J, Merzenich MM. Unintended consequences of white noise therapy for tinnitus-otolaryngology's cobra effect: a review. JAMA Otolaryngol Head Neck Surg. 2018; 144(10):938–943

[50] Folmer RL. No evidence of broadband noise having any harmful effect on hearing. JAMA Otolaryngol Head Neck Surg. 2019; 145(3):291–292

[51] Henry JA, Manning C, Griest S. No evidence of broadband noise having any harmful effect on hearing. JAMA Otolaryngol Head Neck Surg. 2019; 145(3):292

[52] Dawes P, Emsley R, Cruickshanks KJ, et al. Hearing loss and cognition: the role of hearing AIDS, social isolation and depression. PLoS One. 2015; 10(3):e0119616

[53] Hoare DJ, Stacey PC, Hall DA. The efficacy of auditory perceptual training for tinnitus: a systematic review. Ann Behav Med. 2010; 40(3):313–324

[54] Roberts LE, Bosnyak DJ. Auditory training in tinnitus. In: Textbook of tinnitus. Springer; 2011:563–573

[55] Searchfield GD, Morrison-Low J, Wise K. Object identification and attention training for treating tinnitus. Prog Brain Res. 2007; 166:441–460

[56] Bees K, Guan D, Alsarrage N, Searchfield G. The effects of auditory object identification and localization (AOIL) training on noise acceptance and loudness discomfort in persons with normal hearing. Speech Lang Hear. 2017; 22(2):1–8

[57] Searchfield GD, Kobayashi K, Hodgson S-A, Hodgson C, Tevoitdale H, Irving S. Spatial masking: development and testing of a new tinnitus assistive technology. Assist Technol. 2016; 28(2):115–125

[58] Hauptmann C, Williams M, Vinciati F, Haller M. Technical feasibility of acoustic coordinated reset therapy for tinnitus delivered via hearing aids: a case study. Case Rep Otolaryngol. 2017; 2017:5304242

[59] Perreau A, Tyler R. Tinnitus relief using high-frequency sound via the HyperSound audio system. Int Tinnitus J. 2018; 22(2):133–142

9 The Clinical Relevance of Apps for Tinnitus

Ann Perreau, Elizabeth Fetscher, and Michael Piskosz

Abstract

Smartphones have impacted our daily lives including at home and at the workplace. The millions of applications, or "apps" available on smartphones, provide valuable tools that are used in various ways. It has been reported that over half a billion smartphone users use a health or wellness app, a number that will rise exponentially over time. In recent years, there has also been a rise in the development of apps for tinnitus, including assessment and management of tinnitus. With all these available options, it may be an overwhelming task for the audiologist to know which apps are helpful, and not helpful, for patients with tinnitus. This chapter describes the usefulness and clinical relevance of smartphone apps for tinnitus assessment and management and report safety and security concerns related to FDA and HIPAA regulations. Although there are many benefits of using apps for tinnitus assessment and management, this technology should not replace the individual counseling and support that is needed from the audiologist to help patients manage their tinnitus.

Keywords: smartphone apps, healthcare apps, tinnitus, tinnitus management

9.1 Introduction

The invention of the smartphone has changed the way billions of people operate in day-to-day life, including at home and at the workplace. Today, smartphones contain millions of applications, or "apps," that consumers can use in a variety of ways. Smartphones not only allow for instant access and convenience to many services, such as digital banking, online shopping, and the Internet, but users can also download apps that are designed for health care or wellness.[1] Smartphone apps are being implemented into clinical practice. Huckvale et al[2] reported that approximately half a billion smartphone users (including both physicians and patients) use a health or wellness app, a number that is expected to increase dramatically in upcoming years.

There are many reasons for implementing apps in health care and audiology fields. For example, health care providers can use mobile phone apps

as a method for teaching, for collecting data from patients, for record-keeping, and for assessing and treating patients. Apps also allow patients to monitor their own health status. For instance, apps allow patients to monitor their symptoms, and physicians can use apps to prescribe medications.[3,4] In audiology, an emergence of apps has also been observed in recent years. For example, there are many apps available to screen and diagnose hearing loss, including *AudCal* (audiometric testing), *EarTrumpet* (audiometric testing), and *CellScope* (otoscopy), and even more apps available for the intervention and rehabilitation of hearing loss, including *Ear Machine* and *PocketLab* (both for sound amplification). Similarly, there has been a rise in apps to help tinnitus patients, including apps for tinnitus assessment and management. Despite the availability of apps for tinnitus, we emphasize the important role of the audiologist in providing patient-centered care and offer these as additional tools for the audiologist and their patient.

With all these available options, it may be an overwhelming task for the clinician to know which apps are helpful, and not helpful, for tinnitus patients. Therefore, the purpose of this chapter is to determine the usefulness and clinical relevance of smartphone apps for tinnitus. Specifically, we will (a) evaluate apps available for the assessment and the management of tinnitus, (b) describe apps that provide education and information about tinnitus, (c) explore apps that offer assistive tools such as wellness, and (d) review the limitations and risks associated with smartphone apps in the hearing health care field.

9.2 Apps for Tinnitus Assessment and Management

Apps for tinnitus assessment and management can be useful for targeting multiple audiences, including audiologists, patients and their partners, and audiology students in a variety of ways. Audiologists can use smartphone apps to identify helpful information for patients, communicate with patients, and assess and treat a hearing loss and/or tinnitus. Keep in mind the difference in the reliability and accuracy of the use of an app compared to standard audiometric testing. Apps can serve as excellent resource tools for patients, providing information about tinnitus and hearing loss, relaxation tools such as imagery or deep breathing techniques, and/or detecting a potential hearing loss prior to seeing the audiologist. Apps are also available for sound therapy to provide background sounds for masking tinnitus. These apps have the potential and ability to drastically improve the quality of life for our patients by providing helpful tools and learning strategies to manage tinnitus.

To better understand the apps available, a unique framework was proposed by Paglialonga et al[5] that categorized apps in audiology: (a) screening and assessment, (b) intervention and rehabilitation, (c) education and information, and (d) assistive tools. At the time of their research, Paglialonga et al[5] found 203 apps that had relevance to audiology, and 17% of those apps applied to screening and assessment, 52% for intervention and rehabilitation, 24% for education and information, and 7% for assistive tools. Each of these categories provides a means to classify apps based on their clinical relevance and will be used as we consider various apps for tinnitus assessment and management. It is important to note that many apps have frequent updates, launching newer versions that offer users access to new content and features. These updates also allow app platforms to operate more efficiently following the new operating system updates, and can include firmware, architectural, and user-interface (UI) updates. The most current version of an app can be located in the smart device's corresponding app store.

There are many apps focused on the self-assessment of tinnitus in a variety of ways, including helping patients measure their tinnitus severity and reactions to tinnitus and performing basic tinnitus pitch and loudness matching (*Tinnitus Measurer*). Deshpande and Shimunova[6] reported that of the 91 apps for tinnitus on an Apple or iOS platform (excluding apps that provide misinformation), 17.6% allow for screening or assessment of tinnitus. Likewise, of the 248 apps for tinnitus on the Android platform, 7.2% apply to screening or assessment.

Some studies have been conducted to evaluate the usefulness of apps for screening and assessment of tinnitus. For example, Wunderlich et al[7] investigated tinnitus pitch and loudness matching methods using their own developed app and conventional psychoacoustic techniques using an audiometer in a sound-treated booth. The app utilized a recursive two-interval forced choice test (RIFT) to identify the participants' approximate

frequency and intensity of their tinnitus. In the study, 17 participants completed tinnitus pitch and loudness matching using conventional methods in a sound-treated booth presented by the audiologist and using the smartphone app with an iPod independently. Each procedure was completed twice to compare the reliability of each method. There were differences in the tinnitus pitch and loudness values between the two methods. More specifically, the smartphone app produced lower tinnitus pitch matches compared to conventional psychoacoustic testing. However, participants noted that it was easier to use the app, even though the conventional method was faster to administer. It was also found that the app-based measurements were just as reliable as conventional methods when comparing results across trials using each method.[7] Although the app developed by Wunderlich and colleagues was not specifically named, there are apps available that follow a similar RIFT protocol. For example, the *Tinnitus Sound Finder* app by Desyncra follows the two-interval forced choice model for tinnitus pitch and loudness matching. Once the app user has completed the assessment, they are provided with a short description of their tinnitus. If the results from the tinnitus assessment indicate that the tinnitus is tonal, users are given an estimated pure-tone frequency of the tinnitus. Listeners can also be directed to audiology clinics located within a certain distance of the user for further tinnitus support by a hearing care professional.

In addition, tinnitus questionnaires can be administered using apps, which has been done previously by Henry et al[8] using the Tinnitus Functional Index. In that study, the questionnaire was administered via the app as a preliminary step to obtaining an appointment with the audiologist. These studies suggest that apps can be used to assess tinnitus using psychometric testing methods and questionnaires, and that they might be a convenient way for patients to learn more about their tinnitus and know when to seek the help of the audiologist for tinnitus management.

The vast majority of apps for tinnitus are focused on tinnitus management, which would apply to the intervention and rehabilitation category as described by Paglialonga et al.[5] Indeed, the study by Deshpande and Shimunova[6] found that 85.2% of apps for tinnitus on an Apple or iOS platform and 86.7% of Android platforms relate to the management of tinnitus. The functionality of these apps ranges from sound therapy using a variety of sounds including nature or environmental sounds (e.g., waterfall, ocean waves, and forest), physiological sounds (e.g., heartbeat), and static sounds (e.g., white noise, pink noise, and Brownian noise) to providing counseling on thoughts and emotions about tinnitus, coping skills, and relaxation exercises to manage reactions to tinnitus.

A study by Sereda et al[9] generated a list of 55 apps that were used by 120 respondents to self-treat their tinnitus, and the majority applied to sound therapy. The 18 most cited apps (e.g., *White Noise Free, Headspace, Relax Melodies, ReSound Relief, Sleep Pillow*) were evaluated using the mean Mobile Apps Rating Scale (MARS) score as well as based on the features or content of the app. The MARS score is calculated from the average of 23 items using a five-point scale that assesses the quality of health apps in categories like engagement, functionality, and information. Sereda et al[9] reported that sound generation was the most popular feature among all apps for tinnitus management with options like recording and looping your own sounds (*White Noise Free*), importing or downloading additional sounds (*myNoise, ReSound Relief*), and purchasing sounds from the App library or your own library (*Sleep Pillow, Oticon Tinnitus Sound and Tinnitus Balance*). For example, the *Phonak Tinnitus Balance* app allows patients to select a pre-recorded sound, such as ocean or campsite, or music from the smartphone's music library. Hearing aid users who also have tinnitus can benefit from these apps. In fact, many hearing instrument manufacturers allow for Bluetooth streaming of apps today. The sounds produced from these apps can be delivered directly to the hearing aid instead of via traditional headphones or earbuds.

In addition, Sereda et al[9] found that 14 apps were specifically designed for tinnitus, and targeted areas such as sound therapy for relief (e.g., *Tinnitus Therapy Lite, Tinnitus Therapy Tunes, ReSound Relief*), whereas others implemented tinnitus management plans (Tinnitus Retraining Therapy using *iTinnitus*, Progressive Tinnitus Management using *Tinnitus Balance*, and Zen Therapy using *Widex Zen, Tinnitus Management*). This study highlighted the number of apps available for tinnitus management including sound therapy or a combination of sound therapy plus tinnitus management, most of which are implemented as self-treatment options for patients.

One such app, *ReSound Relief*, incorporates multiple tools for tinnitus management and education through sound therapy, informational counseling, and relaxation exercises. *ReSound Relief* works to divert the patient's attention away from their tinnitus, by reducing the contrast between their tinnitus and the background sound. A variety of sounds are offered including environmental sounds (ocean waves, rain, crickets), music, and static sounds (white noise, pink noise), and users can combine up to five sounds to customize their desired soundscape. The informational counseling provides basic education about tinnitus, including causes, treatments, and how to change thoughts about tinnitus, which was developed in collaboration with Dr. Henry from the National Center for Rehabilitative Auditory Research (NCRAR) and Dr. Tyler and Shelley Witt at the University of Iowa Hospitals and Clinics. Finally, the relaxation section of the app contains multiple modules including deep breathing exercises, imagery, and activities to focus away from tinnitus as well as guided meditations by clinical psychologist, Dr. Jennifer Gans who focuses on Mindfulness-Based Tinnitus Stress Reduction (MBTSR) and Dartmouth College. Efficacy of the *ReSound Relief* app has been evaluated by researchers after 3 and 6 months of use.[10] Results from a group of tinnitus patients revealed significantly lower scores on the Tinnitus Functional Index (~15 points lower) and the Tinnitus Handicap Inventory (~19 points lower), indicating that the *ReSound Relief* app is a helpful self-management tool for patients with tinnitus.

Henry et al[11] developed a Tinnitus Coach App that included content from Progressive Tinnitus Management[12] to help patients with bothersome tinnitus learn to cope and manage their symptoms. The app was tested using focus groups and field testing with 25 patients with bothersome tinnitus. Subjective responses from the participants were favorable regarding content of the app; however, many participants reported that app structure and navigation made it difficult to use.[11] Most participants used a learning section of the app, rather than the actual management sections of the app, suggesting that some features need to be easily accessible in management apps in order for these functions to be fully utilized by patients. The Tinnitus Coach App research is a good example of how user-driven research can be beneficial in the building of apps, by allowing clinicians and researchers to better understand the needs and wants of the users.

Kim et al[13] evaluated use of a smartphone app that provided a customized, notched music therapy for 26 patients with chronic tinnitus. The participants used the notched music (i.e., classical music) for 30 to 60 minutes daily for 3 months using their smartphone app. In addition, all participants received Gingko tablets (i.e., Ginexin-F 80-mg, twice a day) during the trial. The primary outcome measure was the Tinnitus Handicap Inventory (THI)[14] and the secondary outcome included visual-analog ratings for loudness, annoyance, effect on daily life, and noticeable time, which were collected pre- and posttreatment. Although posttreatment total THI scores and the emotional subscale scores were significantly improved by as much as 10 points, all other outcomes were not significantly affected.[13] In addition, no control group was used in the study design and results were confounded by the Gingko biloba administration, making it hard to know the degree to which the smartphone app reduced THI scores. Although this study indicates some improvement using a smartphone app, more controlled studies are needed.

9.2.1 Apps for Education and Information on Tinnitus

General education and information regarding tinnitus is a feature of some apps, which varies between 8.3% (on Android platforms) and 37.4% (on Apple or iOS platform) depending on the type of smartphone.[6] Many apps that provide general education will often explain tinnitus (*What is tinnitus?*), describe the most common causes for tinnitus (e.g., aging, noise, etc.), and review management strategies, including the most common treatments (i.e., sound therapy, counseling, and hearing aids).

The *Starkey Relax* app serves as a management tool for tinnitus and also provides educational tools and resources. Within the app, users can choose from an assortment of sounds (e.g., wind chimes, running water, thunderstorm). The app provides a brief tutorial to help the user acclimate to the app and demonstrates how to adjust the loudness, pitch, and modulation of each sound. This allows the user to create a sound that is both soothing to the listener and helpful with masking their tinnitus. The app also has a sleep timer so the masker can phase out gradually without disrupting the sleep pattern of the app user. The Learn section within the app provides educational tools on tinnitus, its symptoms and possible causes, as well as lifestyle modifications, and treatment options for tinnitus.[15]

Finally, sound-level meter apps can be helpful to educate patients about sound exposure and dangerous noise levels. Many of these apps not only report the overall sound level of the environment (in dB) but also indicate if hearing protection is necessary. This can be a very helpful feature for patients with tinnitus and/or hyperacusis as they learn how to reduce bothersome reactions to sound and when to use hearing protection. However, we need to have a clear understanding of how accurate these apps are. Nast et al[16] compared five sound-level meter apps (*DB volume, Advanced Decibel, SPLnFFT Noise Meter, SPL,* and *SoundMeter*) to traditional sound-level meters to investigate the reliability of apps in sound measurement. Statistical analysis revealed that the five apps reported the sound pressure level significantly higher than the actual sound measurement using a sound-level meter, and only one app was within 5 dB of the traditional sound-level meter.[16] As a reminder, if an error occurs using a sound-level meter, it is typically within 1 to 2 dB of the actual loudness of the environment, implying that the apps are not as accurate as they should be. This study also found differences within A-weighted and C-weighted levels, in that C-weighted measurements typically yielded more accurate loudness levels because of the limited filtering used in C-weighting. McLennon et al[17] found similar results in a more recent study when comparing the accuracy of sound-level apps, on iOS and Android platforms, to traditional sound-level meters. These results suggest that smartphone apps used to measure overall sound levels have not drastically improved. When reference signals were presented at 90 dBA, the smartphone apps underreported the actual sound level, specifically apps on the Android platforms.[17] Smartphones may be a convenient way to measure sound levels; however, their reliability needs to be improved. Despite these limitations, sound-level meter apps may be helpful to educate patients about noise levels and encourage use of hearing protection. In addition, native operating system apps (apps that do not need to be downloaded), such as Apple's Health app, records and monitors headphone audio levels, providing the user with helpful information to better understand how loud and prolonged audio signals can affect one's hearing.

9.2.2 Apps for Wellness

There are a variety of apps that provide assistive tools for wellness, including apps for meditation and mindfulness, relaxation, and hypnosis. In the review by Sereda et al,[9] a total of five apps were identified as focusing on meditation and mindfulness (*Beltone*

Tinnitus Calmer, Headspace, Relax Melodies, ReSound Relief, and *Zenways*). All five apps mentioned above provide guided meditation, and several apps (*Beltone, ReSound*) offer imagery techniques as well. Some apps are specifically designed for meditation (*Headspace, Zenways*), whereas other apps incorporate the meditation and mindfulness techniques alongside other modules for tinnitus.[9] All five apps received acceptable MARS scores (>2.0), suggesting that they are of sufficient quality to recommend to tinnitus patients for mindfulness and meditation.

Some apps (*Beltone Tinnitus Calmer, Oticon Tinnitus Sound,* and *ReSound Relief*) contain relaxation or breathing exercises that may be helpful for patients with tinnitus.[9] Specifically, *ReSound Relief* guides individuals through deep breathing exercises by using a visual aid to prompt breathing in and out (i.e., draws a circle as inhale and exhale is completed). Also, the *Oticon Tinnitus Sound* app reviews progressive muscle relaxation, a great technique to tense and relax major muscle groups of the body, which is more fully described in Chapter 10. *Sleep Well Hypnosis,* an app that provides a 25-minute guided hypnosis audio session by a hypnotherapist, was found to have a low MARS score, which may need to be considered when recommending this app to patients.[9]

9.2.3 Limitations and Risks Associated with Smartphone Apps

Despite the number of apps available for tinnitus management, the overall use of apps within the health care field is not widespread. There is high variability among app users and the health care fields that actually utilize apps. Many younger providers use apps in clinical practice, and research shows that more experienced providers use apps far less. Franko and Tirrell[18] found that about 70% of residents who participated in their study used apps in practice while only 40% of attending physicians with over 15 years of experience used apps. The gap in app use can be attributed to the age of each physician, in that older physicians do not find it necessary to use apps in clinical practice, mostly because they did not have access to this kind of technology while they were in school.[18]

There are a multitude of reasons why health care providers are skeptical about implementing apps into their clinical practice. When a smartphone user purchases an app from the store within their smartphone platform, it cannot be easily returned. Many apps that could be suitable for use in practice have an added expense, and health care providers may be hesitant to make a purchase if they are unsure the app will serve its intended purpose. The price of some health care apps can equate to the price of a reference book that will provide the same information. At this point, many health care providers may opt to purchase the textbook because it can be examined prior to purchase.[18] The quantity of apps available can also be problematic for health care professionals. When using search terms such as "anatomy" or "surgical tools," irrelevant apps such as games can be some of the first to appear. Within the scope of tinnitus apps, there seems to be a smaller proportion of apps deemed irrelevant across searches for apps in the iOS, Android, and Windows platforms. A recent study found that only 72% of apps using the search term, "tinnitus," were relevant to the topic on the Android platform, and that percentage increased to 87% and 95% in the iOS and Windows platforms, respectively.[6] It is also important to note that the apps deemed irrelevant featured ringtones, jewelry, and music bands that can be easily ruled out by app users looking for tinnitus management apps.[6]

Even though most mobile phone platforms have an assortment of relevant apps for tinnitus management, there are a multitude of reasons for nonuse. Sereda et al[9] summarized the reasons for nonuse among 643 individuals with tinnitus. An overall lack of awareness of apps available for tinnitus management was the most common reasons for nonuse; 75% of respondents noted they had not used an app and 59.3% of those respondents were not aware apps were available for tinnitus management. Additional reasons for nonuse included limited knowledge of smartphone technology, difficulty locating an app that would be helpful for them, and lack of a device that would support tinnitus apps.[9]

These findings highlight the importance of introducing patients to apps for tinnitus management and even providing demonstrations of such apps. Multiple resources should be made available to patients to address their tinnitus, including the use of smartphone apps. Clinicians should be prepared to direct their patients to apps that can be used to manage tinnitus which can ultimately address the concern of app nonuse.[6] Factors that encouraged patients to use apps included the ease of use, the source of the recommendation for the app (i.e., from hearing care professional or family member/friend), and the name of the app. Clinicians can serve as the bridge between app use for tinnitus management by providing recommendations that specifically address the needs of the individual.[9]

As previously noted, a deterrence to the use of health care apps among physicians was the cost of apps. However, Deshpande and Shimunova[6] found no significant difference in the number of features available in free tinnitus apps and paid apps. The features available across free vs. paid apps included sound generation, meditation and mindfulness, relaxation exercises, elements of cognitive behavior therapy, and information and education.[9] The number of these features was *not* significantly different between paid and free apps, indicating that users do not need to purchase an app to utilize the same functions available within free apps.[6] The overall cost of apps does not lead to more features when compared to less expensive paid apps. There was no significant difference in the number of features available within one app, whether that app costs 20 dollars or less than 1 dollar.[6] These results indicate that individuals with tinnitus do not have to purchase an app to have multiple features for managing tinnitus and that the cost of the app should not be considered a valid factor for app nonuse.

Safety and security of apps remains a consideration in the use of smartphone apps for health and wellness. The growing market for smartphone apps in the health care field leads to a growing market to intercept private medical information of smartphone users. In general, the Food and Drug Administration (FDA) and the Health Insurance Portability and Accountability Act (HIPAA) regulate medical practices in terms of privacy and treatment to protect patients. Due to the newer technology made available, the FDA and HIPAA have created their own set of regulations to monitor health care apps. However, there are still gaps in the legislation that can disrupt the protection of health-related app users.[19] The FDA can only regulate apps that "constitute medical devices and/or pose significant risks to patients."[19] However, in 2019, the FDA re-released its policy on smartphone apps. This document includes regulations that relate directly to audiology.

The role of the FDA is to oversee the safety and effectiveness of smartphone apps. There is a greater focus on apps that present risks to patients if it does not function as it is intended, or performs a similar function that is typically completed by a traditional medical device. This ruling applies to audiology because apps used to measure hearing status by serving as an audiometer, or apps used to adjust hearing aids and cochlear implants would fall into this category for FDA oversight and governance. Regulation for these apps are important because if sound levels become too loud, it can lead to damage to the auditory system.[20] At this time, tinnitus maskers are considered medical devices, and manufacturers creating new maskers are required to submit a premarket notification to the FDA so that the apps can be monitored. However, tinnitus masker apps are not explicitly listed as software functions that FDA has chosen to regulate; so, it is unclear if tinnitus masker apps are regulated by the FDA.[20] There are also apps available within the app store that can be used as a tinnitus masker but were created to serve a different function; therefore, these apps would not be regulated by the FDA. In general, apps that constitute a medical device, but are deemed "low risk," are only regulated by the FDA at their discretion. FDA can choose not to enforce its regulations over these apps.[19] The apparent gaps within the FDA's regulation of health care apps have the potential to cause medical complications or security breaches. For example, apps that are considered "low risk" can still provide medical recommendations and send user information to outside parties and typically are exempt from FDA regulation.[19]

Furthermore, smartphone apps are exempt from HIPAA compliance rules, unless the app distributes patient information to third-party companies. Although this constitutes a smaller number of apps, some apps send private information to third-party companies. This results in a breach of security that many app users may not recognize. According to HIPAA, the only health care information that must be concealed are "covered entities" that include health plans, health care clearinghouses (used for billing), and health care providers who transmit health information in electronic form.[19] As long as these apps do not distribute any identifying information, the app developers do not need to abide by HIPAA.

The nature of these apps allows them to escape stringent regulation of the FDA and HIPAA, making them vulnerable to security breaches. Huckvale et al[2] found that many health care apps have limited security measures because "low-risk" apps do not need high-security measures. In their cross-sectional assessment of 79 apps labeled as "safe," many apps do not have full safety measures in place that would prevent outside users from intercepting confidential patient information.[2] Of the 79 apps that were assessed during the study, 89% transmitted personal information online. There were no apps that store personal information on a local server. Of the 35 apps that sent identifying information over the Internet, 66% did not use encryption, which protects confidential information. According to the study, 78% of the apps that acknowledge sending information over the Internet did not disclose the nature of the information sent.[2] Apps may be very susceptible to hacking because of the lack of security measures employed by app developers. The type of information that can be intercepted from apps is also unclear, such as personal information can be viewed without the consent of the user.

Personal data is often available in the public domain and can typically be found by conducting a search for that person online. Sensitive personal data, however, in countries outside the United States have much stricter rules about how that data can be accessed. The European Union (EU) in 2018 passed the General Data Protection Regulation (GDPR), which expands what falls into the Personal Data segment, and the individual's rights over that data. A big part of the legislation is that individuals must give permission to use the data. According to the GDPR, companies developing health-related apps must meet the regulatory requirements set forth within the Medical Devices Regulation (MDR), obtain a CE mark, and cannot collect or use data without the permission of the individual. Furthermore, the more personal the data, the more clearly written the Terms and Conditions need to be. This is very important with the growing biometric data industry, which collects health measures from individuals that can be used to identify that individual, along with sensitive health information.

These security concerns may not be the only factors that inhibit widespread use of apps in health care. The lack of evidence to support the accuracy of each app can determine patient safety. The lack of research can lead to safety concerns for app users. With the limited safety standards in place, excluding security measures, apps have the potential to cause serious medical errors.[21] For example, apps like *Epocrates* that assign dosage and medication to patients have the ability to make errors. These errors can directly affect the lives of patients. The risks that these apps pose need to be fully assessed before they are used to prevent harm to a patient. Many apps are beginning to be peer-reviewed by physicians; however, more research is needed to fully determine the effectiveness and accuracy of these apps.[21] Extensive research is crucial because it can help app developers create effective, reliable apps for use in clinical practice.

Current research reveals similar findings in terms of safety of these apps. Akbar et al[22] examined the overall safety concerns of high- and low-risk health smartphone apps. Some of the faults found within these apps included relaying incorrect information provided to users, faulty alarms that regulate times to take medication, and incorrect outputs for health measurements (i.e., heart rate, blood pressure, blood alcohol concentration). Of the 74 studies reviewed by these authors, 80 safety concerns for apps were found. It was determined that gaps in app development such as limited expert involvement, no evidence-based principles, and poor validation can contribute to these safety concerns.[22] It is apparent that even though the number of health apps continues to increase, safety concerns about their use have not been fully addressed.

In sum, health apps have many limitations that restrict physicians and health care professionals from selecting apps and integrating them into clinical practice. Overall, security concerns are a major factor for these apps; however, people need to consider that security breaches can occur without the presence of an app. Information can be intercepted from a patient's file just the same as it can be from an app. Health care professionals, including audiologists, need to determine if the risk of security breaches outweigh the convenience of the app. Apps can be successfully incorporated into clinical practice when appropriate safety precautions are used or if an app is used primarily as a tool in collaboration with or under the supervision of the health care practitioner. More research is needed on the effectiveness of health and audiology apps, given the sparse number of studies in this area of development.

9.3 Conclusions

We have reviewed a wide range of apps available for tinnitus patients and have focused on the purposes for which these apps would be used, knowing that apps for tinnitus evaluation and management are likely to change with time. Apps for tinnitus management are most commonly used by patients with tinnitus, and include options for sound therapy, education and counseling, and relaxation tools for wellness. Studies have more recently investigated the utility of apps for tinnitus and suggest that free apps are just as beneficial as paid apps, and that apps can be evaluated based on their helpfulness. Though some studies have evaluated the effectiveness of apps in reducing tinnitus severity, more research is needed. Although apps may be helpful for some patients, patients who are bothered by their tinnitus will likely need greater, one-on-one support from their audiologist to manage tinnitus beyond that of an app.

Audiologists should be aware of safety and security issues, especially if patient information is exchanged during app use. Though there is some oversight on apps used in the health care field (i.e., FDA, HIPAA, GDPR), many apps are considered low risk and not subject to oversight. As a new generation of patients emerges with greater technology skills, audiologists should be reminded of the benefits and risks of these apps and have a plan for incorporating apps into their clinical practice for the treatment of tinnitus.

References

[1] Terry M. Medical apps for smartphones. Telemed J E Health. 2010; 16(1):17–22

[2] Huckvale K, Prieto JT, Tilney M, Benghozi PJ, Car J. Unaddressed privacy risks in accredited health and wellness apps: a cross-sectional systematic assessment. BMC Med. 2015; 13(1):214

[3] Vashist SK, Schneider EM, Luong JH. Commercial smartphone-based devices and smart applications for personalized healthcare monitoring and management. Diagnostics (Basel). 2014; 4(3):104–128

[4] Wiechmann W, Kwan D, Bokarius A, Toohey SL. There's an app for that? Highlighting the difficulty in finding clinically relevant smartphone applications. West J Emerg Med. 2016; 17(2):191–194

[5] Paglialonga A, Tognola G, Pinciroli F. Apps for hearing science and care. Am J Audiol. 2015; 24(3):293–298

[6] Deshpande AK, Shimunova T. Comprehensive evaluation of tinnitus apps. Am J Audiol. 2019; 28(3):605–616

[7] Wunderlich R, Stein A, Engell A, et al. Evaluation of iPod-based automated tinnitus pitch matching. J Am Acad Audiol. 2013; 26(2):205–212

[8] Henry JA, Frederick M, Sell S, Griest S, Abrams H. Validation of a novel combination hearing aid and tinnitus therapy device. Ear Hear. 2015; 36(1):42–52

[9] Sereda M, Smith S, Newton K, Stockdale D. Mobile apps for management of tinnitus: Users' survey, quality assessment,

and content analysis. JMIR Mhealth Uhealth. 2019; 7(1): e10353

[10] Kutyba J, Gos E, Jędrzejczak WW, et al. Effectiveness of tinnitus therapy using a mobile application. Eur Arch Otorhinolaryngol. 2021; https://doi.org/10.1007/s00405-021-06767-9

[11] Henry JA, Thielman E, Zaugg T, et al. Development and field testing of a smartphone "App" for tinnitus management. Int J Audiol. 2017a; 56(10):784–792

[12] Henry JA, Thielman EJ, Zaugg TL, et al. Randomized controlled trial in clinical settings to evaluate effectiveness of coping skills education used with Progressive Tinnitus Management. J Speech Lang Hear Res. 2017b; 60(5):1378–1397

[13] Kim SY, Chang MY, Hong M, Yoo S-G, Oh D, Park MK. Tinnitus therapy using tailor-made notched music delivered via a smartphone application and Ginko combined treatment: a pilot study. Auris Nasus Larynx. 2017; 44(5):528–533

[14] Newman CW, Sandridge SA, Jacobson GP. Psychometric adequacy of the Tinnitus Handicap Inventory (THI) for evaluating treatment outcome. J Am Acad Audiol. 1998; 9(2): 153–160

[15] Tyson P. Relax app offers tinnitus relief. Starkey Hearing Technologies; 2015

[16] Nast DR, Speer WS, Le Prell CG. Sound level measurements using smartphone "apps": useful or inaccurate? Noise Health. 2014; 16(72):251–256

[17] McLennon T, Patel S, Behar A, Abdoli-Eramaki M. Evaluation of smartphone sound level meter applications as a reliable tool for noise monitoring. J Occup Environ Hyg. 2019; 16(9): 620–627

[18] Franko OI, Tirrell TF. Smartphone app use among medical providers in ACGME training programs. J Med Syst. 2012; 36 (5):3135–3139

[19] Flaherty JL. Digital diagnosis: privacy and the regulation of mobile phone health applications. Am J Law Med. 2014; 40 (4):416–441

[20] U.S. Food and Drug Administration. Policy for device software functions and mobile medical applications. Washington, DC: Center for Devices and Radiological Health; 2019

[21] Buijink AWG, Visser BJ, Marshall L. Medical apps for smartphones: lack of evidence undermines quality and safety. Evid Based Med. 2013; 18(3):90–92

[22] Akbar S, Coiera E, Magrabi F. Safety concerns with consumer-facing mobile health applications and their consequences: a scoping review. J Am Med Inform Assoc. 2020; 27(2):330–340

10 Distractions, Relaxation, and Peace with Tinnitus: Guided Imagery, Meditation, Mindfulness, and More

Ann Perreau, Courtney Baker, and Richard S. Tyler

Abstract

This chapter explores alternative methods of tinnitus relief including mindfulness and activity-based practices. The purpose of this chapter is to demonstrate how each activity can be utilized in the treatment of a patient with tinnitus. Each section introduces and explains a method aimed to divert the patient's attention away from their bothersome tinnitus, thus providing some relief and increasing the patient's ability to concentrate on other aspects of their lives. To conclude this chapter, additional recommendations for managing tinnitus are provided.

Keywords: activities engagement, art and music therapy, mindfulness, meditation, relaxation, tinnitus

10.1 Introduction

Tinnitus often grabs one's attention and predominates one's thoughts and emotions, making it difficult to concentrate on anything else. We know that as a result of tinnitus, patients will often report problems with emotional well-being, sleep, concentration, and/or communication abilities.[1,2] For some patients, these reactions to tinnitus impact their daily lives significantly, whereas others may be bothered in certain situations only. Indeed, tinnitus produces a broad range of reactions across patients,[3] and we are all unique in our own ways. So how can our tinnitus patients focus on something else, not think about their tinnitus, and carry on with their lives?

As we may well know, there is no one right answer to how we should refocus on other aspects of life. What may work for one individual to take the focus off tinnitus might not work for another, or work in the same way. That being said, there are many recommended activities that have beneficial effects for tinnitus patients, most of which are self-guided and do not require involvement of a health care professional or therapist beyond a first introduction. In fact, with the availability of apps and podcasts, today's tinnitus patient has many options to begin a self-guided regimen for relaxation or distraction from their tinnitus.

There are a variety of approaches that can help tinnitus patients to put their worries in the background, enjoy the moment, and look forward to a future activity. This is good for all of us, not just our tinnitus patients. In this chapter, we describe several options that can be used to help our tinnitus patients, which includes meditation, mindfulness, guided imagery, biofeedback, progressive muscle relaxation, art therapy, music therapy, exercise, and exploration of new hobbies. Where available, we also reference research and clinical reports in which these specific approaches have been implemented, noting particular strategies specifically for tinnitus.

It should be appreciated that there is no agreement for the precise definition and application of many of these terms related to mindfulness and meditation. These terms also get modified or combined, and new additional terms are invented, sometimes for marketing purposes. Our intent here is to provide a broad perspective of different approaches to the best of our abilities while using terminology that is relevant and current.

10.2 Meditation

Meditation involves much focused contemplation on only one thing, reflecting on it in a very calm and relaxed manner. It involves learning to work with the mind and is categorized into various types that include transcendental and Zen meditation. In transcendental meditation, there is no concentrating or monitoring of one's thoughts, or taking control or emptying the mind. The Cambridge dictionary defines this type of meditation as "the act of giving your attention to only one thing, either as a religious activity or as a way of becoming calm and relaxed."

Meditation is practiced typically for 20 minutes, one or two times a day. The patient should wear loose clothing in order to breathe easily, and lie or sit on the floor using carpet, rug, and cushions to be comfortable. Patients may close their eyes lightly, or gaze at an object in distant view during meditation (▶ Fig. 10.1).

10.3 Mindfulness

The use of mindfulness has become more and more popular over the years. Mindfulness is defined as a mental state achieved by focusing one's attention on the present moment, while acknowledging without

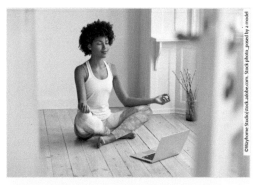

Fig. 10.1 Example meditation position. (Source: ©Wayhome Studio/stock.adobe.com. Stock photo. Posed by a model.)

judgment and accepting one's feelings, thoughts, and bodily sensations.[4] For tinnitus patients, focusing on thoughts and bodily sensations might be a daunting task because they are reluctant to focus on their tinnitus any more than they already do. However, a number of studies have shown promising results using mindfulness meditation with tinnitus patients and with a variety of different protocols.[5,6]

Mindfulness is a general ability or skill involving the body, the breath, and the mind that can be practiced through a variety of approaches. To start practicing mindfulness, one must be familiar with the basic principles—to stay focused and in the present. If patients find their thoughts drifting to the future or the past, they are encouraged to gently bring themselves back to the present moment. The other main principle of mindfulness is to remain nonjudgmental throughout the process. This means recognizing a feeling, emotion, or sensation when it arises, but not labeling it with a name or connotation.[7]

Mindfulness meditation can take many forms, but a particularly useful meditation for tinnitus patients, especially those with insomnia, is to do a body scan meditation and quick replay of the day right before bed while laying down.[8] The mindfulness session is completed as follows:

Start by taking a few deep breaths (e.g., five breaths), in and out, to relax the body. Be aware of your breath and note any thoughts without criticizing or judging them. Become aware of your physical sensations and work to relax your body with each breath. Note your weight distribution from right to left, and any discomfort you feel. From your laying position, adjust your body as necessary to be more comfortable. Return your focus to your breath. If you hear any sounds including your tinnitus,

acknowledge them. Bring your awareness to these sounds momentarily, but then redirect your focus back to your breath. Now imagine that you are taking a tour of your body, starting with your toes and ending with the top of your head. Scan your body from toe to head and observe any tension or tightness in your muscles. Be aware of any areas that are relaxed. You can scan several times, noting any changes in your body as you repeat the body scan. Do not focus extensively on any part of the body, even if you feel tension there. Note the sensations that you feel and move on to the next part of the body. Breathe throughout this body scan, and note the changes in your breath. Is your breath deep, shallow, long, or short? Note these changes in your breath as you scan your body, but resist judging or evaluating your breath. As your mind wanders during this meditation, slowly bring it back to your breath. Pay attention to your inhales and exhales. Next, review your day from morning to night. Begin with the first moment that you can remember in the day, that is, when you first woke up. Using a focused and relaxed "fast-forward" approach, revisit each moment of the day in order that you can easily remember. Consider this as someone who would watch your day as if it were played on video, where you are observing these moments in your day without evaluating or judging them. Do not linger on any part of the day, and avoid thinking about each part of the day in detail. Your replay of the day should take a few minutes (e.g., 2–3 min maximum). If you find yourself replaying a difficult interaction or conversation, remember you are here to visit it and then move on. Keep going to the next part of your day if this happens. Refocus on your breath for a few moments if you feel distracted during your quick replay. Once finished, bring yourself back to the present moment.

This mindfulness session should help to relax the body and prepare for sleep. It is not intended for the patient to be asleep by the end of the meditation, rather to provide a mindfulness moment, or break for the mind, to prepare the body for sleep. It is important to instruct patients with tinnitus that they should acknowledge their tinnitus, but pass no judgment on it.[7] Mindfulness experiences encourage patients to acknowledge the uncomfortable emotional or bodily sensations, but then let them pass.

In recent years, several research groups have applied mindfulness techniques to the treatment of patients with tinnitus. One such treatment program is Mindfulness-Based Cognitive Therapy (MBCT) which has been adopted from a similar approach for clinical depression. The changes in programming are evident in the psychoeducation portion of the therapy sessions where researchers have substituted tinnitus education information in place of the original depression information.[9]

MBCT is a structured 8-week program with weekly sessions where patients continue to learn and practice aspects of mindfulness in relation to their tinnitus symptoms. Several studies have demonstrated successful outcomes with MBCT as measured through tinnitus acceptance and handicap questionnaires.[4,9,10,11] For example, McKenna et al[12] found that MBCT was more effective in reducing tinnitus severity and loudness for 39 tinnitus patients compared to a group receiving relaxation therapy ($n = 36$). Though both treatment groups reported improved tinnitus symptoms, MBCT was more successful than relaxation therapy.[12] Though MBCT typically is provided from a professional, it can be learned through self-help books, podcasts, and CDs, making this form of CBT readily available to tinnitus patients.

10.4 Guided Imagery

Guided imagery is an example of a mindfulness activity that specifically focuses on calming the senses. In this technique, patients are guided through an experience where they imagine and visualize sights and sounds that they find relaxing.

In Tinnitus Activities Treatment,[13] pictures are used to create a visual image for this activity. One example provided is a beach with waves and palm trees. An image can serve as a starting point for patients to begin their visualization, but they should be encouraged to make their experience personal and meaningful to them. For example, a patient may report that the forest is their favored relaxation scene, and the trees, moss, and sky can be visualized to begin the mindfulness activity. Following is a sample script to guide a patient through a guided imagery exercise (▶ Fig. 10.2). This particular activity uses the beach example mentioned initially above. However, remember that you can modify this script to suit the patient's desired location, and substitute any particular situation that is more appropriate for your patient. A demonstration of this exercise is accessible through the companion website in the supplemental video section for this chapter.

First, close your eyes. Get comfortable in your seat or laying down. We are going to start by thinking of a relaxing scene. For this particular example, we will use the beach. Try to imagine the scene as clearly as you can, maybe a particular beach that you visited recently or as a child. Visualize the

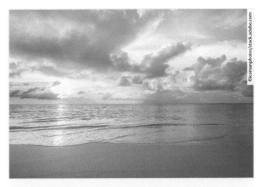

Fig. 10.2 Illustration for visual imagery using the example of a beach. (Source: ©icemanphotos/stock.adobe.com)

beach, including the blue water and sky, the birds flying overhead, and the sand underneath you. Note the smell of the air around you, the smell of the saltwater. Then focus your attention to your feet. They are in the warm sand, move your feet around, dig them into the sand. Notice the feeling of the sand as it moves across your feet, notice the warmth. Listen to the sound of the waves crashing, of the birds that are flying, or the noises of other activities going on. Can you taste the salt from the ocean? Allow yourself to relax as you explore the location in your mind, making special note of the sensory sensations around you. Pay attention to all five senses, sight, smell, touch, hearing, and taste.

When you are ready to return, slowly open your eyes again. Take a moment to reorient yourself to your surroundings.

Guided imagery helps to create a calming sensory experience to control one's reactions to tinnitus and provides a method for self-coping. Henry and Wilson[14] applied imagery training to patients with tinnitus and we have since implemented their approach in our counseling program, Tinnitus Activities Treatment.[13] By involving as many senses in the guided imagery exercise, the sensory experience is enriched, allowing for greater relaxation and enjoyment for the patient.[14]

10.5 Biofeedback

Biofeedback is a process used to gain more control over changes and sensations within the body by reducing the patient's reactiveness to stressors.[15] Biofeedback involves monitoring physiological functions of the body through electrical equipment. Specifically, the sympathetic nervous system, the part of our autonomic nervous system which controls our heart rate, blood flow, breathing, muscle activity, and produces the "fight or flight" response, is monitored during biofeedback. As the sympathetic nervous system engages in response to a trigger (such as bothersome tinnitus), the patient's heart rate may increase, their brain rhythms change, their muscle activity increases, and skin temperature drops, which can be recorded by the equipment.[16] The information collected from the equipment is then displayed to the patient in real time to help improve the patient's awareness and increase their control over these physiological changes.[17] Physiological systems monitored by biofeedback include heart rate, breathing patterns, brainwaves through electroencephalography (EEG), skin temperature, muscle tension, among others. The patient is attached to the electrodes and other monitoring devices which connect to a monitor. The patient then works to manipulate and control the body function, focusing their attention on the feedback from their body system monitors.[17]

Tinnitus patients can benefit from biofeedback as a coping mechanism to ease psychological stress and anxiety associated with tinnitus. Landis and Landis[15] found that the use of exercises such as deep breathing, progressive muscle relaxation, and autogenic relaxation was effective for seven tinnitus patients while using biofeedback monitoring methods. The patients in that study reported that biofeedback helped them cope with their tinnitus and that they would recommend it to fellow tinnitus patients.[15] All three exercises are relaxation techniques that can be used on their own, but when paired with biofeedback technology, the patient is able to objectively see the effects of the exercise on their body. After a few sessions using the biofeedback monitors, patients will then be able to feel the physiological change during the activities, without needing to see the feedback on a monitor.[17] Specific details on biofeedback in the management of tinnitus is provided in "Biofeedback training in the treatment of tinnitus," a chapter in the *Tinnitus Handbook*.[18]

10.6 Progressive Muscle Relaxation

Another approach is to teach the patient to systematically tense and relax groups of muscles, termed "progressive muscle relaxation."[19] With practice, patients can control and focus on their tensed muscle or a relaxed muscle. Though it might sound counterintuitive, tensing a muscle brings one's attention to the muscular tension. Then, after conscious attention is directed to the tension, the patient engages actively in relaxing that same muscle, a practice that produces deep muscle, and hopefully mental, relaxation. There are two steps involved in progressive muscle relaxation, which include deliberately applying tension to certain muscle groups and then stopping the tension and focusing on how the muscles feel as they relax. We use the progressive muscle relaxation technique outlined by Henry and Wilson[14] that focuses on five major muscle groups starting with the arms and ending with the legs and feet. Here is a sample script to begin progressive muscle relaxation (▶ Fig. 10.3). A demonstration of this exercise can also be found on the companion website in the supplemental video section for this chapter.

Begin with deep breathing—take five deep breathes—to achieve a relaxed state. Think the word "relax" as you breathe deeply in and out. Then focus on the physical sensations of your body, and start with your arms. Begin by making a fist and tensing both arms. Think the word "tense" as you tense and hold this for 15 seconds. Then release the tension as you breathe deeply and pay attention to the sensation of your arms relaxing. You may think of the word "relax" as you breathe out and release. Progressive muscle relaxation continues while you tense and relax the following muscle groups in order: (a) both arms; (b) face, neck, and throat; (c) shoulders and chest; (d) back and stomach; and (e) both legs and feet. Try the exercise with your eyes closed and repeat the exercise as desired. When finished, release any remaining tension in your body.

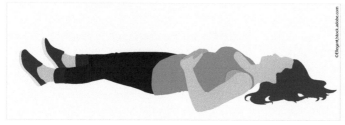

Fig. 10.3 Position for progressive muscle relaxation. (Source: ©Ellegant/stock.adobe.com)

Progressive muscle relaxation can be completed daily to help manage reactions to tinnitus that cause stress, anxiety, or other emotional reactions. During our clinical sessions, we recommend and teach patients how to perform progressive muscle relaxation using this modified approach by Henry and Wilson.[14] As with guided imagery, we have also implemented this approach of progressive muscle relaxation with patients who have hyperacusis, which has been received well.[20] Interested readers can learn more about hyperacusis in Chapter 13.

10.7 Art Therapy

Art is present all around us every day, from the designs of our buildings to the painting hanging on an office wall. The process of creating art is therapeutic in nature; the images or products often reflect the personal conflicts or symbolize the struggle of the artist. Many times, the artist is the only one that can explain the deeper meaning that is portrayed. For that reason, art can be used as constructive therapy, or a way to process difficult feelings. Art therapy actively engages the individual in a variety of artistic endeavors; for example, drawing or painting, with the goal of providing emotional release.[21]

Art therapy also provides an opportunity for self-expression and self-exploration. This is helpful for patients who feel overwhelmed with a variety of emotions or for those who are unsure or uncertain about how they feel. There are a variety of approaches to art therapy, and each individual must make the decision on which approach and therapist best fits their needs. Sessions can use a direct approach to confront certain feelings in an upfront manner, or be more indirect by allowing a free space for creation in an attempt to explore one's feelings.[22] Often having a specific task or goal provided by a professional, such as an art therapist, can help focus one's attention on the particular feelings or thoughts that may be troublesome. There are endless opportunities to the materials that can be used in art therapy. The most common supplies are often easy-to-use craft materials such as paint, markers, paper, and clay. For example, one study by Nan and Ho[23] reported that clay art therapy was more beneficial for patients compared to nondirective art such as handicrafts.

Studies have found benefits of art therapy for patients with other chronic illnesses similar to tinnitus, including trauma[24] and depression.[23] For example, Blomdahl et al[25] conducted a randomized control clinical trial to compare art therapy to treatment as usual (or control) for 79 patients with depression. Results revealed that art therapy resulted in lower depression ratings than the treatment as usual, suggesting that it is beneficial for patients with depression. For tinnitus and hyperacusis patients, art therapy techniques can be used to manage their symptoms. In our clinic, we have directed patients to express their feelings about tinnitus and hyperacusis visually (▶ Fig. 10.4). This could be a painting that represents their tinnitus or hyperacusis as an object, animal-form, or as an abstract concept.

Patients can take this assignment and use it to help them portray what is most troublesome about their tinnitus, whether that be a specific activity affected by tinnitus, an emotional reaction from their tinnitus that they would like to change, or specific challenge or limitation. We encourage patients to use a variety of materials, colors, and simply create what makes sense to them. One patient, in particular, created an intricate painting of the effect of tinnitus on her life. She participated in several research studies using electrical stimulation to control tinnitus, and in response to the positive outcome from the study, drew a painting of a cochlea and lightning bolt (to symbolize her tinnitus) that hangs in the University of Iowa Hospitals and Clinics today.[26] We are also pleased to share the cover art of this book entitled Scream Mosaic, by Liam Haskill. Liam has tinnitus and

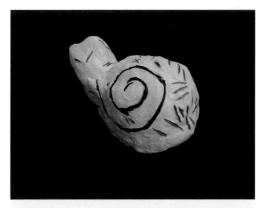

Fig. 10.4 Sculpture portraying the cochlea and hyperacusis. (Courtesy of Liam Haskill.)

hyperacusis and was inspired by the work of Edvard Munch to illustrate how tinnitus and hyperacusis affect his life.

10.8 Music Therapy

Music, just like other art modalities, has healing and calming qualities. Many of us use music as a coping mechanism, perhaps even every day, without even realizing it. Do you listen to music when you are working, studying, and/or exercising? In addition to having music accompany us while completing an activity, music can also easily distract us from other sounds, negative feelings, or difficult situations. Using this logic, many individuals listen to comforting, engaging music to relax or wind down. This practice can be applied directly to our patients with tinnitus. Adding a pleasant auditory signal, such as music, helps the tinnitus to be less prominent because the brain has more difficulty detecting the tinnitus percept and specifically, distinguishing the neural input of tinnitus from that of the music. In addition, many tinnitus patients report low-level music to be calming and relaxing when added to the environment[27] (▶ Fig. 10.5). This can be done through the use of sound machines, maskers, or formal music therapy.

Music therapy is a structured approach that uses music for therapeutic means to treat symptoms of psychological or physiological disease.[28] It can involve creating music, listening to music, singing, and even moving to music with the purpose of relieving the burden of one's symptoms. One specific model of music therapy, the Heidelberg Model on Music Therapy, has been developed and researched specifically for the treatment of tinnitus.[29] The Heidelberg Model uses a structured, neuromusic

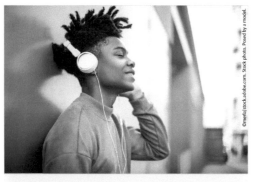

Fig. 10.5 Music can be used for sound therapy and for relaxation. (Source: ©merla/stock.adobe.com. Stock photo. Posed by a model.)

therapy provided through individualized, hour-long sessions over the course of days or weeks.[30] Therapy often consists of four modules that include counseling, resonance training, neuroauditive cortex training, and tinnitus reconditioning.[29] Multiple studies have shown significant reductions in tinnitus severity,[29] tinnitus pitch, loudness, and annoyance,[31,32] and emotional problems such as depression[28] following the use of music therapy. Further, music therapy has been associated with cortical reorganization due to increased gray matter volume in sites of the brain dedicated to sound identification in tinnitus patients.[32]

The Heidelberg Model is a standardized process and requires the involvement of a specially trained professional with expertise in music therapy. Each of the modules addresses general areas of music therapy: vocal exercise, active music therapy, and receptive music therapy, respectively.[30] With this knowledge, we can better inform our patients on the types of music therapy that can be beneficial to their tinnitus treatment.

10.9 Exercise

Exercise is certainly good for all of us and our general health. It can also improve sleep as our bodies fatigue at night following physical exertion during the day. Many individuals who exercise benefit from group activities or classes, where we have to be focused on the group leader or instructor. Awareness that members of the group are exercising along with us helps focus us on the activity, rather than focusing on our worries, concerns, or even tinnitus. Other individuals prefer to exercise on their own, creating a frequent routine to keep them in good health and focused on the physical nature of their exercise. Some examples of group exercise include Pilates, yoga, Tai Chi, weight training, and cross-training classes, whereas individual exercise includes walking, running, swimming, and biking (▶ Fig. 10.6). Yoga is often recommended for patients with tinnitus and other chronic illnesses to engage their bodies in a physical sense, and relax their mind and distract from their tinnitus or condition.[16] Hatha yoga is a practice that can be done on a daily basis and starts with elementary poses and builds to more advanced exercises as needed. Yoga practice often begins with Savasana, or deep breathing exercises, and can be practiced in a group setting or individually. Many individuals practice yoga in groups to both encourage and challenge themselves with

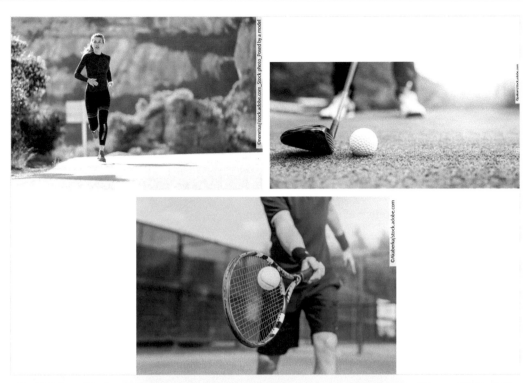

Fig. 10.6 Examples of exercise. (Source: *Top left*: ©nenetus/stock.adobe.com. Stock photo. Posed by a model; *top right*: ©pakorn/stock.adobe.com; *bottom*: ©Akaberka/stock.adobe.com)

help from the instructor, and also practice individually to relax their mind and body on a daily basis.

Individuals can feel good about exercising! Specific to tinnitus, exercise provides many different opportunities to get away from tinnitus. In group exercise, it is possible to make new friends. With a regular group activity, there is the experience of being engaged with others in a healthy activity. One can focus on the instructor, the tasks, others in the group, and not on the tinnitus. When you are active, your mind can be distracted from the tinnitus. And of course, feeling good about doing something healthy provides many benefits to the tinnitus patient.

10.10 A New Hobby

Life has challenges for all of us and we are always changing with respect to our interests and activities in life. For example, after retirement, we may find ourselves with more time in each day, and perhaps need to engage in a new set of activities to fill the void from the busy work day. We can meet new friends and observe different activities while we engage others. In Tinnitus Activities Treatment, we specifically recommend refocusing on other activities in life to help reduce negative thoughts and emotions that may result from tinnitus. We often suggest that patients keep a tinnitus diary (see companion website, Chapter 4 for an example) to consider new hobbies. Keeping a diary can help patients to modify their lifestyle and explore alternate activities where tinnitus is less noticeable or bothersome. As we know, but sometimes hesitate to do, trying a new activity in life can be good for all of us. There are a wide variety of activities to choose from, including book clubs, writing, and pottery, among others. Engaging in an activity that can focus one's attention for extended periods of time has the added advantage of putting tinnitus in the background or refocusing away from tinnitus.

Moreover, for the individual with tinnitus, starting a new and engaging activity can captivate one's attention. The hobby often requires focusing, mindfulness, and being with and learning from others. Starting a new hobby typically requires a new perspective, something very different and apart from the tinnitus. Discussing these benefits with a tinnitus patient, often with the aid of a tinnitus diary, helps to put the tinnitus in the background and improve their enjoyment in life.

10.11 Conclusions

Maybe we are all too busy! Our mind is constantly occupied. We often are stressed, overwhelmed, and anxious. It would be good for all of us to take some time to relax and remove ourselves from the stress and challenges of everyday life. Of course, we have to make time for this, but maybe it can be done in a car, an airplane, taxi, train or bus—some daily activity.

We, like our patients, are all different. We suggest several options here, but of course there are many, many more (yoga, Tai chi, horse-back riding… and on and on). Sometimes, we even ask the client to draw a picture of their tinnitus that can be used to explore emotional reactions to tinnitus, and restructure negative thoughts about tinnitus (e.g., a child drew a picture of their tinnitus as the "Tin-monster"[33]).

Tinnitus can be captivating for the patient. Most tinnitus patients report during the day that they do not notice or are less bothered by their tinnitus. You can ask them to keep a diary and note these activities. It is good for all of us to explore new activities and to refocus on other aspects of life. These activities are healthy for our mind and our body. And, they can certainly put the tinnitus in the background. As we sometimes tell our patients, "The more you think about your tinnitus, the more you think about your tinnitus."

To conclude, here are some specific recommendations that can be made to help patients manage their tinnitus:

- Focus on one sensory experience at a time (i.e., reduce all other sensations).
- Explore our world and senses carefully in great detail.
- Do not judge your thoughts and emotions.
- Provide times when we can focus away from the stress in your life (including tinnitus).
- Remember that we have control over our reactions.
- Create times when we are at peace with our situation and life.
- Know that we can experience life positively while having tinnitus.

To demonstrate mindfulness exercises for tinnitus and hyperacusis, we have created a video available on the companion website. This video will provide information on mindfulness to manage tinnitus and hyperacusis with specific relaxation exercises and practice.

References

[1] Noble W, Tyler R. Physiology and phenomenology of tinnitus: implications for treatment. Int J Audiol. 2007; 46 (10):569–574

[2] Tyler RS, Baker LJ. Difficulties experienced by tinnitus sufferers. J Speech Hear Disord. 1983; 48(2):150–154

[3] Tyler RS, Noble W, Coelho C, Roncancio ER, Jun HJ. Tinnitus and hyperacusis. In: Katz J, Chasin M, English K, Hood L, Tillery K, eds. Handbook of clinical audiology. 7th ed. Baltimore, MA: Lippincott Williams & Wilkins; 2015:647–658

[4] Gans J, Cole M, Greenberg B. Sustained benefit of mindfulness-based tinnitus stress reduction (MBTSR) in adults with chronic tinnitus: a pilot study. Mindfulness. 2015; 6(5):1232–1234

[5] Arif M, Sadlier M, Rajenderkumar D, James J, Tahir T. A randomised controlled study of mindfulness meditation versus relaxation therapy in the management of tinnitus. J Laryngol Otol. 2017; 131(6):501–507

[6] Kreuzer PM, Goetz M, Holl M, et al. Mindfulness-and body-psychotherapy-based group treatment of chronic tinnitus: a randomized controlled pilot study. BMC Complement Altern Med. 2012; 12(1):235

[7] Davenport J, Koch LC, Rumrill PD. Mindfulness-based approaches for managing chronic pain: applications to vocational rehabilitation and employment. J Vocat Rehabil. 2017; 47(2):247–258

[8] Calistoga Press. Mindfulness made simple. New York: Fall River Press; 2014

[9] Husain FT, Zimmerman B, Tai Y, et al. Assessing mindfulness-based cognitive therapy intervention for tinnitus using behavioural measures and structural MRI: a pilot study. Int J Audiol. 2019; 58(12):889–901

[10] McKenna L, Marks EM, Vogt F. Mindfulness-based cognitive therapy for chronic tinnitus: evaluation of benefits in a large sample of patients attending a tinnitus clinic. Ear Hear. 2018; 39(2):359–366

[11] Philippot P, Nef F, Clauw L, de Romrée M, Segal Z. A randomized controlled trial of mindfulness-based cognitive therapy for treating tinnitus. Clin Psychol Psychother. 2012; 19(5):411–419

[12] McKenna L, Marks EM, Hallsworth CA, Schaette R. Mindfulness-based cognitive therapy as a treatment for chronic tinnitus: a randomized controlled trial. Psychother Psychosom. 2017; 86(6):351–361

[13] Tyler RS, Gogel SA, Gehringer AK. Tinnitus activities treatment. Prog Brain Res. 2007; 166:425–434

[14] Henry JL, Wilson PH. Tinnitus: a self-management guide for the ringing in your ears. Boston, MA: Allyn & Bacon; 2002

[15] Landis B, Landis E. Is biofeedback effective for chronic tinnitus? An intensive study with seven subjects. Am J Otolaryngol. 1992; 13(6):349–356

[16] Slater R, Terry M. Tinnitus: a guide for sufferers and professionals. New York: Sheridan House, Inc.; 1987

[17] Thabrew H, Ruppeldt P, Sollers JJ, III. Systematic review of biofeedback interventions for addressing anxiety and depression in children and adolescents with long-term physical conditions. Appl Psychophysiol Biofeedback. 2018; 43(3):179–192

[18] Young DW. Biofeedback training in the treatment of tinnitus. In: Tyler RS, ed. Tinnitus handbook. San Diego, CA: Singular Publishing Group; 2000:281–295

[19] Davison GC, Neale JM. Abnormal psychology. 3rd ed. New York: Wiley; 1982

[20] Perreau AE, Tyler RS, Mancini PC, Witt S, Elgandy MS. Establishing a group educational session for hyperacusis patients. Am J Audiol. 2019; 28(2):245–250

[21] Fleshman B, Fryrear JL. The arts in therapy. Chicago: Nelson-Hall; 1981

[22] Van Lith T. Art therapy in mental health: a systematic review of approaches and practices. Arts Psychother. 2016; 47:9–22

[23] Nan JKM, Ho RTH. Effects of clay art therapy on adults outpatients with major depressive disorder: a randomized controlled trial. J Affect Disord. 2017; 217:237–245

[24] Hass-Cohen N, Bokoch R, Clyde Findlay J, Banford Witting A. A four-drawing art therapy trauma and resiliency protocol study. Arts Psychother. 2018; 61:44–56

[25] Blomdahl C, Guregård S, Rusner M, Wijk H. A manual-based phenomenological art therapy for individuals diagnosed with moderate to severe depression (PATd): a randomized controlled study. Psychiatr Rehabil J. 2018; 41(3):169–182

[26] Rubinstein JT, Tyler RS. Electrical suppression of tinnitus. In: Snow J, ed. Tinnitus: theory and management. Hamilton, Canada: B.C. Decker; 2004:326–335

[27] Tyler RS, Ed. The consumer handbook on tinnitus. 2nd ed. Sedona, AZ: Auricle Ink Publishers; 2016

[28] Gutiérrez EOF, Camarena VAT. Music therapy in generalized anxiety disorder. Arts Psychother. 2015; 44:19–24

[29] Argstatter H, Grapp M, Plinkert PK, Bolay HV. Heidelberg neuro-music therapy for chronic-tonal tinnitus: treatment outline and psychometric evaluation. Int Tinnitus J. 2012; 17 (1):31–41

[30] Argstatter H, Grapp M, Hutter E, Plinkert PK, Bolay HV. The effectiveness of neuro-music therapy according to the Heidelberg model compared to a single session of educational counseling as treatment for tinnitus: a controlled trial. J Psychosom Res. 2015; 78(3):285–292

[31] Hutter E, Grapp M, Argstatter H, Bolay HV. Music therapy for chronic tinnitus: variability of tinnitus pitch in the course of therapy. J Am Acad Audiol. 2014; 25(4):335–342

[32] Krick CM, Grapp M, Daneshvar-Talebi J, Reith W, Plinkert PK, Bolay HV. Cortical reorganization in recent-onset tinnitus patients by the Heidelberg Model of Music Therapy. Front Neurosci. 2015; 9:49

[33] Kentish RC, Crocker SR. Scary monsters and waterfalls: tinnitus narrative therapy for children. In: Tyler RS, ed. Tinnitus treatment: clinical protocols. New York: Thieme; 2006:217–229

11 Tinnitus in Children

Mohamed Salah Elgandy and Claudia Coelho

Abstract

Tinnitus assessment and treatment in children has not been studied sufficiently to date. Among audiologists and clinicians, there is no consensus regarding the management of tinnitus in children. Tinnitus counseling can be considered as one of the most basic tools among therapeutic options of tinnitus in children. In this chapter, management of tinnitus in children will be highlighted through a review of the available literature. Also, we will provide a full description of tinnitus for children with regard to etiology, clinical investigation, and possible treatment options.

Keywords: tinnitus, children, pediatrics, etiology, treatment

11.1 Introduction

Tinnitus assessment and treatment in children is often more complicated than in adults; in part because children are often not as vocal or clear about the problems that they are experiencing.[1] Some children might consider their tinnitus as trivial, or because they think they have always had it, it is "normal." As a result, children often do not report tinnitus as a symptom to their parents, and that may lead to a delay in management. Older children with a later onset will face similar challenges as adults do. Many children, however, will not be able to share their symptoms and concerns clearly.

Children who experience tinnitus often suffer in a similar way as adults with tinnitus. Difficulty in thoughts and emotions, concentration, sleeping, and hearing are the most frequent complaints associated with tinnitus in children.[2,3,4] Many will also experience hyperacusis (see Chapter 13).

The symptoms might affect many kinds of leisure activities such as sports,[2] as well as decrease in school performance.[5] These symptoms can significantly interfere with a child's life, in general, which can inevitably affect their entire family and the family dynamic as well.

11.2 Prevalence

In children, most of the data concerning tinnitus has been obtained by means of questionnaires completed by parents. It is difficult to obtain an accurate estimate of the prevalence of tinnitus in children due to difficulties in interviewing children and obtaining reliable information. Children rarely discuss symptoms that are not associated with pain.[6] They may perceive their tinnitus as a familiar experience, some children can be more easily distracted by events of the external environments such as playing, sports practice, and videogames, for example,[7] and some might not perceive the symptom as a health issue.[8] Tinnitus is less frequent among those children with severe hearing loss, and more frequent in children with mild and moderate hearing loss[9] (▶ Table 11.1).

Many different factors may have contributed to the discrepancies between the results of the different studies[10,11,12,13,14] that have been published. These include the criteria for tinnitus, the criteria for hearing loss criteria, the age range of the participants, cultural issues, and various methodological factors.[14]

11.3 Etiology of Tinnitus in Children

Tyler and Smith[15] have suggested certain terms, congenital versus acquired and middle ear versus

Table 11.1 The prevalence of tinnitus in children of different ages and from different countries

Author	Place of study	Number of patients	Age	Diagnostic tool	Prevalence
Nodar[10]	U.S.A.	2,000	10–18	Questionnaire	13.3% normal hearing and 58.6% impaired hearing
Stouffer et al[11]	Canada	161	7–12	Interview	13% in normal hearing and 29% in impaired hearing
Holgers[12]	Sweden	964	7	Questionnaire	13% in normal hearing and 8.8% in hearing impaired
Aksoy et al[13]	Turkey	1,020	6–16	Questionnaire	9.2% tinnitus perception and 5.8% tinnitus annoyance
Coelho et al[14]	Brazil	506	5–12	Interview	37.7% tinnitus perception with normal hearing, 50% hearing impaired and tinnitus annoyance 19% with normal hearing, 17.8% hearing impaired

sensorineural tinnitus, as useful etiological classifications:

- Congenital tinnitus occurs when the tinnitus onset was at birth or infancy, and it is not diagnosed until later in life, perhaps during a conversation with a friend who does not have tinnitus. Graham[16] proposed that a child with congenital tinnitus could habituate to it early.
- Acquired tinnitus develops later in life, and for children, they are often aware that tinnitus represents a change that was not there before. The experience for a child with acquired tinnitus is similar to that of adults in terms of the severity of tinnitus. Many forms of hearing loss, as common as excessive cerumen and otitis media, can cause transitory tinnitus.
  Another approach to classifying tinnitus is to parallel the way we classify hearing loss—conductive versus sensorineural.
- Conductive tinnitus results from obstruction or damage to the outer or middle ear, preventing sound from being conducted to the inner ear.

Nearly all children experience at least one episode of otitis media. Occurrence of tinnitus due to middle ear infection is debatable. One theory is that conductive hearing loss caused by a middle ear effusion attenuates external sounds that normally mask low-level tinnitus. Attenuation of these external sounds "unmasks" an already existing, low-level tinnitus.[17]

Beyond otitis media, other middle ear disorders can result in tinnitus in children. The list of these disorders is long, and includes all tinnitus-inducing middle ear problems of adults (see Chapter 2). As in adults, some forms of middle ear tinnitus represent a more general health problem, such as intracranial tumors. In these cases, treatment of the underlying health condition can alleviate the tinnitus.

Middle ear tinnitus in children can be classified as follows:

Pulsatile middle ear tinnitus includes venous hums, transmitted bruits, glomus tumors, hydrocephalus, and vascular malformation (e.g., dural arteriovenous fistula, dehiscent jugular bulb, aberrant carotid artery, and persistent stapedial artery). Middle ear myoclonus (presumed secondary to abnormal movement of the tensor tympani or stapedius muscles) is usually characterized as a rhythmic, regular or irregular, continuous or intermittent form of pulsatile tinnitus.

Nonpulsatile middle ear tinnitus includes tympanic perforation, ear infections, patulous Eustachian tube, temporomandibular joint disorders, and familial tinnitus.

- Sensorineural hearing loss tinnitus results from damage of the hair cells, the stria vascularis, the cochlear synapses, the spiral ganglion neurons, or more proximal auditory structures. Any change compromising the auditory system in any location can lead to tinnitus.

Tinnitus can also be associated with sensorineural hearing loss from any cause. This is true in adults as well as in children. Children with moderate hearing loss tend to present tinnitus more frequently than children with severe and profound hearing loss according to Coelho et al.[14] Common causes of sensorineural hearing loss in children include head trauma, noise exposure, sudden hearing loss, ototoxic drugs, autoimmune hearing loss, metabolic disorders (including type 2 diabetes or prediabetes), dyslipidemias (high-serum low-density lipoprotein), nutrients deficiency, and malabsorption syndromes (such as celiac disease and lactose intolerance).

- Somatosensory tinnitus is suspected clinically when at least one of the following occurred before the onset of tinnitus: a history of head or neck trauma; recurrent pain in the head, neck, and/or shoulder region; tinnitus occurrence with some manipulations of teeth, jaw, or cervical spine; inadequate posture during rest, sleep walking, and working; or intense periods of bruxism (clench or grind the teeth) during day or night.[18]

The integration of auditory and somatosensory afferents nerves occurs early in the auditory pathway occurs the cochlear nucleus (CN) which is suggested to be a possible site for somatosensory tinnitus modulation.

- Ototoxicity:

Ototoxic drugs such as antibiotics (gentamicin and vancomycin) are sometimes prescribed to children, including newborns. Similar to adults, ototoxic drugs are associated with a risk for hearing loss and tinnitus. Although drug dose is adjusted for small body size, children may be particularly at risk for tinnitus. We have no guarantee against hearing loss and accompanying tinnitus due to ototoxic drugs.

- Recreational noise and music-induced tinnitus:

Children can acquire hearing loss and tinnitus from recreational noise, such as videogames, snowmobiles, water jet skis, gunfire, toys, and/or fireworks.[19] In addition, children are often at risk for music-induced tinnitus as either players or listeners if they are exposed to intense music (> 80 dBA) for long time periods (> 2 or 3 hours) on a routine basis (> 3 or 4 days a week). Segal et al[20] reviewed a retrospective study of 53 cases and stated that 25% of the children (n = 13) who sought health care after being exposed to noise from toys and firecrackers were complaining from tinnitus.

• Musicians:

Hearing loss and tinnitus are not problems solely for rock musicians; they can also develop in classical musicians as well. There is increased risk for hearing loss and tinnitus when the musician is playing next to the sound source, such as another instrument or a loudspeaker, and when they are exposed for several hours over an extended time period. Generally, sound must be above 80 dBA for over 8 hours per day to be considered potentially damaging to hearing. Exposure at higher levels for shorter durations can also cause hearing loss. In fact, single bursts of very intense sound are sufficient to damage hearing and produce tinnitus. It should be appreciated that different children will have different degrees of susceptibly to sound-induced tinnitus, as with adults.[21]

• Concert listeners:

Hearing loss and tinnitus can occur in children who regularly attend or are exposed to loud sounds at concerts and dances, or through personal wearable or nonwearable sound playback systems. Loud concerts can certainly produce damaging noise levels that last for several hours. Yassi et al[22] reported that 60% of attendees reported tinnitus immediately after a concert. Wearable headphones also produce high sound levels that can produce a temporary threshold shift (TTS) and tinnitus.[23]

11.4 Factors that may Promote Tinnitus in Children

Identification of risk factors such as age, hearing loss and noise exposure, plays an important role in understanding the etiology of tinnitus, and might help in understanding the symptoms and develop strategies for the prevention of tinnitus.

11.4.1 Age

Research suggests that, among children, tinnitus loudness and tinnitus annoyance increase with age

by 1.1 times each year.[14] Nodar[10] found that age increases the risk for tinnitus occurrence by 1.2 times. Aksoy et al[13] reported a progressive increase in tinnitus incidence around the age of 13 to 14 years.

11.4.2 Gender

Unlike tinnitus in adults, most epidemiological studies among children showed that there is a higher prevalence of tinnitus among girls with a higher prevalence of anxiety and depressive symptoms.[24] This observation could be related to these findings:
• Girls present a higher tendency to express symptoms than boys, including those related to affective mood disorders[25];
• Spontaneous otoacoustic emissions are more frequent among females[26] and that might be considered as a possible cause of tinnitus;
• Genetic differences among genders are associated with neurotransmitter expressions pursuing an action in the auditory pathway, including serotonin and female reproductive hormones that affect GABA receptors in the brain.[27]

11.4.3 Hearing Loss

Hearing loss, even on a mild degree, could promote tonotopic reorganization of the auditory cortex. Coelho et al[14] reported that tinnitus occurred in 50% of children with slight to mild hearing loss, and in 23.5% of cases with moderate to profound hearing loss. Bothersome tinnitus was classified in 33.8% of the children with minimum to mild hearing loss and in 18.8% with moderate to profound hearing loss. The results suggested that mild hearing loss was a risk factor for tinnitus, with the odds ratio of 1.8 for tinnitus sensation, and 2.4 for bothersome tinnitus. Moderate-to-profound hearing loss was also considered a risk factor, with an odds ratio of 0.5 for tinnitus sensation and 1.1 for bothersome tinnitus.[14] These results suggest that mild hearing loss represents a greater risk to the occurrence of tinnitus sensation and bothersome tinnitus when compared to moderate to profound hearing loss.

11.4.4 Temporary Threshold Shifts

Holgers and Petterson[28] have reported that individuals with TTSs from noise exposure had an odds ratio of 1.4 to present spontaneous tinnitus and 2.0 to noise-induced tinnitus. When comparing participants who sometimes experienced TTS to participants who did not have TTS, the odds ratio was 2.8 to present spontaneous tinnitus and 8.4 to noise induced tinnitus. This indicates that individuals that develop temporary threshold shifts from noise exposure have a higher risk to develop spontaneous and noise-induced tinnitus.

Coelho et al[14] reported that a history of noise exposure was a risk factor for both tinnitus sensation and tinnitus suffering with odds ratio of 1.8 and 2.8, respectively. They found that firecrackers were the most frequent kind of noise exposure. Segal et al[19] stated that exposure to high levels of noise from toys and firecrackers were reported by 25% of children who sought medical care because of noise trauma.

It is clear that noise exposure can cause reorganization on the tonotopic map of the primary auditory cortex. Moreover, activation of the neural plasticity appears to cause tinnitus following noise-induced trauma.[29]

11.4.5 Motion Sickness

Motion sickness was found to be a risk factor for tinnitus sensation with an odds ratio of 1.8. In children, motion sickness has been highly associated with migraine and vestibular symptoms.[30]

11.4.6 Hyperacusis

Tyler and Conrad-Armes[31] described that hyperacusis and tinnitus are related symptoms. Coelho et al[14] showed that hyperacusis was the highest risk factor for tinnitus in children, with an odds ratio of 4.2, but tinnitus was not a risk factor for hyperacusis.

11.5 Criteria of Tinnitus in Children

A variety of terms have been used by children to describe the quality of their tinnitus. They include "ring," "buzz," "hum,"[13] "wheezing," "peeping" or as a "murmur" or "humming," "swishing," and "whistling."[1]

11.6 Impact of Tinnitus on Children and Parents

There is limited literature examining the effects of tinnitus on the health and wellbeing of children. Children often lack the ability to describe their tinnitus. One particular child interpreted his tinnitus

as the sound of a robot and would often incorporate this sound into his play.

Common symptoms reported by children include headache,[3] dizziness and vertigo,[13] interference with sleep,[13] and difficulty with attention and concentration at home and at school.[32] Tiredness was also reported as the precipitating factor for tinnitus in just under half of the children.[13]

Kentish et al[33] reported parental concerns that the tinnitus might be a sign of hearing loss or might cause a hearing loss. They also worried that it might be an indicator of mental health problems, brain tumors, or another neurological condition.

11.7 Evaluation

In general, the evaluation of children with tinnitus parallels that of an adult (see Chapter 12). One exception is that children are frequently less verbal about their health conditions, and on questioning they may attempt to please the health care provider. Therefore, open communication and caution should be exercised during the examination. Children are more likely to omit relevant facts rather than give inaccurate information. However, children can provide accurate information to open-ended questions.[34] Even if the information obtained from a child is segmented, it can help to develop a full picture over time.

11.7.1 History

The presence of tinnitus as with any other auditory symptom should be evaluated fully. It is sometimes thought that asking children specifically about their tinnitus could stir up symptoms that do not bother them. Therefore, allowing tinnitus to be discussed without considering it a distressing issue can be advantageous.

The interview should be conducted in a child-friendly approach and setting. The key is for the professionals to be able to match their interviewing mode and manner to the cognitive and linguistic level of the child. The initial discussion with the child and parent should focus on the child's beliefs and concerns, if they have any, regarding the tinnitus. The child could be encouraged to give a visual representation of the tinnitus such as drawings that can also be informative. Probing questions can help to gather important history about the child and their tinnitus, as described in ▶ Table 11.2.

A systematic review through case history is salient as it can be a great diagnostic tool. For example, if a

Table 11.2 Questions relating to history and possible answers guiding to diagnosis[33]

Questions related to tinnitus	Possible guided answers
What do they sound like?	Buzzing, ringing, wheezing, peeping
What do you do when you have the noise?	Ignoring, consider it normal, play, or sleep
How does the noise affect you?	No effect, headache, vertigo, lack of sleep, tiredness
When is it worse?	For example, at school or home, what about the time of day
Where do you hear the sounds?	In one/both ears or in the head
How long have you heard these sounds?	Chronic tinnitus or recent one

Table 11.3 Maneuvers used for somatic testing[18]

Jaw maneuvers	
Clench teeth together	Performed by the child
Open mouth with restorative pressure	
Protrude jaw with restorative pressure	
Slide jaw to left with restorative pressure	
Slide jaw to right with restorative pressure	

Head and neck maneuvers	
Resist pressure applied to forehead	All performed by the examiner
Resist pressure applied to occiput	
Resist pressure applied to vertex	
Resist pressure applied under mandible	
Resist pressure applied to right temple	
Resist pressure applied to left temple	
Pressure to right zygoma with head turned right	
Pressure to left zygoma with head turned left	
Pressure to left temple with head turned right and tilted to left (left sternocleidomastoid muscle)	
Pressure to right temple with head turned left and tilted to right (right sternocleidomastoid muscle)	

child presents with headache, visual changes, and dizziness, this might guide the physicians and medical team to the diagnosis of a congenital arteriovenous malformation. Patients with fluctuating tinnitus, hearing loss, and vertigo in form of attacks indicate that the child should be seen by a physician for exclusion of Meniere disease. The association of tinnitus to headaches and dizziness could indicate the presence of vestibular migraine. Cranial nerve deficits indicate the possibility of a skull base tumor (i.e., vestibular schwannoma). A history of bloody otorrhea, otalgia, paroxysmal hypertension, and sweating all suggest a diagnosis of glomus tumors (tumors involving the middle ear cavity).

11.7.2 Physical Examination

A complete head and neck examination along with a full neurological evaluation is required when evaluating a child with tinnitus. The tympanic membrane should be inspected thoroughly with examination of movement with respiration to exclude patulous Eustachian tube and myoclonic activity in cases of palatal myoclonus.

Involvement of the middle ear space could indicate aberrant carotid artery (pale red mass located anteriorly behind tympanic membrane), jugular veins (dark blue mass located posteriorly), and vascular middle ear tumors like glomus tympanicum tumors. Fundus examination is critical with associated papilledema in cases of benign intracranial hypertension. Cranial nerve examination with comment on palatal elevation, vocal cord mobility, and

shoulder and neck movement are important items in the diagnosis of glomus jugulare tumors. Finally, changes to the child's posture; presence of tenderness on head, neck, and face muscles as well as temporal mandibular joint (TMJ) with dental inspection and occlusion would raise the hypothesis of somatosensory modulation of tinnitus.[35]

Somatosensory tinnitus can be diagnosed by asking patients to perform a specific movement or resist a pressure applied against their head, shoulders, and jaw. Ralli et al[18] described some maneuvers used for somatic testing and evaluation of tinnitus (see ▶ Table 11.3).

Auscultation of the ear canal including the pre- and postauricular regions, orbit, and neck also are needed to exclude certain conditions such as carotid bruit, jugular venous hums, and arteriovenous malformation.

11.7.3 Audiological

Pure-tone audiometry should be performed to determine presence and nature of a hearing loss. However, this may need to be sensitively performed for those children whose tinnitus is aggravated by a quiet environment (sound-attenuating booth), whose tinnitus is made worse by sound, or who have hyperacusis.

If abnormalities in audiometric studies appear, that should lead us to further diagnostic tools to identify the source of tinnitus. Otoacoustic emission testing can confirm the integrity of outer hair cells whereas the auditory brainstem response tests may indicate more central pathology.

Tympanometry and stapedial reflex testing provide the status of the middle ear and its function, and a distal aspect of the auditory pathway to the superior olive. If middle ear function is normal, stapedial reflex could be considered as a normal stapedial reflex indicating that the lower brainstem is intact. If a stapedius reflex is desirable, then caution should be taken, as loud sounds can make the tinnitus worse, and the child might have hyperacusis.

Assessing loudness discomfort levels (LDLs) may be important in the tinnitus evaluation for a child, as tinnitus is associated to hyperacusis. LDL testing will diagnose the presence of loudness hyperacusis. Normal thresholds in children are around 90 dBHL from 250 to 6000 Hz.[36] Again, caution should be taken, as loud sounds can make the tinnitus worse, and the child might have hyperacusis.

11.7.4 Laboratory Evaluations

A complete laboratory evaluation might be helpful to diagnose some types of tinnitus including:
- Complete blood count (anemia).
- Lipid profile: Total cholesterol, HDL cholesterol, LDL cholesterol, and triglycerides (hyperlipidemia).
- Blood glucose screening: For a youth who is overweight, sedentary with a family history of diabetes and other risk factors, order one of the following tests: Fasting glucose and 2-hour oral glucose tolerance test (OGTT) (in case you have a high suspicious). Hemoglobin A1C also helps to monitor nutritional therapies for the glucose/ insulin resistant youth.
- Chemistry panel: Iron, ferritin, vitamin B12, vitamin D3 and Zinc, sodium and potassium, blood (BUN), creatinine, urine analysis, and thyroid function test: TSH and Free T4.
- Virology work-up: Tinnitus is a frequent symptom associated to sudden hearing loss. A work-up for viral infection should be performed on an individual basis according to the history and clinical findings. ESR, CRP, cytomegalovirus, Rubella, Herpes simplex, Epstein-Barr, HIV, and Lyme disease.[37]
- Serological test: Screening for congenital neurosyphilis through Venereal Disease Research Laboratory (VDRL).

- Autoimmune investigations: If a child presents tinnitus associated to a progressive bilateral and asymmetrical sensorineural hearing loss (SNHL), with threshold fluctuations, developing between 3 and 90 days, an immune-mediated investigation is mandatory. Screening tests for autoimmune disorders include erythrocyte sedimentation rate (ESR), C-reactive protein (CRP), serum immunoglobulins (IgM, IgG, IgA, and IgE), rheumatoid factor (RF), antithyroid antibodies, antinuclear antibodies (ANA), antineutrophil cytoplasmic antibody (ANCA), and antiphospholipid/anticardiolipin antibodies.[38]

11.7.5 Radiological

Tinnitus is a challenging diagnostic dilemma, particularly in the pediatric population. In the adult population, the American Academy of Otolaryngology-Head and Neck Surgery Foundation (AAO-HSNF) guidelines[39] are clear on when imaging is recommended, specifically in cases of pulsatile tinnitus, unilateral hearing loss with tinnitus, and the presence of focal neurological symptoms.[39] Unfortunately, for children with tinnitus, there is little evidence to guide the clinician on the need for imaging studies. Performing a magnetic resonance imaging (MRI) in children with tinnitus is unclear as it may require the use of sedation or anesthesia, and therefore it is costly and involves some risk.

Levi et al[40] reported a study on 34 children with tinnitus and found that among the 25 children with normal hearing thresholds, there were no specific abnormal MRI findings, and in the 9 children with abnormal audiograms, 4 had abnormal MRI findings (44%).

Kerr et al[41] assessed 102 pediatric patients with tinnitus; 53 of them had imaging studies. Twenty of the children with normal hearing thresholds had no inner ear anomalies; thus, no specific MRI findings to suggest inner ear pathology. On the other hand, in children with hearing loss, there was significant incidence of inner ear anomalies (18.2%). Therefore, there is high incidence of abnormal imaging tests in children with tinnitus and hearing loss, suggesting that imaging should be conducted in the evaluation of pediatric patients with tinnitus.

Hegarty and Smith[42] presented a schematic approach regarding the radiological investigation of children with tinnitus:
- Nonpulsatile tinnitus in children with unilateral or bilateral hearing loss could suggest a congenital defect in the cochlea-vestibular

apparatus, such as cochlear dysplasia. Therefore, computed tomography (CT) of temporal bone should be mandatory.

- The absence of any developmental anomalies via a CT with nonpulsating tinnitus might suggest the need for an MRI of the brainstem. This could be diagnostic for an acoustic neuroma associated with neurofibromatosis type 2.
- Children with pulsatile tinnitus, a normal audiogram, and normal otological results should be evaluated with a CT of the head to rule out hydrocephalus.
- Children with pulsatile tinnitus, and otoscopic examination showing a retrotympanic mass diagnosis should be done through CT and MRI which can guide to glomus tumors, aberrant internal carotid artery, persistent stapedial artery, and high riding jugular bulb.
- Patients with nonpulsatile tinnitus and otoscopic and physical examination showing retrotympanic mass might suggest cholesteatoma.

11.8 Preventing Tinnitus in Children

Of course, the prevention of tinnitus is more desirable than treating it. There are at least two causes of tinnitus in children that can be preventable: drug-induced and noise-induced tinnitus. Use of ototoxic mediations should be carefully monitored using drug-specific parameters and we should try to encourage children to report changes in hearing or the onset of tinnitus when acquiring a drug treatment. The potentially harmful consequences of exposure to loud music and noise (continuous and impulse) can be minimized through education on the importance of hearing protection. Modeling the judicious use of hearing protection by siblings, peers, and parents is beneficial. Children who are at risk also can be warned of the implication of the onset of tinnitus; it may be the harbinger of permanent noise-induced hearing loss.

11.9 Treatment Options

11.9.1 Medical Treatment

Unfortunately, there are no magic pills that can cure tinnitus, and no safe medication has been shown to help large numbers of tinnitus patients in controlled investigations.[43] Drug trials have not been performed in children.

The AAO-HNSF guidelines stated that[39] clinicians should not recommend Ginkgo biloba, melatonin, zinc, or other dietary supplements for treating patients with persistent, bothersome tinnitus. However, there are different subtypes of patients that may benefit, which should be appreciated. Several reports in literature described these dietary supplements, for example:

- Dietary supplements such as vitamin B, zinc, and iron and magnesium can be helpful in tinnitus.[44] They are indicated in the presence of deficiency which is often associated to malabsorptive conditions such as lactose intolerance and celiac disease.
- Ginkgo biloba is one of the popular complementary and alternative medicines used by many physicians, but it could decrease tinnitus in some patients with a large trial failed to yield definitive success.[45]

Stapedius myoclonus syndrome is rare and severely affects daily activities such as eating, talking, and walking. It may be treated with anticonvulsant agents with very good result obtained through the addition of botulinum toxin A.[46]

11.9.2 Surgical Treatment

Some forms of middle ear tinnitus such as persistent middle ear effusion, cholesteatoma, and more rarely, vascular tumors need a surgical approach.

Myoclonic activity of both tensor tympani muscle and stapedius muscle can be treated surgically through section of the tensor tympani tendon and stapedial tendons through tympanotomy incision. The decision to perform a surgical treatment should be strongly discussed with parents and indicated only in cases where tinnitus is dramatically affecting the child's quality of life.

Patients with dural arteriovenous fistula can be managed surgically through either ligation of the involved vessel or selective embolization of the feeding vessels.

Patients with skull base neoplasm can be managed surgically as in cases of glomus tumors confined to middle ear that can be managed through middle ear and mastoid approach. On the other hand, skull base tumors with extension to jugular foramen or upper neck can be managed through skull base techniques.

11.9.3 Counseling

Treatment for Young Children

The approach to the management of a young child with sensorineural tinnitus would be as follows:

1. Listen to the concerns of the family, provide reassurance to them, and support. You will want to help the family recognize that the tinnitus is a nonthreatening condition affecting many other children.
2. Identify the potential causes of tinnitus that might include noise exposure, medications, or head injuries. In addition, you should identify the common problems experienced by the child and family when tinnitus first presented or was noticed. It is reasonable that there will be worries experienced by the child and family regarding tinnitus-related difficulties either at home or school. Gabriels[47] noted that, in the management of tinnitus in children, the effect of tinnitus on school and social life must be considered. She reported on one 5-year-old child with tinnitus and hyperacusis who attacked a schoolmate because the friend shouted in his ear.
3. Include parents, siblings, and the entire family in the treatment process. It is imperative that the audiologist engage with (or involve) the family because they need to understand the difficulties and problems that the child faces related to their tinnitus. Because tinnitus is usually subjective, in some situations, it can be difficult for parents to accept their child's complaint.[47]
4. Consider amplification if there is hearing loss present for the child. Children with hearing loss of any degree and sensorineural tinnitus should be fitted with hearing aids. Hearing aids help patients with tinnitus and hearing loss in multiple ways. Amplification not only improves communication abilities and reduces the stress of listening (reducing stress helps the patient cope with tinnitus), amplification of some background noise also facilitates masking of the patient's tinnitus (see Chapters 7 and 8).
5. Involve the child's teachers and other relevant professionals to monitor the child's progress at school with understanding that any associated problems provoking or causing tinnitus will need to be addressed. This may involve management of other underlying educational or psychological concerns.
6. Counseling for tinnitus should be presented at a level that the child finds easy to understand. It is usually important to involve the parents in the discussion of the nature of tinnitus by providing clear simple information. For example, by building on coping skills, incorporating the imagination of child, and providing effective strategies to manage the condition, these coping strategies can be discussed at length with younger and older children who are bothered by tinnitus. Moreover, an audiologist should inquire about the activities that the child with tinnitus might choose to do when their tinnitus gets troublesome. Some children like reading a storybook, listening to music of their choice, or drawing a picture.
7. Psychological approaches such as narrative therapy (see Chapter 5).

Narrative therapy is a form of psychotherapy that seeks to help individuals identify their values and the skills, and the knowledge that they have to live these values. This type of therapy can be used in managing tinnitus in children.[48] More specifically, the therapist seeks to help the child coauthor a new narrative about themselves with the condition or tinnitus included in their story. Narrative therapy claims to be a social justice approach to therapeutic conversations, seeking to challenge the dominant discourses that shape people's lives in destructive ways and investigating the history of those qualities. For example, by role-playing or drawing a picture, the child is encouraged to separate him/herself from the tinnitus and to see that the tinnitus is coming from an outside source that is not scary. This process of separation helps relieve the child from negative thoughts, ideas, and feelings. Once the distress or precipitating situation associated with the tinnitus is addressed, the child learns to habituate to the presence of tinnitus.

Treatment of Older Children

Tinnitus treatment for older children is similar to treatment for adults (see Chapters 4 and 5). When a child does complain of tinnitus, this should be taken seriously. Not only can tinnitus be debilitating, but it can also reflect an underlying treatable disease. Treatment for tinnitus that is provided to adults can be easily adopted for older children.

1. Counseling: General counseling (from physicians and audiologists) can be helpful to assist the child in developing successful coping

strategies to reduce distress and modify maladaptive behaviors. The specific problem which compels children to seek help might be the overwhelming anxiety associated with the risk of suffering a mental breakdown as opposed to solely their tinnitus.

2. Relaxation: The aim of relaxation is to control tension and being able to relax when necessary. This can be used (with or without) tinnitus, and also has the benefit of increasing a child's confidence. Examples of relaxation tools include videos using recorded soft music, deep breathing exercises, body scanning for meditation, etc. These are often best provided by trained persons in that field, though there are many tools available including apps, podcasts, etc. See Chapters 9 and 10 for more information on relaxation and apps for tinnitus relief.

3. Cognitive behavioral modification: Cognitive behavioral therapy (CBT) is usually provided by training the child with tinnitus to cope with the condition, and then changing the way the child thinks about his or her tinnitus. By decreasing the negative thoughts about tinnitus, its annoyance can be minimized. This technique alters the psychological response to tinnitus by identifying and reinforcing coping strategies, and relaxation and distraction techniques. Large studies reported benefit in reducing tinnitus-related distress using CBT for many patients who are bothered by their tinnitus.[49]

4. Tinnitus Activities Treatment includes individualized counseling focused on the four primary functions of daily living that are affected by tinnitus (i.e., thoughts and emotions, hearing, concentration, and sleep) (see Chapter 4). The aim of this therapy is to reach a stage in which patients with tinnitus are unaware of their condition for example, within seconds of entering a room, our brain will ignore a noisy refrigerator unless we consciously focus on it.[50]

5. Sound therapy: Sound therapy involves presenting a background sound to reduce the prominence and loudness of the tinnitus (see Chapter 8). This can be achieved either through wearable hearing devices, a combination device of hearing aids with maskers, or nonwearable devices such as the radio, personal listening devices (IPODs), and compact disc players. Some of these devices including white noise generators and music played through a tablet or speakers can be used to help child to get to sleep.

Types of sounds that can be particularly useful for children include:
- Broad band noise such as white noise, pink noise, or low-frequency Brownian noise.
- Music that might be light classical or simple piano music, or another type that they enjoy.
- Nature sounds such as rain, waterfall, or crickets.

6. Refocus therapy[51]: Many patients focus their attention on their tinnitus. They think about their tinnitus much of the day. The more they think about their tinnitus, the worse it gets and the worse it gets, the more they think about it. This negative thought pattern creates a viscous circle. Tinnitus becomes a critical part of their life where the patient spends much of their time thinking about their tinnitus sound, and focuses on fixing or eliminating the sound in their head.

Refocus therapy aims to redirect the patient's attention away from their tinnitus. For most patients, tinnitus is chronic, and will not go away. Therefore, the focus of this therapy is on finding ways to concentrate on other activities, so we should have the desire to manage it. Frank conversation between patients with tinnitus about other activities in their life that they enjoy is often beneficial in relieving tinnitus. Patients could also be encouraged to develop new interests; the clinician's role here is to help them to put the handicap resulting from their tinnitus in perspective, helping them to focus on other activities in their life and to pay attention to things that they enjoy.

Treatment of Somatosensory Tinnitus

Children presenting somatosensory tinnitus need an evaluation through multidisciplinary team (otolaryngologist, neurologist, physiotherapist, and dentist). Various treatment approaches are available to this type of tinnitus in children.

Relaxing Muscle Tension in the Jaw and Neck

Pediatric patients with temporomandibular disorder often present with muscular tension in both the jaw and neck, as well as tinnitus, vertigo/dizziness, and aural fullness. The first aim of treatment for somatosensory tinnitus is the reduction of such muscular tension. That can be done through regular stretching exercises of their suboccipital (located in the back of the neck) muscles at home, as well as rotation movements in the atlanto-occipital joint (which is the bony connection between the cervical spine and the base of the skull) especially to the restricted side, and relaxing exercises involving breathing with the diaphragm.[52] Wright and Bifano[53] reported an 82.5% improvement of tinnitus in patients whose temporomandibular disorders improved with the use of cognitive therapy, bite splints (a dental device commonly used to prevent tooth wear caused by bruxism) and home exercises.

Manual Therapies (Cervical Manipulation)

It seems that some somatosensory tinnitus could be alleviated by correcting the misalignment of the cervical spine through manual therapy (chiropractic or osteopathy), especially in the upper cervical region. Such readjustment might allow the entire spine to reposition itself and possibly readjust the input of the region through the somatosensory pathway on the auditory system.

Alcantara et al[54] described how chiropractic treatment could reduce tinnitus, vertigo, and hearing loss in a patient with cervical subluxation and temporomandibular disorder. Symptoms eventually ceased after some sessions.

Myofascial Trigger Point (MTP) Deactivation

Many techniques dealing with MTP relief have been published, but few of them had been supported by scientific evidence. The most commonly used treatment procedures for myofascial pain syndrome were reviewed by Vernon and Schneider[55] who showed that they were supported by evidence. The duration of relief fluctuates across therapies.

Rocha and Sanchez[56] reported a patient who experienced improvement in tinnitus, dizziness, and chronic facial and cervical pain after having her MTP deactivated by pressure release and after having a home exercise program (muscle stretching, postural guidance, and hot pack).

Tinnitus Modulation Through Repeated Training Exercise

Exercise, in general, may be beneficial because it increases brain-derived neurotrophic factor. Training with repetitive movements generates specific neurophysiological changes through the activation of neural plasticity. Activation of neural plasticity has been proved to have therapeutic effects on many disorders, such as vestibular diseases and tinnitus.[57] Exercises should be encouraged for children with tinnitus.

Treatment of Tonic Tensor Tympani Syndrome

Treatment of Tonic Tensor Tympani Syndrome (TTTS) is an involuntary condition where the centrally mediated reflex threshold for tensor tympani muscle activity is lowered, resulting in a frequent spasm.[58] Symptoms consistent with TTTS can include: a sharp stabbing pain in the ear; a dull earache; tinnitus, often with a clicking,[58] rhythmic or buzzing quality; a sensation of aural pressure or blockage and tympanic flutter.[59] Pain/numbness/burning around the ear, along the cheek and the side of the neck; mild vertigo and nausea; a sensation of "muffled," or distorted hearing[60] and headache. Any of these symptoms could affect children quality of life.

TTTS symptom desensitization can be achieved using a similar approach to hyperacusis treatment, with the addition of CBT strategies to reframe maladaptive beliefs, and manage auditory and TTTS symptom hypervigilance.[61]

11.10 Conclusion

Tinnitus in children may be distressing for some children, but not all. In addition to the primary functions of thoughts and emotions, hearing, sleep, and concentration, children with disturbing tinnitus can also require assistance with social, school, and behavioral issues. Tinnitus in children needs to be addressed and appropriately managed to avoid adverse consequences on a child's health and wellbeing. Tinnitus can often be prevented early with education about the use of hearing protection, and the acknowledgment that some drugs are ototoxic and monitoring the potential for tinnitus could be wise.

To illustrate the experience of children with tinnitus, this chapter also has an interview with a parent of a child with tinnitus, available on the companion website.

References

[1] Aust G. Tinnitus in childhood. Int Tinnitus J. 2002; 8(1): 20–26

[2] Coelho CB, Sanchez TG, Tyler RS. Tinnitus in children and associated risk factors. Prog Brain Res. 2007; 166:179–191

[3] Martin K, Snashall S. Children presenting with tinnitus: a retrospective study. Br J Audiol. 1994; 28(2):111–115

[4] Savastano M. Characteristics of tinnitus in childhood. Eur J Pediatr. 2007; 166(8):797–801

[5] Drukier GS. The prevalence and characteristics of tinnitus with profound sensori-neural hearing impairment. Am Ann Deaf. 1989; 134(4):260–264

[6] Graham J. Tinnitus aurium. Acta Otolaryngol. 1965; Suppl 202:24–26

[7] Viani LG. Tinnitus in children with hearing loss. J Laryngol Otol. 1989; 103(12):1142–1145

[8] Savastano M. A protocol of study for tinnitus in childhood. Int J Pediatr Otorhinolaryngol. 2002; 64(1):23–27

[9] Graham JM. Tinnitus in children with hearing loss. Ciba Found Symp. 1981; 85:172–192

[10] Nodar R. Tinnitus aurium in school age children: a survey. J Aud Res. 1972; 12:133–135

[11] Stouffer JL, Tyler RS, Both JC, Buckrell B. Tinnitus in normal-hearing and hearing-impaired children. In: Aran JM, Dauman R, eds. Tinnitus. Amsterdam/New York: Kugler; 1992:255–259

[12] Holgers KM. Tinnitus in 7-year-old children. Eur J Pediatr. 2003; 162(4):276–278

[13] Aksoy S, Akdogan O, Gedikli Y, Belgin E. The extent and levels of tinnitus in children of central Ankara. Int J Pediatr Otorhinolaryngol. 2007; 71(2):263–268

[14] Coelho CB, Sanchez TG, Tyler R. Tinnitus in children and associated risk factors. In: Langguth B, Hajak G, Kleinjung T, Cacace A, Moller A, eds. Tinnitus: pathophysiology and treatment. Amsterdam: Elsevier, BY; 2007:185–200

[15] Tyler RS, Smith RJ. Management of tinnitus in children. In: Newton VE, ed. Pediatric audiological medicine. Philadelphia, PA: Whurr Publishers; 2002:397–404

[16] Graham JM. Tinnitus in children with hearing loss. In: Vernon JA, Moller AR, eds. Mechanisms of tinnitus. Needham Heights, MA: Simon & Schuster; 1995:51–56

[17] Leonard G, Black FO, Schramm VL. Tinnitus in children. In: Bluestone CD, Stool SE, eds. Pediatric otolaryngology. Philadelphia: WB Saunders; 1983:271–277

[18] Ralli M, Greco A, Turchetta R, Altissimi G, de Vincentiis M, Cianfrone G. Somatosensory tinnitus: current evidence and future perspectives. J Int Med Res. 2017; 45(3):933–947

[19] Rytzner B, Rytzner C. Schoolchildren and noise: the 4 kHz dip-tone screening in 14391 schoolchildren. Scand Audiol. 1981; 10(4):213–216

[20] Segal S, Eviatar E, Lapinsky J, Shlamkovitch N, Kessler A. Inner ear damage in children due to noise exposure from toy cap pistols and firecrackers: a retrospective review of 53 cases. Noise Health. 2003; 5(18):13–18

[21] Greinwald JH, Taggart TR. Environmentally induced hearing impairment: the impact of genetics. Curr Opin Otolaryngol Head Neck Surg. 2002; 10(5):346–349

[22] Yassi A, Pollock N, Tran N, Cheang M. Risks to hearing from a rock concert. Can Fam Physician. 1993; 39:1045–1050

[23] Lee PC, Senders CW, Gantz BJ, Otto SR. Transient sensorineural hearing loss after overuse of portable headphone cassette radios. Otolaryngol Head Neck Surg. 1985; 93(5):622–625

[24] Holgers K, Svedlund C. Tinnitus in childhood. J Psychosom Res. 2003; 55(2):135

[25] Eley TC, Lichtenstein P, Stevenson J. Sex differences in the etiology of aggressive and nonaggressive antisocial behavior: results from two twin studies. Child Dev. 1999; 70(1):155–168

[26] Burns EM, Arehart KH, Campbell SL. Prevalence of spontaneous otoacoustic emissions in neonates. J Acoust Soc Am. 1992; 91(3):1571–1575

[27] Tremere LA, Jeong JK, Pinaud R. Estradiol shapes auditory processing in the adult brain by regulating inhibitory transmission and plasticity-associated gene expression. J Neurosci. 2009; 29(18):5949–5963

[28] Holgers KM, Pettersson B. Noise exposure and subjective hearing symptoms among school children in Sweden. Noise Health. 2005; 7(27):27–37

[29] Robertson D, Irvine DR. Plasticity of frequency organization in auditory cortex of guinea pigs with partial unilateral deafness. J Comp Neurol. 1989; 282(3):456–471

[30] Uneri A, Turkdogan D. Evaluation of vestibular functions in children with vertigo attacks. Arch Dis Child. 2003; 88(6): 510–511

[31] Tyler RS, Conrad-Armes D. The determination of tinnitus loudness considering the effects of recruitment. J Speech Hear Res. 1983; 26(1):59–72

[32] Davis AC. The prevalence of hearing impairment and reported hearing disability among adults in Great Britain. Int J Epidemiol. 1989; 18(4):911–917

[33] Kentish RC, Crocker SR, McKenna L. Children's experience of tinnitus: a preliminary survey of children presenting to a psychology department. Br J Audiol. 2000; 34(6):335–340

[34] Fitzpatrick G, Reder P, Lucey C. The child's perspective. In: Reder P, Lucey C, eds. Assessment in parenting: psychiatric and psychological contributions. London: Routledge; 1951

[35] Gelb H, Bernstein I. Clinical evaluation of two hundred patients with temporomandibular joint syndrome. J Prosthet Dent. 1983; 49(2):234–243

[36] Coelho CB, Sanchez TG, Tyler RS. Hyperacusis, sound annoyance, and loudness hypersensitivity in children. Prog Brain Res. 2007; 166:169–178

[37] Pitaro J, Bechor-Fellner A, Gavriel H, Marom T, Eviatar E. Sudden sensorineural hearing loss in children: etiology, management, and outcome. Int J Pediatr Otorhinolaryngol. 2016; 82:34–37

[38] Agrup C. Immune-mediated audiovestibular disorders in the paediatric population: a review. Int J Audiol. 2008; 47(9): 560–565

[39] Tunkel DE, Bauer CA, Sun GH, et al. Clinical practice guideline: tinnitus executive summary. Otolaryngol Head Neck Surg. 2014; 151(4):533–541

[40] Levi E, Bekhit EK, Berkowitz RG. Magnetic resonance imaging findings in children with tinnitus. Ann Otol Rhinol Laryngol. 2015; 124(2):126–131

[41] Kerr R, Kang E, Hopkins B, Anne S. Pediatric tinnitus: incidence of imaging anomalies and the impact of hearing loss. Int J Pediatr Otorhinolaryngol. 2017; 103:147–149

[42] Hegarty JL, Smith R. Tinnitus in children. In: Tyler RS, ed. Handbook on tinnitus. San Diego, CA: Singular Publishing Group; 2000:243–261

[43] Murai K, Tyler RS, Harker LA, Stouffer JL. Review of pharmacologic treatment of tinnitus. Am J Otol. 1992; 13(5): 454–464

[44] Baguley D, McFerran D, Hall D. Tinnitus. Lancet. 2013; 382 (9904):1600–1607

[45] Rejali D, Sivakumar A, Balaji N. Ginkgo biloba does not benefit patients with tinnitus: a randomized placebo-controlled double-blind trial and meta-analysis of randomized trials. Clin Otolaryngol Allied Sci. 2004; 29(3):226–231

[46] Liu HB, Fan JP, Lin SZ, Zhao SW, Lin Z. Botox transient treatment of tinnitus due to stapedius myoclonus: case report. Clin Neurol Neurosurg. 2011; 113(1):57–58

[47] Gabriels P. Children with tinnitus. In: Reich GE, Vernon JA, eds. Proceedings of the Fifth International Tinnitus Seminar. Portland, OR: American Tinnitus Association; 1996: 270–274

[48] Sween E. The one-minute question: what is narrative therapy? Some working answers. In: Denborough D, White C, eds. Extending narrative therapy: a collection of practice-based papers. Adelaide: Dulwich Centre Publications; 1999:191–194

[49] Zachriat C, Kröner-Herwig B. Treating chronic tinnitus: comparison of cognitive-behavioural and habituation-based treatments. Cogn Behav Ther. 2004; 33(4):187–198

[50] Berry JA, Gold SL, Frederick EA, Gray WC, Staecker H. Patient-based outcomes in patients with primary tinnitus undergoing tinnitus retraining therapy. Arch Otolaryngol Head Neck Surg. 2002; 128(10):1153–1157

[51] Tyler RS, Erlandsson S. Management of the tinnitus patient. In: LuXon LM, Furman JM, Martini A, Stephens D, eds. Textbook of audiological medicine. London: Martin Dunitz; 2003:571–578

[52] Björne A. Assessment of temporomandibular and cervical spine disorders in tinnitus patients. Prog Brain Res. 2007; 166:215–219

[53] Wright EF, Bifano SL. Tinnitus improvement through TMD therapy. J Am Dent Assoc. 1997; 128(10):1424–1432

[54] Alcantara J, Plaugher G, Klemp DD, Salem C. Chiropractic care of a patient with temporomandibular disorder and atlas subluxation. J Manipulative Physiol Ther. 2002; 25(1):63–70

[55] Vernon H, Schneider M. Chiropractic management of myofascial trigger points and myofascial pain syndrome: a systematic review of the literature. J Manipulative Physiol Ther. 2009; 32(1):14–24

[56] Rocha CACB, Sanchez TG. Tinnitus modulation by myofascial triggers points and its disappearance by treatment of the myofascial pain syndrome: an interesting result. In: Langguth B, ed. Abstracts of the Second Meeting of Tinnitus Research Initiative. Monaco: University of Regensburg; 2007: 49

[57] Vaynman S, Gomez-Pinilla F. License to run: exercise impacts functional plasticity in the intact and injured CNS by using neurotrophins. Neurorehabil Neural Repair. 2005; 19:283–295

[58] Klockhoff I. Tensor tympani syndrome: a source of vertigo. Uppsala, Sweden: Meeting of Barany Society; 1978

[59] Ellenstein A, Yusuf N, Hallett M. Middle ear myoclonus: two informative cases and a systematic discussion of myogenic tinnitus. Tremor & Other Hyperkinetic Movements (N Y), 2013:3

[60] Riga M, Xenellis J, Peraki E, Ferekidou E, Korres S. Aural symptoms in patients with temporomandibular joint disorders: multiple frequency tympanometry provides objective evidence of changes in middle ear impedance. Otol Neurotol. 2010; 31(9):1359–1364

[61] Westcott M. (2010). Hyperacusis: a clinical perspective on management. Tinnitus Discovery: Asia and Pacific Tinnitus Symposium, Auckland, 123, 1311

12 Measuring Tinnitus and Reactions to Tinnitus

Ann Perreau, Patricia C. Mancini, and Richard S. Tyler

Abstract

Tinnitus outcome measures are useful in clinical settings to guide treatment decisions, demonstrate the impact of tinnitus on everyday functioning, and monitor effectiveness of intervention. This chapter outlines how to measure tinnitus using psychoacoustic measures and reactions to tinnitus using questionnaires of tinnitus severity. We also emphasize use of open-ended questionnaires and diaries to document patient-specific concerns. We conclude with a review of quality-of-life scales and specific questionnaires on problems related to tinnitus such as depression, anxiety, and sleep. Given the vast number of tinnitus measurements available to the audiologist or clinician, the selection of the "optimal" measurement tool depends on the intended purposes of the test and more than one tool is often needed. By incorporating multiple measurement tools, we can have a comprehensive understanding of the patient's tinnitus and its related problems.

Keywords: tinnitus, questionnaires, tinnitus assessment, psychoacoustic measurement, quality-of-life scales

12.1 Introduction

As audiologists, we are trained to measure hearing. It is often the first skill we learn in graduate school—conducting a hearing test. Therefore, we often begin treatment for a patient with hearing loss by measuring hearing thresholds, testing word recognition ability, etc. Likewise, in the area of tinnitus management, audiologists often want to begin their therapy by first measuring their patient's tinnitus. Though measurement of tinnitus is important, it is not always clear where we should begin, and how to apply these results to the treatment of tinnitus. This chapter will outline methods of measuring tinnitus and reactions to tinnitus and provide a general framework for assessing tinnitus in a clinical setting.

One of the first questions to be asked is: Why is measurement important? Though we know the reasons for conducting a hearing test that include treatment planning, providing a diagnosis, and disease monitoring, the rationale for measuring tinnitus and its reactions in the clinic can be less clear to audiologists who are unfamiliar with these procedures. These reasons for conducting measurements of tinnitus are similar, and include[1]:

- To guide treatment decisions (e.g., hearing aid vs. tinnitus sound generator).
- To show the patient and partners that tinnitus is real.
- To demonstrate the acoustic characteristics of the patient's tinnitus.
- To understand the problems associated with tinnitus and identify areas to address.
- To track the effectiveness of treatment.

Our research indicates that tinnitus is not often discussed by patients with their partners.[2] Measuring the tinnitus and sharing that with partners provides validation of the problems reported by the tinnitus patient. In addition, tinnitus may be a problem in the patient's life that exists in a larger context of other challenges. By administering a questionnaire to the patient, we will know what problems they are experiencing, and how we might be able to help them. It is our recommendation that tinnitus measures be administered pre- and post-treatment by establishing a baseline, and repeating the measurement (i.e., 3 or 6 mo later). By obtaining measurements before and after intervention (often at multiple intervals such as every 1–2 months during therapy), the audiologist can monitor patient progress and demonstrate evidence of treatment effectiveness. This can be powerful to patients, partners, and will be one means of securing insurance reimbursement going forward. In our own clinical experience, we incorporate multiple methods of tinnitus measurement for a given patient. By using more than one measurement of tinnitus, we are more likely to have a comprehensive understanding of the patient's tinnitus and their problems related to tinnitus. Lastly, tinnitus measurements may vary across patients for many reasons. However, it is advised that audiologists select the appropriate measures and be consistent in their administration to develop a standardized procedure in the tinnitus clinic.

Four broad areas of measurement will be covered in this chapter: (a) differentiating and evaluating methods of tinnitus measurement (e.g., psychoacoustic measures) and the patient's reactions to

Table 12.1 Measurements of tinnitus, reactions to tinnitus, quality of life, and related problems

Area of measurement	Method of measurement	Procedure/Questionnaire
Measuring tinnitus	Psychoacoustic measures	Pitch matching
		Loudness matching
		Minimum masking level (MML)
		Residual inhibition
	Tinnitus magnitude estimation	Tinnitus qualities rated using a numerical, categorical, or visual analog scale
Measuring reactions to tinnitus	Established questionnaires	Tinnitus Questionnaire
		Tinnitus Handicap Questionnaire
		Tinnitus Reaction Questionnaire
		Tinnitus Handicap Inventory
		Tinnitus Functional Index
		Tinnitus Primary Functions Questionnaire
	Open-ended	Tinnitus Problems Questionnaire
		Client Oriented Scale of Improvement in Tinnitus (COSIT)
	Other	Patient Diary
		Tinnitus intake questionnaire (U of Iowa)
Measuring quality of life	Generic	EQ-5D
		SF-36
		WHO DAS 2.0
		Meaning of life
Measuring related problems	Specific	Beck Depression Inventory
		State-Trait Anxiety Inventory
		Pittsburgh Quality Sleep Index
		Insomnia Severity Index

tinnitus (e.g., questionnaires of tinnitus severity or handicap); (b) analyzing the advantages of open-ended questionnaires and patient diaries in tinnitus management; (c) comparing generic questionnaires that assess quality of life; and (d) reviewing specific questionnaires on tinnitus-related problems such as depression, anxiety, and sleep. ▶ Table 12.1 displays these four areas of tinnitus measurement and the specific assessments associated with each broad area of measurement.

12.2 Measuring Tinnitus

A discussion about tinnitus measurement should start with a review of psychoacoustics. Sound has four physical characteristics that correlate with four perceptual characteristics measured using different scales. For example, sound frequency (Hz) relates to its pitch (mels), duration relates to the perceived duration (msec) of sound, sound intensity (dB) relates to loudness (phons, or sones when equated to a 1000-Hz tone presented at 40 dBSPL),

and spectral aspects of the sound relate to its quality. These aspects of sound are important to consider in tinnitus measurement because the internal tinnitus sound that patients hear will vary along these four dimensions. The pitch, onset, loudness, and quality of tinnitus will be unique for each patient. Performing psychoacoustic measurements of tinnitus will determine these aspects of the patient's tinnitus that can be used for clinical decision-making or for counseling.

It is important to recall that our perception of sound is influenced by many factors, including the method of presentation (i.e., headphones vs. sound field), the testing method used to assess hearing (e.g., bracketing procedure), and specific listener variables (e.g., mental state, motivation). These factors affect the responses gathered from a patient, and ways to control variability and develop standardized procedures for tinnitus measurement are encouraged. We have developed psychoacoustic procedures for measuring tinnitus, which are described here.

12.2.1 Psychoacoustic Measurements

The psychoacoustic measurements include pitch matching, loudness matching, the minimum masking level, and residual inhibition. We perform these four psychoacoustic measurements in a sound-treated booth using a clinical audiometer. It is advisable to have a high-frequency audiometer and headphones because many patients have high-frequency tinnitus extending above 8000 Hz that cannot be measured with traditional TDH or insert earphones. Psychoacoustic measurements should generally be obtained in the ear in which the patient experiences tinnitus, to avoid differences between ears (e.g., diplacusis). If the patient has bilateral tinnitus that is similar across ears, we often present the test signals in one ear (i.e., the right ear) based on time constraints in a clinical setting. The choice of presenting to one or both ears, of course, depends on the purpose of the measurements.

Regarding pitch matching, some patients will relate their tinnitus to a pure tone signal, though not all. For patients whose tinnitus is not like a pure tone, tinnitus still often has a distinct pitch or prominent pitch that is heard.[1] Tinnitus pitch can be measured using a pure-tone stimulus (1000 Hz) presented at a supra-threshold level (e.g., 50 dBHL for normal hearing listeners). We use pulsed tones for measuring tinnitus pitch because the pitch of a sound is influenced by the duration of the sound. Longer tones may change the pitch percept; shorter signals such as pulsed tones are desired for tinnitus measurements. Potential loudness adaptation can also influence the pitch match. We also use a bracketing procedure for measuring tinnitus pitch ascending or descending in ½ octave steps (Hz), similar to bracketing a hearing threshold. Patients respond in a clear manner during the test by saying "my tinnitus is lower" or "my tinnitus is higher" than the tone. We stop the procedure when there is a tone that is closest to the patient's perceived pitch. The last frequency presented that is reported as lower than their perceived tone is recorded as the pitch match. Because tinnitus pitch may be variable, we have suggested repeating this measurement up to six times to establish a reliable pitch match.[3]

Like pitch matching, the loudness of the patient's tinnitus can be matched using a bracketing procedure. Here, we present a pulsed, 500-Hz tone at the patient's hearing threshold in the right or left ear and the pulsed tone is increased in 2-dB steps until the patient reports that their tinnitus is softer than the presented tone. Patients respond to each presentation by either saying "my tinnitus is louder" or "my tinnitus is softer" than the tone. We have emphasized the importance of measuring the patient's hearing threshold for the masking stimuli, especially if the results of loudness balancing are reported in sensation level.[3] Other methods for quantifying tinnitus loudness include converting the loudness of the tinnitus to sones.[3]

For measuring the maskability of tinnitus, the minimum masking level can be determined using the procedure here, or the one outlined by Searchfield (see Chapter 8). Briefly, we first measure the patient's hearing threshold for a pulsed, speech-shaped noise (not a pure tone like for pitch or loudness matching). The speech-shaped noise is then presented at hearing threshold, and an ascending method of limits using 2-dB steps is used to determine the level (in dBHL) where tinnitus is masked. Patients respond to the stimulus by saying "I can hear my tinnitus" or "I cannot hear my tinnitus." We do not exceed 80 dBHL because, for some patients, tinnitus cannot be masked.[4]

Due to the variability in the patient's tinnitus and how their tinnitus interacts with the stimuli, it is recommended that tinnitus measurements be replicated using several trials.[3] For tinnitus pitch matching, loudness matching, and the minimum masking level, the measurements are often collected three times, and the average of all three trials is computed. As described by Tyler et al,[3] the audiologist might consider recording the results of each trial in the patient's chart to illustrate the variability in these measurements. If the first trial is an outlier compared to the consecutive trials, a fourth trial is completed and the average is calculated based on the final three trials with the outlier excluded.

Prior to measuring the residual inhibition for a masker, we determine the masking effect for both ears, which is helpful for measuring residual inhibition. Using a broadband masking signal, such as speech-shaped noise, we measure the amount of residual inhibition of the patient's tinnitus for one minute. The level of the noise is set approximately 10 dBHL above the patient's minimum masking level to ensure adequate masking of the tinnitus with a high-level masker.[4] Residual inhibition is measured by asking the patient if their tinnitus sounds the same or different after presentation of the masker. If different, we categorize the patient's response into one of five postmasking effects. Tyler et al[4] reported that there were five different postmasking responses for the 10 subjects tested: (a) tinnitus immediately returned to its premasker loudness, (b) a partial suppression of tinnitus that gradually returned to its premasker loudness, (c) a complete suppression of tinnitus that gradually returned to its premasker level, (d) a complete suppression of tinnitus that returned to its premasker loudness more abruptly, and (e) an increase in tinnitus loudness that gradually returned to its premasker loudness. Finally, we also assess the timeline over which the tinnitus changed (e.g., how many minutes and seconds for the tinnitus to return to its premasker loudness). These results can be particularly useful in determining who might benefit from sound therapy based on if the patient's tinnitus can be masked and/or a partial to complete suppression of tinnitus occurs when a broadband masker is presented.

The four psychoacoustic measures are typically conducted by audiologists during a tinnitus evaluation and can be reimbursed by many U.S. insurance carriers using the Current Procedural Terminology (CPT) code 92625: Assessment of Tinnitus.[3] Because there is no standardized procedure for evaluating tinnitus, it is difficult to obtain reliable data across tinnitus patients and clinics.[5] Therefore, in addition to describing our procedures, we provided a rationale to explain why we conduct psychoacoustic measurements of tinnitus using this protocol to facilitate a more unified approach. See Appendix 12.1 for clinician instructions on performing and recording these psychoacoustic measurements.

The perceptual qualities of tinnitus pitch, loudness (i.e., the most common), annoyance, etc., can be also assessed by obtaining magnitude estimations using single questions. For example, a patient could complete a single question on the loudness of their tinnitus and rate the loudness using a numerical rating scale from 0 = very faint to 100 = very loud. For single questions, we suggest a numerical rating scale from 0 to 100 because it provides a large range for adequate resolution and is closely related to familiar scales to patients such as dollars/cents. In a numerical scale from 0 to 100, patients will often use 5- or 10-point intervals for rating qualities that produces 21 distinct points. Other scales implemented are ordinal scales that use categories (e.g., "yes," "no," "sometimes"), or a visual analog scale where the patient marks on a line (however, this requires measurement of the distance along a 10-point line). We prefer interval scales that have less linguistic ambiguity ("sometimes" may not be interpreted similarly for all patients and the difference between "yes" and "sometimes" might not be the same value as between "sometimes"

and "no")[6] and more intervals rather than fewer for better resolution.[7]

12.2.2 Measuring Reactions to Tinnitus

The clinical practice guidelines for managing patients with tinnitus[8] strongly recommend that audiologists distinguish between patients who have bothersome tinnitus from those with non-bothersome tinnitus. Though we might debate what constitutes bothersome versus nonbothersome tinnitus, the point of this recommendation is that audiologists should incorporate established questionnaires into their clinical practice to measure their patient's reactions to tinnitus and take action (e.g., make a referral to a psychologist). We know that tinnitus can cause sleep disturbances, emotional problems, hearing and communication difficulties, and problems with concentration.[9] These effects vary from patient to patient. Knowing the areas that are impacted and the severity of the problem is important to provide adequate treatment to the patient. There are many validated, established questionnaires available for measuring a patient's reactions to tinnitus (a review can be found in Newman et al).[5] ▶ Table 12.2 lists several established questionnaires that are easily available to audiologists.

- The Tinnitus Questionnaire (TQ)[10] was designed to assess the psychological effects of tinnitus for patients who might benefit from cognitive behavioral therapy. The TQ has 52 items that spread over five factors relating to tinnitus distress (see Chapter 6 by McKenna for a review). A three-point ordinal scale ("true," "partly true," "not true") is used to score the patient's responses. The TQ is useful for screening patients who are seeking services at a tinnitus or hearing clinic,[11] though it was not intended to be a measurement of tinnitus handicap or coping strategies. The TQ has been translated into several languages, including German, and psychometric evaluation studies suggest it is a valid, reliable measure of tinnitus-related distress.[12,13]
- Tinnitus Handicap Questionnaire (THQ; see Appendix 12.2)[14] measures emotional, behavioral, and general health effects of tinnitus. There are a few items that relate to beliefs about tinnitus in a more general sense. The THQ consists of 27 items and has a high reliability of 0.94. A total score is derived from the average of all 27 items, and three subscale scores can also

Table 12.2 Questionnaires to measure the patient's reactions to tinnitus

Questionnaire	Purpose	Items and subscales	Rating scale
Tinnitus Questionnaire[10]	To assess psychological effects of tinnitus	52 items (sleep disturbance, emotional distress, auditory perceptual difficulties, inappropriate or lack of coping skills)	Level of agreement to each statement (true = 2 points; partly true = 1 point; not true = 0 points). Score range: 0–104 points with higher scores reflecting greater tinnitus complaints
Tinnitus Handicap Questionnaire[14]	To assess tinnitus severity	27 items in 3 factors: Factor 1 (physical, emotional, social consequences of tinnitus); Factor 2 (effects on hearing); and Factor 3 (patient's view of tinnitus)	Level of agreement to each statement (0–100; 0=completely disagree; 100=completely agree). Mean scores calculated with higher scores reflecting greater handicap (need to invert scores from items 25 and 26)
Tinnitus Reaction Questionnaire[16]	To assess emotional effects	26 items in 6 domains (distress consequences including anger, confusion, annoyance, help-lessness, activity avoidance, and panic)	Five-point scale (0=not at all; 4=almost all of the time) Score range: 0–104 with higher scores reflecting greater distress
Tinnitus Handicap Inventory[20]	To assess tinnitus severity and impact on daily life	25 items in 3 subscales (functional, emotional, and catastrophic)	Response to each statement with yes (4 points), sometimes (2 points), or no (0 points) Higher scores reflect greater handicap
Tinnitus Functional Index[22]	To assess the negative impact of tinnitus as well as to meas-ure treatment-related changes (responsiveness)	25 items in 8 subscales (intru-sive; sense of control; cognitive; sleep; auditory; relaxation; quality of life; emotional)	11-point scale (0–10) with anchors varying per item All responses are summed, divided by number of questions answered, and multiplied by 10 Score range: 0–100
Tinnitus Primary Functions Questionnaire[23]	To evaluate the primary func-tions affected by tinnitus	12 items and 4 subscales (thoughts and emotions, hearing, sleep, and concentration)	Level of agreement to each statement (0–100; 0 = completely disagree; 100 = completely agree) Higher scores reflect greater tinnitus complaints

be calculated. The subscales relate to the physical, emotion, social consequences of tinnitus, and hearing-related changes. The THQ is typically completed by most patients in 5 to 10 minutes. The psychometric validation study found that the THQ correlated moderately high with similar measures of tinnitus distress, including tinnitus loudness magnitude (0–100 rating scale), average hearing thresholds, and scales of life satisfaction, depression, and health status.[14] The test-retest reliability of the THQ was independently tested and found to be high[15] for the total score, and Factor 1 and 2 subscales.

• Tinnitus Reaction Questionnaire (TRQ)[16] also measures the emotional effects of tinnitus. It consists of 26 items that are rated on a five-point ordinal scale ("not at all" to "almost all of the time"), and though the TRQ emphasizes emotional distress and the ability to cope with

tinnitus, it contains items on cognitive effects, avoidance, handicap, and sleep. The TRQ has high test-retest reliability ($r = 0.88$), and though some of the item-total correlations were low (0.44), it has moderate to high correlations with other measures including the State-Trait Anxiety Inventory[17] and the Beck Depression Inventory.[18] There are some patients who have a negative reaction to some of the TRQ items such as "tinnitus has led me to think about suicide."[19]

• Tinnitus Handicap Inventory (THI)[20] was developed to determine the impact of tinnitus symptoms on a tinnitus patient's daily life. The THI is one of the most commonly used tinnitus questionnaires internationally because it has been translated into at least 15 languages (including Spanish, French, and Chinese). The THI has 25 items and three subscales that relate to functional impairments (e.g., limitations in social and physical functioning), emotional distress (e.g., anger, frustration, depression, annoyance), and catastrophic response (e.g., desperation, loss of control, inability to cope). The THI uses a three-point ordinal scale for scoring patient's responses (e.g., "yes," "sometimes," "no") and the total score indicates the severity of the tinnitus handicap ranging from no handicap to severe. The THI was shown to have high reliability (0.93), but weak correlations with other measures such as the Beck Depression Inventory,[18] the Modified Somatic Perception questionnaire,[21] and pitch and loudness magnitude estimations.[20]

- Tinnitus Functional Index (TFI)[22] was designed to measure tinnitus severity and the negative consequences of tinnitus, and to assess outcomes from treatment. The TFI was developed by a group of tinnitus researchers and clinicians and tested across multiple US tinnitus clinics. The TFI includes 25 items with eight subscales: intrusive, sense of control, cognitive, sleep, auditory, relaxation, quality of life, and emotions, and is scored on a numerical scale from 0 to 10. The TFI is a highly reliable questionnaire; it has strong validity with similar measures of tinnitus handicap (THI)[20] and depression.[18] One advantage of the TFI is that effect sizes are available as well as clinically meaningful differences to compare outcome scores over time. More research is needed to determine the usefulness of the TFI in research clinical trials and with more racially diverse populations.[22]

- Tinnitus Primary Functions Questionnaire (TPFQ)[23] measures the effect of tinnitus on primary functions or activities of daily living. The TPFQ consists of 12 items with four subscales: emotion, hearing, sleep, and concentration that relate to the four areas that are typically affected in tinnitus patients. A total score can be calculated from the average of all items and has been shown to be a reliable measure (0.89) of tinnitus. There is a full, 20-item version of the TFPQ, though the sensitivity of 12-item version was tested and found to be similar in reliability and validity to the full version. Pre- to post-treatment scores from the TFPQ 12-item version were evaluated for 100 participants at University of Iowa Tinnitus Research program after providing counseling for tinnitus. There was a 13 to 14% improvement in post-treatment total scores for the TPFQ and the THQ, suggesting good sensitivity in changes related to tinnitus function after treatment. Subscale scores (e.g., hearing, sleep) also decreased after treatment, showing how this questionnaire is clinically useful in determining how tinnitus impacts the patient's lifestyle. Further descriptions of the TPFQ are available in other chapters (Chapters 8 and 4).

These established questionnaires have been psychometrically evaluated and are reliable, valid tools for assessing patients' reactions to their tinnitus.[5] It is important that audiologists use a standardized, psychometrically validated questionnaire that has good internal consistency and test-retest reliability, good construct validity, and published normative data.[24] This provides a proper means to document treatment effectiveness and minimizes variabilities in outcomes across clinics. However, tinnitus questionnaires vary based on the content of a closed-set of questions (i.e., TQ and THQ = emotional, cognitive, and health effects are assessed vs. THI = tinnitus severity) and the scaling method used to quantify the patient's response (THI and TRQ = ordinal vs. THQ and TPFQ = interval). As suggested by Meikle et al,[25] smaller interval scales using five-point responses do not provide adequate resolution to document treatment-related changes. Moreover, audiologists should determine the barriers such as time constraints and problems with interpretation of scores that prevent them from administering questionnaires. Screening versions of some of the established questionnaires (e.g., 12-item TFPQ[23]; 10-item THI)[26] have similar factor structures and high reliability and validity as the original versions. Screening versions take less than 5 minutes to complete and can be easily incorporated into a busy audiology or tinnitus clinic.

In addition, use of open-ended questionnaires should be considered because patients might not identify with the situations presented in established questionnaires. Open-ended questionnaires have the advantage that they assess the most important problem reported by the patient, ensuring patient-centered care is provided. Furthermore, using questions that are not applicable to some individuals may result in missing or ambiguous answers that are difficult to interpret. For example, the Tinnitus Problems Questionnaire[9] asks the patient to list the difficulties that are associated with their tinnitus. Patients list the problems in the order of importance and note as many difficulties as they can. Data from the 72 participants from a tinnitus self-help group found that tinnitus contributed to four broad areas including lifestyle changes (93%; e.g., getting to sleep), emotional problems (69.4%; e.g., depression, annoyance), hearing difficulties (52.7%; e.g., understanding speech), and health effects (55.6%; e.g., drug dependence).

The Client Oriented Scale of Improvement for Tinnitus (COSIT)[19] was modified from the Client Oriented Scale of Improvement[27] and can be used for identifying problems associated with tinnitus, setting goals of therapy, and determining treatment effectiveness. See Chapter 8 for a more detailed description of the COSIT. We use COSIT similarly to Searchfield[19] by asking patients to identify three to five problem areas associated with tinnitus that serve as goals for the therapy, and measure progress in achieving these goals overtime. Searchfield[19] compared the responses from the COSIT to those from the THQ, the THI, and the TFI for 122 adult patients and research participants at a university hearing and tinnitus clinic. Results revealed that there was moderate convergent validity with the COSIT to the established questionnaires. The five most common treatment goals were to: (a) improve hearing, (b) reduce emotional effects and lessen depression, (c) better cope or control one's tinnitus, (d) manage the effect of the environment such as improved relaxation, and (e) improve sleep. The problems from the COSIT[19] were similar to the problems reported by patients on the Tinnitus Problems Questionnaire,[9] indicating that the newly developed COSIT has good validity. In sum, the COSIT and Tinnitus Problems Questionnaire may serve as helpful tools to determine the specific problems of a patient, and to create goals for tinnitus treatment.

In addition, another tool that can be used in tinnitus treatment is the tinnitus diary. Patients often benefit from a specific assignment to assist them in learning to cope with their tinnitus. For example, completing a tinnitus diary may help patients to (a) identify their negative thoughts about tinnitus and find ways to neutralize these thoughts, (b) document the activities where tinnitus is better or worse and modify their lifestyle accordingly, or (c) determine background sounds that make tinnitus less prominent to use sound therapy more effectively. In Tinnitus Activities Treatment (see Chapter 4), we provide instructions on creating a tinnitus diary, examples of tinnitus diaries, and ideas for tracking and making changes based on the diary results. In Chapter 6, McKenna provided details on creating a sleep diary for patients with insomnia and tinnitus that has been used successfully in tinnitus management. Tinnitus diaries can

be maintained using paper and pencil, though there are a number of Apps available to log a journal entry as well. Whatever the method used, it is recommended that patients stop journaling about their tinnitus after 2 weeks. The intent is not to concentrate on tinnitus, as constant journaling will bring tinnitus to the patient's conscious attention and reduce the ability to ignore it.[28] Rather, patients should be encouraged to make modifications and adjustments in their daily life to improve their reactions to tinnitus based on the information logged in their diary during the first few weeks of therapy.

Finally, a well-designed tinnitus intake questionnaire is helpful in determining specific aspects of the patient's tinnitus (e.g., duration and location of tinnitus), the patient's experiences with tinnitus, and potential causes of tinnitus and related problems including hyperacusis or decreased sound tolerance. An example of a Tinnitus Intake Questionnaire is shown in Appendix 12.3. Other researchers have proposed screening questionnaires for assessing problems related to tinnitus, hearing loss, and hyperacusis for clinical use.[29]

12.3 Measuring Quality of Life

According to the WHO model, a patient's quality of life may be impacted if the patient is not able to fully engage or participate in their everyday activities due to impairments in bodily function or structure[30] (see Chapter 8 for a review). Quality-of-life scales are classified as general health instruments because they measure the health and well-being of an individual as opposed to condition-specific questionnaires that measure specific aspects of function (i.e., THQ, TPFQ, THI that measure reactions to tinnitus). Health-related quality-of-life scales may be used to determine treatment effectiveness or to compare treatments. In addition, some researchers and governments have used results from quality-of-life scales to direct appropriate funding for health-related problems (e.g., for patients with bilateral cochlear implants (CIs)).[31] Most quality-of-life scales include general assessments of functional ability, health status, psychological well-being, social networks and social support, and life satisfaction and morale.[32,33,34]

The SF-36 (Medical Outcomes Study 36-Item Short-Form Health Survey)[32] was developed for clinical practice and research, and has been implemented in health policy evaluations and general population surveys. Eight dimensions of health are assessed via self-report with the SF-36: vitality, physical functioning, bodily pain, general health perceptions, physical functioning, emotional functioning, social functioning, and mental health. Patient responses are scored using a magnitude estimation interval scale from 0 to 100. The SF-36 is widely used because it has been translated into many languages and applied to over 200 health conditions.[35] In addition, the SF-6D[33] and the EQ-5D (The EuroQol Group)[34] are screening versions derived from SF-36 that measure health-related quality of life. However, there are no specific questions on hearing, hearing loss, or tinnitus in the SF-36, SF-6D, and EQ-5D that may limit their usefulness with patients with hearing loss and/or tinnitus.[36]

By comparison, the WHO Disability Assessment Schedule (WHODAS 2.0)[37] covers six domains of functioning: cognition, mobility, self-care, getting along, life activities, and participation. Under the cognition domain, understanding and communication are evaluated, but only one question assesses the "generally understanding of what people say." The Health Utilities Index Mark 3 (HUI3)[38] is part of a health status classification system that evaluates health on eight attributes: vision, hearing, speech, ambulation, dexterity, emotion, cognition, and pain and includes some questions on hearing ability.

Finally, we developed a Meaning of Life questionnaire (refer to Appendix 12.4) at the University of Iowa that has 23 items covering a broad range of health and well-being.[39] We include some questions on specific abilities like hearing, talking, and sleeping. The questionnaire is scored numerically on a 0 to 100 interval scale similarly to the THQ and TPFQ. We conducted a preliminary analysis of self-report data from the Meaning of Life questionnaire

with 116 adult tinnitus patients and 196 adult patients with CIs. Four factors were prominent based on a factor analysis: friendship, physical health, hearing and mental health, and positive outlook.

We found that the mean total score for the CI participants was 76.8% and for tinnitus participants, 76.9%, which was not statistically significant. The highest item rating was for item 8, "I eat and drink with ease" (e.g., 94% for CI participants and 95% for tinnitus participants) that suggests little to no difficulty in eating or swallowing (▶ Fig. 12.1).

Comparatively, the lowest item mean rating (48% for CI and tinnitus patients) on the Meaning of Life questionnaire was found for item 1, "I hear well in any situation." For tinnitus patients, these lower ratings may indicate that the communication problems associated with tinnitus are difficult to distinguish from hearing loss.[9] Ratings of approximately 60% for items 22 ("I never feel depressed, sad or anxious") and 23 ("I never experience pain or discomfort") suggest moderate emotional or physical difficulties for tinnitus and CI patients alike. Hearing loss and tinnitus can contribute to social isolation, loneliness, frustration, and dependence on a caregiver. Finally, the tinnitus patients reported significantly more sleep difficulties compared to the CI patients based on results from item 5 ("I sleep well"). Sleep disturbance has long been recognized as the single most important complaint among adults with tinnitus.[9,40]

In summary, there are many quality-of-life scales available for clinical use, though most quality-of-life scales do not assess communication or hearing directly and may not be sensitive enough to communication or hearing-related

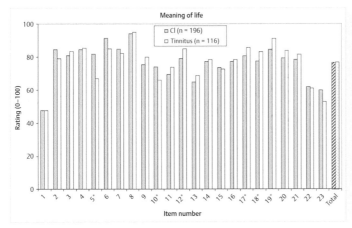

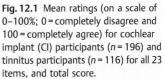

Fig. 12.1 Mean ratings (on a scale of 0–100%; 0 = completely disagree and 100 = completely agree) for cochlear implant (CI) participants (n = 196) and tinnitus participants (n = 116) for all 23 items, and total score.

issues.[41] Our published Meaning of Life questionnaire was found to be sensitive to differences between groups with hearing loss and tinnitus, and includes items on communication, sleep, and cognition that relate to hearing disorders including tinnitus. Efforts are being made to adopt a universally accepted quality-of-life measure in the United States for hearing-related issues that may also be applied to tinnitus patients.[42]

12.3.1 Measuring Related Problems

Tinnitus is often associated with other related problems for many patients, including depression, anxiety, and sleep disturbances.[43] There are many scales that are administered to patients to assess the severity of these conditions. However, our purpose in reviewing these questionnaires is not to encourage audiologists to administer them. Rather, we want audiologists to be aware of these scales that measure related problems to tinnitus in hopes that this will better facilitate care as audiologists interact with psychologists and mental health professionals.

- Beck Depression Inventory (BDI)[18] is a widely used scale of depression. The BDI contains 21 multiple-choice items that assess the severity of the patient's depression. For each item, patients are asked to indicate which choice is most representative of their feelings, and then their response is scored numerically from 0 to 3 to calculate a total score ranging from 0 to 59. A higher BDI score represents a higher level of depression.
- State-Trait Anxiety Inventory measures the general state or feelings of a person. It consists of 40 items; 20 items for assessing trait anxiety and 20 for state anxiety. Each item is assigned a number from 1 to 4 by the patient that represents how they feel about themselves. The responses are added together to produce a total score from 20 to 80. A higher total score represents a higher level of anxiety.
- Pittsburgh Quality Sleep Index (PSQI)[44] assesses the patient's sleep habits. There are 24 items total, 5 of which are completed by a patient's bed partner. As described in Chapter 6 (McKenna), the seven component scores are added to create a total score. Higher PSQI scores represent severe sleep difficulties.
- Insomnia Severity Index (ISI)[45] also measures insomnia, and includes seven items. See Chapter 6 (McKenna) for a description of this scale.

12.4 Conclusions

Regarding measures of tinnitus, the audiologist has many options to assess a patient's tinnitus and their reactions to it. The selection of the "optimal" measurement tool largely depends on the intended purposes of the test, and in most cases, more than one tool will be needed. A complete list of suggested tinnitus outcome measures is in Appendix 12.5. In this chapter, we emphasized the clinical aspects of performing psychoacoustic measures of tinnitus, administering self-report questionnaires of tinnitus, health-related quality of life, and related problems, and even maintaining a patient diary during the first few weeks of therapy. Moreover, it is important to recognize that these measures are implemented in tinnitus research studies to measure patient outcomes from treatment and to guide decisions about effectiveness.[8] We have previously recommended the use of both primary (i.e., established tinnitus questionnaires) and secondary measures (e.g., tinnitus magnitude estimation) to assess benefit from a given treatment in tinnitus research.[7] Likewise, we encourage audiologists to implement several measures including questionnaires to assess patient reactions to tinnitus and psychoacoustic measures of tinnitus. In this chapter, we presented helpful tools to determine the specific problems of a tinnitus patient, and to create goals for treatment. As a final note, we must be cautious of different scaling procedures, the sensitivity and validity of these measures, and patient-specific variables such as related problems (e.g., depression, anxiety) that may affect the results.

We have created a video available on the companion website which demonstrates the psychoacoustic tests to measure tinnitus pitch, loudness, minimum masking level, and residual inhibition.

References

[1] Tyler RS. The psychoacoustical measurement of tinnitus. In: Tyler RS, ed. Tinnitus handbook. San Diego, CA: Singular Thomson Learning; 2000:149–179

[2] Mancini PC, Tyler RS, Smith S, Ji H, Perreau A, Mohr AM. Tinnitus: how partners can help? Am J Audiol. 2019; 28(1): 85–94

[3] Tyler RS, Noble WG, Coelho C, Roncancio ER, Jun JH. Tinnitus and hyperacusis. In: Katz J, ed. Chasin, English, Hood, & Tillery, Handbook of clinical audiology. 7th ed. Philadelphia, PA: Wolters Kluwer; 2014

[4] Tyler RS, Conrad-Armes D, Smith PA. Postmasking effects of sensorineural tinnitus: a preliminary investigation. J Speech Hear Res. 1984; 27(3):466–474

[5] Newman CW, Sandridge SA, Jacobson GP. Assessing outcomes of tinnitus intervention. J Am Acad Audiol. 2014; 25(1):76–105

[6] Stevens SS. On the theory of scales of measurement. Science. 1946; 103(2684):677–680

[7] Tyler RS, Noble W, Coelho C. Considerations for the design of clinical trials for tinnitus. Acta Otolaryngol Suppl. 2006; 126: 44–49

[8] Tunkel DE, Bauer CA, Sun GH, et al. Clinical practice guideline: tinnitus. Otolaryngol Head Neck Surg. 2014; 151 (2) Suppl:S1–S40

[9] Tyler RS, Baker LJ. Difficulties experienced by tinnitus sufferers. J Speech Hear Disord. 1983; 48(2):150–154

[10] Hallam RS, Jakes SC, Hinchcliffe R. Cognitive variables in tinnitus annoyance. Br J Clin Psychol. 1988; 27(3):213–222

[11] McKenna L, Hallam RS, Hinchcliffe R. The prevalence of psychological disturbance in neurotology outpatients. Clin Otolaryngol Allied Sci. 1991; 16(5):452–456

[12] Hiller W, Goebel G. A psychometric study of complaints in chronic tinnitus. J Psychosom Res. 1992; 36(4):337–348

[13] Hiller W, Goebel G, Rief W. Reliability of self-rated tinnitus distress and association with psychological symptom patterns. Br J Clin Psychol. 1994; 33(2):231–239

[14] Kuk FK, Tyler RS, Russell D, Jordan H. The psychometric properties of a tinnitus handicap questionnaire. Ear Hear. 1990; 11(6):434–445

[15] Newman CW, Wharton JA, Jacobson GP. Retest stability of the tinnitus handicap questionnaire. Ann Otol Rhinol Laryngol. 1995; 104(9 Pt 1):718–723

[16] Wilson PH, Henry J, Bowen M, Haralambous G. Tinnitus reaction questionnaire: psychometric properties of a measure of distress associated with tinnitus. J Speech Hear Res. 1991; 34(1):197–201

[17] Spielberger CD, Gorsuch RL, Lushene R. Manual for the state-trait anxiety inventory. Palo Alto, CA: Consulting Psychologists Press; 1970

[18] Beck AT, Ward CH, Mendelson M, Mock J, Erbaugh J. An inventory for measuring depression. Arch Gen Psychiatry. 1961; 4:561–571

[19] Searchfield GD. A Client Oriented Scale of Improvement in tinnitus for therapy goal planning and assessing outcomes. J Am Acad Audiol. 2019; 30(4):327–337

[20] Newman CW, Jacobson GP, Spitzer JB. Development of the Tinnitus Handicap Inventory. Arch Otolaryngol Head Neck Surg. 1996; 122(2):143–148

[21] Main CJ. The Modified Somatic Perception Questionnaire (MSPQ). J Psychosom Res. 1983; 27(6):503–514

[22] Meikle MB, Henry JA, Griest SE, et al. The tinnitus functional index: development of a new clinical measure for chronic, intrusive tinnitus. Ear Hear. 2012; 33(2):153–176

[23] Tyler R, Ji H, Perreau A, Witt S, Noble W, Coelho C. Development and validation of the Tinnitus Primary Function Questionnaire. Am J Audiol. 2014; 23(3):260–272

[24] Bentler RA, Kramer SE. Guidelines for choosing a self-report outcome measure. Ear Hear. 2000; 21(4) Suppl:37S–49S

[25] Meikle MB, Stewart BJ, Griest SE, Henry JA. Tinnitus outcomes assessment. Trends Amplif. 2008; 12(3):223–235

[26] Newman CW, Sandridge SA, Bolek L. Development and psychometric adequacy of the screening version of the tinnitus handicap inventory. Otol Neurotol. 2008; 29(3):276–281

[27] Dillon H, James A, Ginis J. Client Oriented Scale of Improvement (COSI) and its relationship to several other measures of benefit and satisfaction provided by hearing aids. J Am Acad Audiol. 1997; 8(1):27–43

[28] Henry JL, Wilson PH. The psychological management of chronic tinnitus: a cognitive-behavioral approach. Needham Heights, MA: Allyn and Bacon; 2001

[29] Henry JA, Griest S, Zaugg TL, et al. Tinnitus and hearing survey: a screening tool to differentiate bothersome tinnitus from hearing difficulties. Am J Audiol. 2015; 24(1):66–77

[30] World Health Organization. International classification of functioning, disability and health: ICF. Geneva: World Health Organization; 2001

[31] Quentin Summerfield A, Barton GR, Toner J, et al. Self-reported benefits from successive bilateral cochlear implantation in post-lingually deafened adults: randomised controlled trial. Int J Audiol. 2006; 45(1) Suppl 1:S99–S107

[32] Ware JE, Jr, Sherbourne CD. The MOS 36-item short-form health survey (SF-36). I. Conceptual framework and item selection. Med Care. 1992; 30(6):473–483

[33] Brazier J, Roberts J, Deverill M. The estimation of a preference-based measure of health from the SF-36. J Health Econ. 2002; 21(2):271–292

[34] EuroQol Group. EuroQol—a new facility for the measurement of health-related quality of life. Health Policy. 1990; 16(3): 199–208

[35] Garratt A, Schmidt L, Mackintosh A, Fitzpatrick R. Quality of life measurement: bibliographic study of patient assessed health outcome measures. BMJ. 2002; 324(7351):1417–1421

[36] Barton GR, Bankart J, Davis AC. A comparison of the quality of life of hearing-impaired people as estimated by three different utility measures. Int J Audiol. 2005; 44(3): 157–163

[37] World Health Organization. In: Üstün TB, Kostanjsek N, Chatterji S, Rehm J, eds. Measuring health and disability: manual for WHO disability assessment schedule (WHODAS 2.0). Geneva, Switzerland: WHO Press; 2010

[38] Feeny D, Furlong W, Boyle M, Torrance GW. Multi-attribute health status classification systems. Health Utilities Index. PharmacoEconomics. 1995; 7(6):490–502

[39] Tyler R, Perreauf A, Mohr AM, Ji H, Mancini PC. An exploratory step toward measuring the "Meaning of Life" in patients with tinnitus and in cochlear implant users. J Am Acad Audiol. 2020; 31(4):277–285

[40] McKenna L. Tinnitus and insomnia. In: Tyler RS, ed. Tinnitus handbook. San Diego, CA: Singular; 2000:59–84

[41] Granberg S, Dahlström J, Möller C, Kähäri K, Danermark B. The ICF Core Sets for hearing loss—researcher perspective. Part I: Systematic review of outcome measures identified in audiological research. Int J Audiol. 2014; 53(2):65–76

[42] National Institutes on Health [Internet]. Bethesda, MD: National Institute on Deafness and Other Communication Disorders (NIDCD) 2017–2021 Strategic Plan; [updated 2008 Aug 8; cited 2019 Oct 24]. https://www.nidcd.nih.gov/about/strategic-plan/2017-2021-nidcd-strategic-plan/

[43] Andersson G, Baguley DM, McKenna L, McFerran D. Tinnitus: a multidisciplinary approach. London, England: Whurr; 2005

[44] Buysse DJ, Reynolds CF, III, Monk TH, Berman SR, Kupfer DJ. The Pittsburgh Sleep Quality Index: a new instrument for psychiatric practice and research. Psychiatry Res. 1989; 28 (2):193–213

[45] Bastien CH, Vallières A, Morin CM. Validation of the Insomnia Severity Index as an outcome measure for insomnia research. Sleep Med. 2001; 2(4):297–307

Appendix 12.1 Data Sheet

Tinnitus Pitch*

Date:
Patient Name:

Location of tinnitus   Left   Right   Binaural   Head

1. Fit the participant with inserts and face the participant away from the audiologist.
2. Present the stimulus in the ear in which the participant experiences tinnitus. If the participant has binaural tinnitus, present the pitch in the right ear. If you are unable to test one ear (tone is too loud or not loud enough), test the other ear and report this in the "comments" section on the data sheet.
3. Start by explaining the test: **Now we are going to do a test of your tinnitus. This test can be difficult and exhausting, and that's okay as I will help you along the way. I am going to play a series of tones into your [right/left] ear. I want you to tell me if the most prominent pitch of your tinnitus is higher or lower than the pitch of my tone. Try to ignore the loudness or the volume of the tone, and just focus on the pitch. I need you to respond each time by using one of the following phrases "My tinnitus is higher than the tone," or "My tinnitus is lower than the tone."**

4. Start with a 1000-Hz pulsed tone and use a bracketing procedure. The presentation level should be adjusted to 50 dBHL for normal hearing listeners. Present a tone. If the participant says, "My tinnitus is higher," go up a half octave. If the participant says, "My tinnitus is lower," go down a half octave. Stop when the tinnitus pitch is bracketed and record the last test frequency. (For example: 1000 Hz = "higher," 1500 Hz = "higher," 2000 Hz= "lower." Stop, record 2000 Hz.) Repeat the trial two more times. If the first trial seems to be an outlier compared to the consecutive two trials, perform a fourth trial.
5. It is important that the participant respond with the phrase "My tinnitus is higher," or "My tinnitus is lower." If they do not respond with the correct phrase, prompt them to do so. If they say "That is the pitch of my tinnitus," prompt them to use one of the phrases, "My tinnitus is higher," or "My tinnitus is lower," present the stimulus again, and ask them to rephrase their response.

Threshold at 1000 Hz: dB HL

Trial 1	Trial 2	Trial 3	Average

COMMENTS:

Tinnitus Loudness

Date:
Patient Name:

Location of tinnitus   Left   Right   Binaural   Head

1. Present the stimulus in the ear in which the participant experiences tinnitus. If the participant has binaural tinnitus, present the pitch in the right ear. If you are unable to test one ear (tone is too loud or not loud enough), test the other ear and report this in the "comments" section on the data sheet.
2. Explain the next phase of testing; **"Now we are going to continue testing your tinnitus. I will present a sound to your [right/left] ear. After**

you hear the sound, I need you to tell me if your tinnitus is louder or softer than the loudness of my tone. At this point, try to focus only on the loudness, or volume of the tone, and try not to pay attention to the pitch. Respond each time by using the following phrases, "My tinnitus is louder than the tone," or "My tinnitus is softer than the tone."

3. Present a 500-Hz pulsed tone at the participant's hearing threshold and use a bracketing procedure. If the participant says, "My tinnitus is louder," go up 2 dB. If the participant says, "My tinnitus is softer," go down 2 dB. Stop when the tinnitus loudness is bracketed and record the last test intensity (dBHL). (For example: Threshold at

500 Hz = 60 dBHL; 60 dBHL = "my tinnitus is louder," 62 dBHL = "my tinnitus is louder," 64 dBHL = "my tinnitus is softer." Stop, record 64 dBHL). Repeat the trial two more times. If the first trial seems to be an outlier compared to the consecutive two trials, perform a fourth trial.

4. It is important that the participant respond with one of the phrases "My tinnitus is louder," or "My tinnitus is softer." If they do not respond with the correct phrase, prompt them to do so. If they say "That is the volume of my tinnitus," prompt them to use one of the phrases "My tinnitus is louder," or "My tinnitus is softer." Present the stimulus again, and ask them to rephrase their response.

Threshold at 500 Hz: dB HL

Trial 1	Trial 2	Trial 3	Average

COMMENTS:

Minimal Masking Level (MML)

(Test each ear individually if tinnitus is binaural)

Date:
Patient Name:

Location of tinnitus	Left	Right	Binaural	Head

1. Explain the next test procedure to the participant. **"Next, I will be playing a sound to your [right/left] ear that sounds like a whooshing fan noise. I need you to tell me if you can hear your tinnitus above my noise. Respond using the phrase, "I can hear my tinnitus," or "I cannot hear my tinnitus."**

2. With a pulsed (three long, manual pulses), speech-spectrum shaped noise, measure the threshold and minimum level required to mask the tinnitus in each ear. Use an ascending method of limits. For MML, present the noise at threshold. If the participant says, "I can hear my tinnitus," go up 2 dB. Stop when the tinnitus is masked and record the last test level (dBHL). Do

not exceed 80 dBHL; rather, accept that if you reach 80 dBHL, their tinnitus cannot be masked. Repeat the trial two more times. If the first trial seems to be an outlier compared to the consecutive two trials, perform a fourth trial. You can accelerate the process by increasing the dBHL steps to 10 dB increments until you are within 10 dB of the previous trial for MML.

3. Then, ask the participant, **"Does the masking noise mask tinnitus in one ear or both ears?"** If the participant complains that the noise is too loud, or the tinnitus cannot be masked, record this on the data sheet.

4. Repeat on the other ear if participant has binaural tinnitus.

RIGHT Noise threshold: dBHL

Trial 1	Trial 2	Trial 3	Average

*If binaural tinnitus, ask if masking noise masked tinnitus in one ear or both.

Masking affected: _____ right ear only; _____ left ear only; _____ both ears
Check here if the noise was too loud _____ Check here if the tinnitus could not be masked _____
COMMENTS:_____
_____

LEFT Noise threshold: dBHL

Trial 1	Trial 2	Trial 3	Average

*If binaural tinnitus, ask if masking noise masked tinnitus in one ear or both.
Masking affected: _____ right ear only; _____ left ear only; _____ both ears
Check here if the noise was too loud _____Check here if the tinnitus could not be masked _____
COMMENTS:_____
_____

Residual Inhibition

Date:
Patient Name:

Location of tinnitus	Left	Right	Binaural	Head

1. Start by asking the participant **"Is your tinnitus normal today?"** If not, make a note that the tinnitus is different than an average day. Then, explain the next test to the participant. **"I am going to put some noise in one ear for approximately one minute to see how your tinnitus reacts to it. You can just sit and listen to the noise and you do not have to respond in any way. Once the noise is turned off, I want you to tell me how your tinnitus reacted to the noise."** Then play the noise at 10 dBHL above MML in the loudest trial for one minute using a personal timer. Continue instruction,

   "Now that the noise is turned off, does your tinnitus sound the same or different? If different, how is it different?"
2. Record exactly what the participant says: different, how it is different, and the timeline over which it changed.
3. Sometimes the participant will not experience any change, other times they will say their tinnitus is softer or louder. If their tinnitus is softer, explain, **"We will wait, tell us when the tinnitus returns."** Then record the participant's response as to when their tinnitus returned and record the time on the data sheet.

MML **RIGHT** ear: Presentation level **RIGHT** ear:

MML **LEFT** ear: Presentation level **LEFT** ear:

If tinnitus changed for a period of time   Minutes   Seconds
in **RIGHT** ear, how long did this last?

If tinnitus changed for a period of time   Minutes   Seconds
in **LEFT** ear, how long did this last?

Noise in RIGHT ear (circle one):

Noise in LEFT ear (circle one):

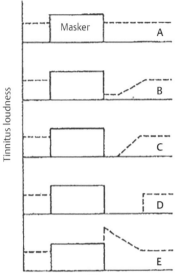

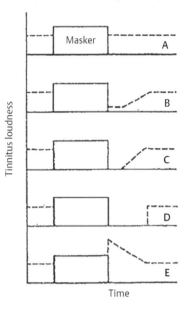

Appendix 12.2 Tinnitus Handicap Questionnaire

Patient Name: _____

Date: _____

INSTRUCTIONS: This questionnaire has 27 questions. Please indicate **0** if you strongly disagree (up to) **100** if you strongly agree. Please do not skip any questions.

#	Item	Your rating
1	I do not enjoy life because of tinnitus.	
2	My tinnitus has gotten worse over the years.	
3	Tinnitus interferes with my ability to tell where sounds are coming from.	
4	I am unable to follow conversation during meetings because of tinnitus.	
5	Tinnitus causes me to avoid noisy situations.	
6	Tinnitus interferes with my speech understanding when talking with someone in a noisy room.	
7	I feel uneasy in social situations because of tinnitus.	
8	The general public does not know about the devastating nature of tinnitus.	
9	I cannot concentrate because of tinnitus.	
10	Tinnitus creates family problems.	
11	Tinnitus causes me to feel depressed.	
12	I find it difficult to explain what tinnitus is to others.	
13	Tinnitus causes stress.	
14	I am unable to relax because of tinnitus.	
15	I complain more because of tinnitus.	
16	I have trouble falling asleep at night because of tinnitus.	
17	Tinnitus makes me feel tired.	
18	Tinnitus makes me feel insecure.	
19	Tinnitus contributes to a feeling of general ill health.	
20	Tinnitus affects the quality of my relationships.	
21	Tinnitus has caused a reduction in my speech understanding ability.	
22	Tinnitus makes me feel annoyed.	
23	Tinnitus interferes with my speech understanding when listening to the television.	
24	Tinnitus makes me feel anxious.	
25	I think I have a healthy outlook on tinnitus.	
26	I have support from my friends regarding my tinnitus.	
27	I feel frustrated frequently because of tinnitus.	

Note: Kuk FK, Tyler RS, Russell D, Jordan H. The psychometric properties of a tinnitus handicap questionnaire. Ear Hear 1990;11(6):434–442.

Appendix 12.3 Tinnitus Intake Questionnaire

Patient Name: _____

Date: _____

1	What is your gender?	Female Male

2   What is your age?   _____ years

3   Please rate, using a scale from 0–100, whether sounds that others   _____ (0–100)
believe are moderately loud are *too* loud to you. (0 = strongly
disagree; 100 = strongly agree)
Please list sounds that are too loud to you:

4   Where is your tinnitus? (Please choose only ONE answer.)

a) Left ear	a) In the head, but no exact place
b) Right ear	b) More in the right side of head
c) Both ears, equally	c) More in the left side of head
d) Both ears, but worse in left ear	d) Outside of head
e) Both ears, but worse in right ear	e) Middle of head

If you hear more than one sound or a different sound in each ear, answer the following questions with regard to the one most annoying sound.

5   Describe the most prominent *PITCH* of your tinnitus on a scale
from 1 to 100, where 1 is like a *VERY LOW* pitch fog horn, and 100   _____ (1–100)
is like a *VERY HIGH* pitch whistle.

6   Does the *PITCH* of the tinnitus vary from day to day?   a. No
                                                       b. Yes

7   Describe the *LOUDNESS* of your tinnitus using a scale from 0–100.   _____ (0–100)
(0 = *VERY FAINT*; 100 = *VERY LOUD*)

8   Does the *LOUDNESS* of the tinnitus vary from day to day?   No
                                                       Yes

9   Describe the typical *ANNOYANCE* of your tinnitus using a scale from   _____ (0–100)
0–100. (0 = *NOT ANNOYING AT ALL*; 100 = *EXTREMLY ANNOYING*)

10   Which of all these qualities *BEST* describes your tinnitus? (Please circle only ONE.)

a) Ringing or whistling	a) Humming
b) Cricket-like	b) Hissing
c) Roaring, "Shhh," or rushing	c) OTHER, PLEASE SPECIFY:
d) Buzzing	_____

11   During the time you are awake, what percentage of the time is your tinnitus present? For example, 100% would indicate that your tinnitus was present all the time, and 25% would indicate that your tinnitus was present ¼ of the time.
         _____% (Please write in a single number between 1 and 100.)

12   On the average, how many days per month are you bothered by   _____ days
your tinnitus?

13   How many months or years have you had tinnitus?   _____ months OR

    _____ years

14   When you have your tinnitus, which of the following makes it *WORSE*?

a) Alcohol
b) Being in a noisy place
c) Being in a quiet place
d) Caffeine (coffee/tea/cola)
e) Drugs/medicine
f) Eye movement
g) Food (please specify) _____
h) Moving your head or neck
i) Physical activity
j) Relaxation
k) Touching your head

a) Wearing a hearing aid
b) When you first wake up in the morning
c) Being tired
d) During your menstrual period
e) Emotional or mental stress
f) Lack of sleep
g) Shooting guns, rifles, etc.
h) Smoking
i) Nothing makes it worse
j) OTHER, PLEASE SPECIFY _____

15   Which of the following *REDUCES* your tinnitus?

a) Alcohol
b) Being in a noisy place
c) Being in a quiet place
d) Caffeine (coffee/tea/cola)
e) Drugs/medicine
f) Eye movement
g) Food (please specify) _____
h) Moving your head or neck

a) Physical activity
b) Relaxation
c) Touching your head
d) Wearing a hearing aid
e) When you first wake up in the morning
f) Nothing makes it better
g) OTHER, PLEASE SPECIFY _____

16   What do you think originally caused your tinnitus? (Select up to THREE choices)

a) Aging
b) Autoimmune disease
c) Brain Tumor
d) Cochlear implant, after surgery
e) Cochlear implant, after switch on
f) Cochlear implant, unknown
g) Deafness from birth, genetic
h) Deafness from birth, syndromic
i) Deafness from birth, unknown
j) Diabetes
k) Electrical trauma
l) Head injury
m) Medication/drug
n) Meniere Disease
o) Middle ear, blood vessel
p) Middle ear, muscle

a) Middle ear, unknown
b) Noise exposure
c) Noise exposure (non-gunfire, impulsive)
d) Noise exposure (hunting/gunfire)
e) Noise exposure (military service)
f) Otosclerosis
g) Problems with teeth or jaw
h) 8th nerve tumor (acoustic neuroma)
i) Sudden hearing loss
j) Surgery
k) Thyroid
l) Unknown
m) Other (please specify)_____
n)

17   In which ear do you wear hearing aids?   Left
    Right
    Both
    None

18   Do you have any legal action or compensation claim pending in relation to your   No
tinnitus, or are you planning legal action?   Yes

Appendix 12.4 Meaning of Life and Happiness Questionnaire

Patient Name: _____

Date: _____

INSTRUCTIONS: Please indicate your agreement with each statement on a scale from 0 (completely disagree) to 100 (completely agree).

Item	Statement	Score
1.	I hear well in any situation.	
2.	I see well in any situation.	
3.	I walk easily in any situation.	
4.	I talk well and am easily understood.	
5.	I sleep well.	
6.	I manipulate things well with my hands.	
7.	I concentrate and focus well.	
8.	I eat and drink with ease.	
9.	I have many friends that I socialize with.	
10.	I always remember things.	
11.	I have many hobbies.	
12.	I have emotional support from many others.	
13.	I participate in several recreational activities.	
14.	In general, I feel very relaxed.	
15.	I am satisfied with my sex life.	
16.	I am satisfied with my financial situation.	
17.	I feel good about my self-image.	
18.	I am very healthy.	
19.	I have close friends or family that I can confide in.	
20.	In general, I get all the pleasure I want out of life.	
21.	I think the future looks very bright.	
22.	I never feel depressed, sad or anxious.	
23.	I never experience pain or discomfort.	

Note: Tyler R, Perreau A, Mohr AM, Ji H, Mancini PC. An exploratory step toward measuring the "Meaning of Life" in patients with tinnitus and in cochlear implant users. J Am Acad Audiol 2020;31(4):277–285.

Appendix 12.5 Ordered References for Tinnitus Outcome Measures

Psychoacoustic Measures

- *Psychoacoustic Tests*: Tyler RS. The psychoacoustical measurement of tinnitus. In: Tyler RS, ed. Tinnitus handbook. San Diego, CA: Singular Thomson Learning; 2000:149–179.

Tinnitus Magnitude Estimation

- *Rating Tinnitus Qualities*: Tyler RS, Noble W, Coelho C. Considerations for the design of clinical trials for tinnitus. Acta Otolaryngol Suppl 2006;126:44–49.

Established Questionnaires

- *Tinnitus Questionnaire*: Hallam RS, Jakes SC, Hinchcliffe R. Cognitive variables in tinnitus annoyance. Br J Clin Psychol 1988;27(3):213–222.
- *Tinnitus Handicap Questionnaire*: Kuk FK, Tyler RS, Russell D, Jordan H. The psychometric properties of a tinnitus handicap questionnaire. Ear Hear 1990;11(6):434–445.
- *Tinnitus Reaction Questionnaire*: Wilson PH, Henry J, Bowen M, Haralambous G. Tinnitus reaction questionnaire: psychometric properties of a measure of distress associated with tinnitus. J Speech Hear Res 1991;34(1):197–201.
- *Tinnitus Handicap Inventory*: Newman CW, Jacobson GP, Spitzer JB. Development of the Tinnitus Handicap Inventory. Arch Otolaryngol Head Neck Surg 1996;122(2):143–148.
- *Tinnitus Functional Index*: Meikle MB, Henry JA, Griest SE, et al. The tinnitus functional index: development of a new clinical measure for chronic, intrusive tinnitus. Ear Hear 2012;33(2):153–176.
- *Tinnitus Primary Functions Questionnaire*: Tyler R, Ji H, Perreau A, Witt S, Noble W, Coelho C. Development and validation of the Tinnitus Primary Function Questionnaire. Am J Audiol 2014;23(3):260–272.

Open-Ended Questionnaires

- *Tinnitus Problems Questionnaire*: Tyler RS, Baker LJ. Difficulties experienced by tinnitus sufferers. J Speech Hear Disord 1983;48(2):150–154.
- *Client Oriented Scale of Improvement in Tinnitus*: Searchfield GD. A Client Oriented Scale of Improvement in tinnitus for therapy goal planning and assessing outcomes. J Am Acad Audiol 2019;30(4):327–337.

Other Reactions Measurement Questionnaires

- Patient Diary: a
- Tinnitus Intake Questionnaire: b

Measuring Quality of Life

- *EQ-5D*: EuroQol Group. EuroQol—a new facility for the measurement of health-related quality of life. Health Policy 1990;16(3):199–208.
- *SF-36*: Ware JE Jr, Sherbourne CD. The MOS 36-item short-form health survey (SF-36). I. Conceptual framework and item selection. Med Care 1992;30(6):473–483.
- *WHO DAS 2.0*: World Health Organization. In: Üstün TB, Kostanjsek N, Chatterji S, Rehm J, eds. Measuring health and disability: manual for WHO disability assessment schedule (WHODAS 2.0). Geneva, Switzerland: WHO Press; 2010.
- *Meaning of Life*: Tyler R, Perreauf A, Mohr AM, Ji H, Mancini PC. An exploratory step toward measuring the "Meaning of Life" in patients with tinnitus and in cochlear implant users. J Am Acad Audiol 2020;31(4):277–285.

Measuring Specific Related Problems

- *Beck Depression Inventory*: Beck AT, Ward CH, Mendelson M, Mock J, Erbaugh J. An inventory for measuring depression. Arch Gen Psychiatry 1961;4:561–571.
- *State-Trait Anxiety Inventory*: Spielberger CD, Gorsuch RL, Lushene R, et al. Manual for the state-trait anxiety inventory. Palo Alto, CA: Consulting Psychologists Press; 1970.
- *Pittsburg Quality Sleep Index*: Buysse DJ, Reynolds CF III, Monk TH, Berman SR, Kupfer DJ. The Pittsburgh Sleep Quality Index: a new instrument for psychiatric practice and research. Psychiatry Res 1989;28(2):193–213.
- *Insomnia Severity Index*: Bastien CH, Vallières A, Morin CM. Validation of the Insomnia Severity Index as an outcome measure for insomnia research. Sleep Med 2001;2(4):297–307.

13 Hyperacusis

Richard S. Tyler, Ann Perreau, and Patricia C. Mancini

Abstract

Many tinnitus patients also have hyperacusis, a prevalent auditory disorder that can cause significant distress and affects the patient's quality of life. All hyperacusis patients can describe specific sounds in their environment that are troublesome. Patients with hyperacusis may have very different complaints about the sounds and situations that they experience difficulty. There are four main symptoms that can be used to describe patients' hyperacusis experiences: (1) loudness, (2) annoyance, (3) fear, and (4) pain. Many patients will experience more than one of these symptoms, and the types of symptoms will vary from patient to patient. Although there are currently no cures available for hyperacusis, there are several treatment options that can be successful for patients, including counseling, sound therapy, filtered earplugs, medications for related symptoms, and relaxation exercises. The Hyperacusis Activities Treatment is a counseling program that includes education about hyperacusis, counseling on reactions to hyperacusis, and treatments to relieve symptoms such as sound therapy and relaxation exercises.

Keywords: hyperacusis, tinnitus, counseling, therapy

13.1 Introduction

In our early studies of tinnitus, we discovered that many tinnitus patients also have hyperacusis[1] that has been confirmed in later studies.[2,3,4,5] There must have been common mechanisms in these patients with tinnitus who were also reporting symptoms of hyperacusis, though this association is less well understood. Of course, it is also possible to have hyperacusis without tinnitus and tinnitus without hyperacusis. It is, therefore, appropriate to include a chapter on hyperacusis in this book for audiologists providing treatment to tinnitus patients.[6]

Across studies, the prevalence of hyperacusis in patients with tinnitus averages to about 40%.[7,8,9] By comparison, in patients with hyperacusis, the prevalence of tinnitus approaches 86%.[10] Considering the general public, hyperacusis is reported by about 6 to 17% of individuals.[11,12] Certainly, these numbers suggest that hyperacusis is common![13]

13.2 Terminology

The term "hyperacusis" has been used for over 75 years, but recently, several new terms have been used, including hypersensitivity, misophonia, select-sound sensitivity, exaggerated sound response, decreased sound tolerance, phonophobia, to name a few. All hyperacusis patients can describe specific sounds in their environment that are troublesome. As an example, Urnau and Tochetto[14] reported that music, horns, people talking loudly, traffic noise, doors slamming, sudden and loud noises, sinks dripping, restaurant noise, door bells, police sirens, airplanes, plastic bag noise, blenders, and phones ringing were bothersome sounds to patients with hyperacusis.

One important difference between tinnitus and hyperacusis patients is that the problems experienced by tinnitus patients generally decrease over time.[15] However, this is not as common in hyperacusis patients. Perhaps hyperacusis is less easy to adapt to? Or perhaps hyperacusis is more likely to get worse over time?

Because hyperacusis is not well known and new terms are being added, hyperacusis can be confusing to patients, health care professions including audiologists and ENT specialists, and the general population. We suggest that the following four main symptoms be used to describe patients' hyperacusis experiences[16]:

- Loudness hyperacusis: Perceiving moderately loud sounds as very loud compared to what a listener with normal hearing would perceive.
- Annoyance hyperacusis: Having a negative response to sound often manifested as irritation, anxiety, or tension (but not always loud[14]).
- Fear hyperacusis: Anticipating sounds that are uncomfortable and cause fear (but not always loud). Fear hyperacusis results in behaviors such that the individual often takes steps to avoid situations.
- Pain hyperacusis: Perceiving pain at a sound level that is much lower than a listener with normal hearing (but not always intense) would perceive. This can be reported, for example, as a stabbing pain in the ear or the head.

It is important to note that many patients will experience more than one of these symptoms, and the types of symptoms will vary from patient to patient.[17] Also, using this framework or classification can help in determining the treatment plan for each patient. For example, if a patient has loudness or annoyance hyperacusis types, the audiologist may provide counseling and sound therapy that will be adequate to address their needs. Patients report a variety of sounds as being annoying, for example, babies crying, doors slamming, or people chewing. Other patients with pain or fear hyperacusis may need further counseling and medication from a mental health professional. Consider the following examples of dramatic experiences from patients with pain hyperacusis:

- "The sound of putting on clothing feels like lightly blowing on an open wound."
- "My ear feels raw and vulnerable to sound as if it were an open wound."
- "Setting a coffee mug on a wooden table feels like a thumb pressing hard on broken bone, deep in the ear."
- "Walking on gravel feels as if I am pressing the gravel into my wounded ears."

To illustrate the varying nature of hyperacusis, we recorded several interviews with individuals with hyperacusis (and tinnitus), including adult patients and a parent of a child, that are available on our companion website. These interviews also provide helpful perspectives by patients and family members, including their daily experiences with hyperacusis, their reactions to having hyperacusis, and any strategies for managing their hyperacusis.

13.3 Causes

Similar to tinnitus and hearing loss, there are many causes of the different subtypes of hyperacusis[18,19,20] (for reviews, see Tyler et al[16] and Pienkowski et al[21]). For example, excessive noise exposure, Meniere's disease, and head injury are common causes of hyperacusis. Other causes of hyperacusis include Bell palsy, migraines, and genetic disorders and even autism. Interestingly, there might be a genetic cause in a few cases such as that of William syndrome (83.7% as reported by Gothelf et al[22]).

13.4 Mechanisms

There are likely many different causes and mechanisms for hyperacusis similar to what is reported in the tinnitus literature.[23,24, 25] Normally, the coding of loudness when sound intensity increases is thought to result from an increase in electrical activity on an individual nerve fiber and an increase

in the number of nerve fibers that are activated (see ▸ Fig. 13.1).

However, in cases of hyperacusis, there is likely an abnormal auditory gain control.[26] The thought is that the brain searches for electrical activity and magnifies this response. The resulting nerve activity will be high for moderately loud and loud sounds, regardless of the input sound level. There is an abnormal unexpected relationship between the level of the sound and the neural rate and/or overall/phase locked activity of the auditory nerve fibers, which causes this abnormal response observed in hyperacusis.

13.5 Measuring Hyperacusis

Hyperacusis is not closely linked to hearing thresholds, as revealed in numerous studies.[14,27,28,29,30] In fact, many patients with hyperacusis have no worse than a mild hearing loss.[31] Given that the audiogram is not likely to be indicative of hyperacusis, we need to consider other options for measuring hyperacusis.

Loudness hyperacusis can be measured by determining the loudness discomfort levels (LDLs) for the patient.[21,32] Caution must be used when measuring LDLs in patients with hyperacusis. In many patients, presenting pulsed tones at or near their level of discomfort will be difficult and could potentially trigger a hyperacusis episode. We counsel patients carefully about LDL testing and provide many breaks to help them recover. Not all audiologists perform LDLs on the first visit to the clinic to avoid any discomfort to the patient. Rather, this testing can be performed at a subsequent visit after rapport has been established with the patient. One approach to measuring LDLs is as follows:

- Using a pulsed tone, say to the patient: "Assign a number from 0 to 100 that represents the loudness of the tone. A score of 0% would mean that you can't hear the tone. A score of 100% would mean that the tone is uncomfortably loud."
- Start with levels just above threshold and gradually present tones at higher levels, using 5-dB increments. Do not present a signal that produces a rating above 80%. Test at least three times at each frequency and average the trials.
- Test the sound frequencies of 500, 1000, 2000, and 4000 Hz. Because many patients are bothered at high frequencies, consider avoiding 8000 Hz when measuring LDLs.

Again, caution must be used when testing LDLs in some patients! The maximum response for a given patient can be reduced to 70% instead of 80%, so a careful approach by the audiologist is needed.

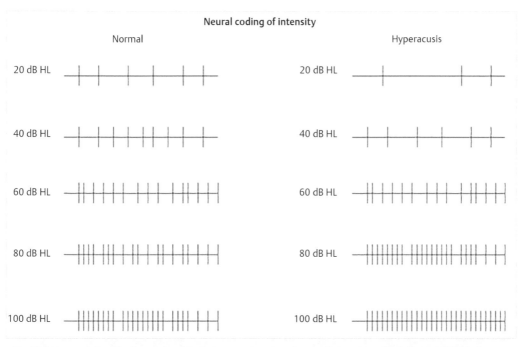

Fig. 13.1 An example of how neural activity increases on a normal nerve fiber as intensity is increased (*left*). One possible mechanism in hyperacusis (*right*) shows that neural activity increases more rapidly as intensity is increased.

13.6 Questionnaires

Like tinnitus, it is important to distinguish the hyperacusis from the reactions to the hyperacusis. A good method for identifying the patient's complaints is to use a self-report questionnaire. In addition, some patients with hyperacusis can have serious reactions to sound exposures, suggesting that the hyperacusis is quite bothersome.[33,34] Likewise, self-report questionnaires are an important tool for determining the severity of the hyperacusis. Indeed, there are several questionnaires available for measuring reactions to and severity of hyperacusis.[4,10,35,36,37,38,39] We have adapted our open-ended tinnitus questionnaire[15] to be inclusive of hyperacusis that is referred to as the Hyperacusis Problems Questionnaire (see Appendix 13.1 Hyperacusis Problems Questionnaire).

As an example, many patients report: "I just don't go to restaurants anymore," or "The sound of the dishes clanging is the worst!" In addition, we use a hyperacusis intake questionnaire for patients who decide to receive counseling and sound therapy in our clinics (see Appendix 13.2 Hyperacusis Intake Questionnaire). This questionnaire collects important information about the duration of their hyperacusis, any known causes of the hyperacusis,

along with things that make the hyperacusis better or worse. We also use the intake questionnaire to determine the type of hyperacusis, including loudness, annoyance, fear, and pain. Finally, the intake questionnaire is helpful in determining what treatments that the patient has tried already to help his/her hyperacusis, as well as the presence of other symptoms like migraines, smell or taste disturbances that may require our attention. Lastly, we often use a hyperacusis handicap scale, which can be used before and after treatments (see Appendix 13.3).

13.7 Treatments

Unfortunately, there are no medications or surgeries that have been shown to cure hyperacusis at this time. However, there are several treatment options that show positive results for patients with hyperacusis. Research is still emerging about the effectiveness of these therapy approaches. First, we recommend counseling for hyperacusis such as Hyperacusis Activities Treatment, which will be described in more detail here. In addition, we recommend sound therapy using background sound to reduce annoyance and/or increase sound tolerance. Counseling and sound therapy approaches are beneficial in managing hyperacusis symptoms, as evidenced through multiple treatment studies of patients with hyperacusis.[31,40,41,42] At our initial sessions, we often recommend that patients purchase customized musician earplugs with noise reduction filters and a standard plug to reduce sound exposure in noisy situations and provide comfort when listening to loud sounds. We also inform patients that medications can be very helpful to manage any related symptoms that patients may experience such as anxiety, depression, and insomnia. We will work closely with the patient's physician, psychologist, or psychiatrist to manage these symptoms and make the necessary referrals when needed. Lastly, we review and demonstrate relaxation exercises in our sessions to provide patients with effective coping strategies after a hyperacusis episode and to lessen fear and anxiety. Chapter 10 on mindfulness outlined relaxation exercises that tinnitus patients find beneficial, that will also be helpful to patients with hyperacusis. Finally, Appendix 13.4 provides an informational brochure on hyperacusis that can be modified for individual clinics and outlines therapy options for patients (also available in our companion website).

Here, we will concentrate on Hyperacusis Activities Treatment to support audiologists providing counseling and sound therapy recommendations to patients with hyperacusis.

13.7.1 Counseling—Hyperacusis Activity Treatment

Our counseling strategy evolved from our Tinnitus Activities Treatment,[43,44] and there is an overlap between the two approaches (see Chapter 4). Though we will concentrate mostly on adults, children with hyperacusis should be considered and assisted in a similar format with a few modifications (see Coelho et al[45] for a review). We prefer to start our patients in a group session (often times with tinnitus patients because many patients have both tinnitus and hyperacusis) before individual counseling sessions begin, although this is not a requirement.[46] Our counseling approach is flexible and patient-centered, developed along with the patients to address their needs. Subjective responses from the hyperacusis intake questionnaire, problems questionnaire, and interviews with the patient will be beneficial in identifying the patient's needs and inform the direction of counseling. See Appendices 13.1 to 13.3 for these questionnaires. Another approach is to use the Client Oriented Scale of Improvement, or COSI,[47] and modify it for the patient with hyperacusis. This tool identifies three to five problem areas for the patient, which can then be used to create goals for the counseling therapy. In Hyperacusis Activities Treatment (refer to Appendix 13.5 for the slides), we provide education about hyperacusis, counseling on reactions to hyperacusis, and review treatments to relieve symptoms such as sound therapy, medications, and relaxation exercises. We typically begin therapy for a new patient with hyperacusis in a one-hour session and review as needed.

We cover the four areas potentially affected, thoughts and emotions, hearing, sleep, and concentration, depending on the patient's specific problems. The picture-based counseling occurs in the clinic (see ▶ Fig. 13.2), by practicing exercises,[39,43,48] and providing homework to practice the strategies and exercises in daily life (refer to Appendix 13.6 for an example handout to provide patients on hyperacusis treatment options). On the return visit, the homework is reviewed, and the next area is introduced. Our initial session on Hyperacusis Activities Treatment slides, including a narrated version, is available as Appendix 13.5 and also on the companion website. Here, we will make some general comments about our experience with patients with hyperacusis and provide specific examples to illustrate our approach.

13.7.2 Introduction

The best place to start is with introductions either with the therapy group or, if it is a one-on-one session, with the patient. We get to know the patient better by discussing their experience with hyperacusis, what brought them to the clinic, and what they are expecting out of treatment. A general explanation of how hearing works, as well as hearing loss and hyperacusis will also benefit the patient(s).

13.7.3 Thoughts and Emotions

The impact of hyperacusis on emotional wellbeing, causing distress, depression, or anxiety is one of the worse effects for many patients. We do our best to connect with the patients and interact with them at their level (see Chapter 5 for a detailed approach of connecting to your patient!). We show patients that we care and that we want to know how they are coping to nurture their expectations and provide a sense of hope. In the process of getting to know the patient well and building rapport, we ask them about their daily experiences with hyperacusis:

- Are there times during the day when you are particularly bothered?

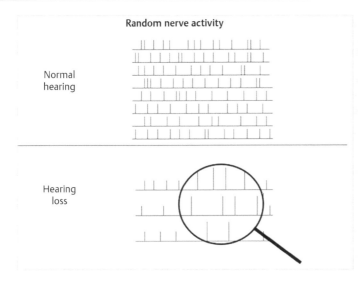

Fig. 13.2 An example of one of the pictures from Hyperacusis Activities Treatment. The brain, with a hearing loss (nerve fibers lost), attempts to magnify the brain activity. It is often helpful to show patients that brain activity is actually responsible for their hyperacusis (see Appendix 13.4).

- Are there times during the day when you are not bothered?
- How long do the episodes typically last after the triggering event?

We share that it is reasonable to be upset and distressed by hyperacusis. We share that everyone experiences challenges in life and hyperacusis often is difficult for many patients. Their concerns are reasonable, and yet, there are many treatments and strategies that patients can try including medications for anxiety, depression, and also relaxation exercises to address the emotional problems created by the hyperacusis. Providing these options and reinforcing their benefits is often received with a sense of relief to many patients with hyperacusis. There are several things that patients can do to make their hyperacusis less problematic, and we are there to help.

13.7.4 Hearing and Communication

Some patients with hyperacusis may have a hearing loss, though not all. However, even in patients with normal hearing, they can have significant problems with hearing and communication as a result of the hyperacusis. For example, some patients with bilateral normal hearing have reported that hyperacusis makes it hard for them tell how loud they are speaking, or that it makes it difficult to focus on conversation or on what people are saying. The strategies for helping a patient with hyperacusis are often the same as more traditional approaches for patients with hearing loss that we would take in aural rehabilitation. This approach includes

making sure you can see the talker's face, reducing background noise, and asking the talker to slow down and speak clearly, for example. In addition, concentrating or engaging fully in the conversation or auditory task, and focusing one's attention away from their hyperacusis will also be beneficial.

13.7.5 Sleep

Many hyperacusis patients are very stressed emotionally that can interfere with their sleep. Other patients will report that while trying to get to sleep, they are disturbed by background noises in their environment or awakened by nearby sounds. Sleep strategies as discussed in Chapter 4 on Tinnitus Activities Treatment, as well as relaxation exercises (see Chapter 10) can be very helpful to alleviate sleep problems. Many patients benefit from playing a low-level background sound in the bedroom such as a fan or soft music to reduce the annoyance of external sounds and relax before bed. For some patients, the same nonwearable sound generators used for tinnitus (see Chapter 8), or even an App for tinnitus relief (see Chapter 9), have additional benefits for relaxing patients at night.

13.7.6 Concentration

When one is worried about and attentive to potential background sounds, it makes it difficult to concentrate. Many hyperacusis patients have difficulty concentrating because they are anticipating being exposed to a loud sound and focusing more on hyperacusis than the task at hand. A variety of techniques can be explored to increase one's concentration abilities, including eliminating distractions in the environment (particularly unwanted noise), staying focused and attentive to a particular task, and shortening the duration of more complex tasks to 20- to 40-minute chunks when concentration is extremely important. We often recommend patients journal or write down their concerns and worries, which can be addressed at certain times of the day, rather than creating anxiety that is experienced regularly and distracts from other tasks. Finally, attention diversion exercises used for tinnitus and reviewed in Chapter 4 are also appropriate for patients with hyperacusis. These exercises promote volitional control of one's attention that is also necessary to cope with emotional distress from hyperacusis. Again, the relaxation exercises (see Chapter 10) can be very helpful for some patients to calm anxieties and fears, and provide better focus away from hyperacusis.

13.7.7 Hearing Protection

Many hyperacusis patients come to our clinics wearing earplugs, or even earmuffs for everyday listening! This, of course, reduces the intensity of sound reaching their cochlea, which helps them cope with their hyperacusis. However, it also reduces the level of speech, affecting their communication negatively and reducing socialization and their quality of life over time. This approach of using earplugs daily, all day long does not improve their hyperacusis, and might even make it worse by degrading sound tolerance over time.[26,49] We explain to patients that constant use of earplugs might result in not allowing their auditory system to be exposed to everyday sounds. Further, the constant use of hearing protection does not let your brain get used to hearing normal sounds. However, we also emphasize the importance to protect our hearing when exposed to loud noise, for example, cutting the grass or vacuuming. We provide earplugs to our patients who do not have a reliable set of hearing protection.

As mentioned earlier, we also recommend the use of musician's earplugs for patients with hyperacusis and fit them at our clinics. Regular, foam earplugs reduce sound levels to effectively manage noise exposures, but often have a negative effect on speech perception for the listener, given their high noise reduction rating. By comparison, musician filtered earplugs do not attenuate sound levels as significantly, and also preserve high frequencies necessary for speech perception. Reducing all frequencies using a filtered earplug by the same amount, but not as severely as a foam earplug, will result in better speech perception for most patients, which is often desired by patients with hyperacusis seeking comfort in noisy situations who will use them often.

Hearing protection devices are available for hunters with very rapid reaction times to reduce impulsive noise. This might be helpful for some hyperacusis patients who are bothered by rapid-onset high-level sounds. Similar to foam earplugs, these devices do not treat the hyperacusis, but can be effective in allowing some patients to function in everyday situations with considerable background noise.

13.7.8 Sound Therapies

There are three general strategies for using sound therapy to manage hyperacusis. Compared to the use of sound therapy for tinnitus (see Chapter 8), there are some similarities in these approaches for hyperacusis. However, there are also important differences that we will review here.

Low-Level Broadband Noise

Hazell[26] and Hazell and Sheldrake[50] based their approach of using low-level background noise on their theory of the brain amplifying and searching for sound. By providing background sound, Hazell and Sheldrake believed that they could reduce the brain's need to provide some central gain to external sounds. They suggested that bilateral noise generators provide continuous exposure to patients using low-level noise. Several publications from Formby's group have shown this approach can improve LDLs for many patients with hyperacusis.[49,51,52,53,54] In some subjects, Formby and colleagues were able to show that the use of sound generators (no counseling) resulted in ~20-dB elevations (or improvement) of LDLs after several weeks of sound therapy.

Successive Approximations with High-Level Broadband Noise

Vernon[55] and Vernon and Press[56] suggested an approach entitled, "Desensitization with Pink Noise." Patients listened to pink noise for about 2 hours per day through traditional earphones. The noise level of the pink noise was gradually increased daily or weekly to approximate each patient's LDLs. Vernon reported success in many patients with hyperacusis using this approach with pink noise. However, results varied significantly in the timeline for these positive outcomes, with some patients requiring 3 months with the noise therapy whereas others 2 years!

Successive Approximations Using Low-Level Sounds

Tyler[57] and Tyler et al,[39] as part of Hyperacusis Activities Treatment, suggested using successive approximations at low levels rather than approaching LDLs to help improve sound tolerance gradually and to avoid any discomfort by the patient. The sounds selected for this treatment include using sounds that produced the hyperacusis response or using relaxing sounds such as enjoyable music, nature sounds, or other noises that patients find pleasant to listen to for an extended time every day. If using the patient's sounds that elicit hyperacusis, successive approximation uses the following steps:

- Identify some of the sounds that produce the hyperacusis.
- Record or produce these sounds.
- Listen to the recorded sounds at a low acceptable level daily for several minutes when the patient is relaxed and has control over the level and duration of listening. They can be performing another activity, such as reading, if they wish.
- Over several weeks or months, gradually increase the duration and level of the sounds (if needed, it is OK to back up and reduce the level and duration).
- Eventually move the listening experience to the location where the actual sounds are produced.
- Switch from the recorded sound to the actual sounds, but the patient still maintains control (progressing from low to high levels, and short to longer durations).
- Have other individuals, such as a close friend or family member, produce the sounds that would have previously been disruptive (progressing from low to high levels, and short to longer durations) to illustrate the benefits with this therapy.

Essentially the same steps would be completed if using pleasant or relaxing sounds. On the companion website, we offer a sound therapy protocol (see Appendix 13.6) and sound diary (see Appendix 13.7) for patients with hyperacusis that utilizes this second approach to successive approximations. The sound therapy protocol assists patients in selecting sounds for their therapy, as well as suggestions for the duration of therapy, and increasing the level of the sound gradually over time. Patients can use the sound diary to record the sound selected, the number of hours of listening, the level of the sound, and any reactions to the sound during the listening session. This data will be informative for the patient and clinician in evaluating progress with the therapy.

13.7.9 Using Hearing Aids to Help with Hyperacusis

In our clinical experience, there are many patients with hyperacusis who also have hearing loss and want to use hearing aids to improve their communication abilities and speech understanding. However, a common complaint among hearing aid users with hyperacusis is that the hearing aids amplify sounds to distressing levels that exasperates their hyperacusis. There are strategies to help patients with hyperacusis using hearing aids, as follows:

- Set the maximum power output (MPO) of the hearing aid below their measured LDLs. Use real ear verification measures to check the MPO as well as subjective input from the patient. The MPO can be increased over time with increased device use, as appropriate.
- Increase the reaction time of automatic gain control to adjust quickly in response to loud sounds.
- Ensure that the user can adjust the volume control on the aid(s) using the controls on the aid, on an App, and/or a remote device.
- Add and encourage use of programs that suppress background noise using adaptive directional microphones and noise reduction to ensure comfort in noisy situations.
- Add and encourage use of programs that combine amplification plus tinnitus sound therapies, including static and modulated sounds, to help mask environmental sounds that are annoying. Start the tinnitus sound at a low level as described previously regarding successive approximations.
- Encourage use of hearing aids for at least 8 hours a day, but recognize that patients with hyperacusis may not use their devices as much compared to patients using hearing aids who do not have hyperacusis.

Sammeth et al[58] proposed a clever approach that involves desensitizing patients with hyperacusis using hearing aids, with or without hearing loss. At first, one might think hearing aids amplify sound for the patient, which should make their situation worse! However, using closed ear pieces with a hearing aid, these devices actually function as earplugs, reducing the level of sound, and therefore, providing a way to manage the patient's hyperacusis. The hearings aids are adjusted to the individual's hearing thresholds, maximizing their speech perception. As suggested previously, the maximum power output of the hearing aids is adjusted to their LDLs so the patient does not experience hyperacusis. This reduction of the dynamic range will likely reduce the patient's speech perception abilities in some situations. However, the advantage here is that hyperacusis is not experienced by the patient. The next step, perhaps over several weeks or even months, is to increase the maximum power output setting gradually over time. The long-term goal with this approach would be to enable the patient to adapt to louder sounds gradually, and experience the full dynamic range of sounds in the environment.

13.8 Conclusion

We know that patients with hyperacusis can be distressed by their daily experiences of sound and that hyperacusis can have a lasting impact on their social interactions with others, emotional well-being, and overall quality of life. There are many different causes for hyperacusis, the most common among these being noise exposure, Meniere's disease, and head injury. The common complaints of patients with hyperacusis are that (1) everyday, moderate-level sounds are too loud and/or annoying that are not bothersome to others around them; (2) they avoid social situations or noisy places to lessen anxiety and fear about sound exposure; and (3) they experience pain with sound exposure that is intense and often debilitating. There are likely many different subtypes and many different mechanisms of hyperacusis that need to be researched. Although there are currently no cures available for hyperacusis, there are several treatment options that can be successful for patients, including counseling, sound therapy, filtered earplugs, medications for related symptoms, and relaxation exercises.

We offer several videos for this chapter on Hyperacusis available on the companion website, including three interviews with hyperacusis patients describing their hyperacusis experience, the challenges in having hyperacusis, and advice for other hyperacusis patients. Also, you will find a narration of Hyperacusis Activities Treatment slides intended for audiologists who counsel patients with hyperacusis.

References

[1] Tyler RS, Conrad-Armes D. The determination of tinnitus loudness considering the effects of recruitment. J Speech Hear Res. 1983; 26(1):59–72

[2] Bläsing L, Goebel G, Flötzinger U, Berthold A, Kröner-Herwig B. Hypersensitivity to sound in tinnitus patients: an analysis of a construct based on questionnaire and audiological data. Int J Audiol. 2010; 49(7):518–526

[3] Chen G, Lee C, Sandridge SA, Butler HM, Manzoor NF, Kaltenbach JA. Behavioral evidence for possible simultaneous induction of hyperacusis and tinnitus following intense sound exposure. J Assoc Res Otolaryngol. 2013; 14(3):413–424

[4] Dauman R, Bouscau-Faure F. Assessment and amelioration of hyperacusis in tinnitus patients. Acta Otolaryngol. 2005; 125 (5):503–509

[5] Deshpande AK, Tyler R. Tinnitus and hyperacusis. In: Valente M, Valente LM, eds. Adult audiology casebook. 2nd ed. New York, NY: Thieme; 2018

[6] Tyler RS. Interest in hyperacusis on the rise. Hear J. 2016; 69 (2):32–33

[7] Bartnik G, Fabijańska A, Rogowski M. Experiences in the treatment of patients with tinnitus and/or hyperacusis using the habituation method. Scand Audiol Suppl. 2001; 30(52): 187–190

[8] Kochkin S, Tyler RS. Tinnitus treatment and the effectiveness of hearing aids: hearing care professional perceptions. Hearing Rev. 2008; 15(13):14–18

[9] Sood SK, Coles RRA. Hyperacusis and phonophobia in tinnitus patients. Br J Audiol. 1998; 41:545–554

[10] Anari M, Axelsson A, Eliasson A, Magnusson L. Hypersensitivity to sound: questionnaire data, audiometry and classification. Scand Audiol. 1999; 28(4):219–230

[11] Andersson G, Lindvall N, Hursti T, Carlbring P. Hypersensitivity to sound (hyperacusis): a prevalence study conducted via the Internet and post. Int J Audiol. 2002; 41(8):545–554

[12] Hannula S, Bloigu R, Majamaa K, Sorri M, Mäki-Torkko E. Self-reported hearing problems among older adults: prevalence and comparison to measured hearing impairment. J Am Acad Audiol. 2011; 22(8):550–559

[13] Blaesing L, Kroener-Herwig B. Self-reported and behavioral sound avoidance in tinnitus and hyperacusis subjects, and association with anxiety ratings. Int J Audiol. 2012; 51(8): 611–617

[14] Urnau D, Tochetto TM. Characteristics of the tinnitus and hyperacusis in normal hearing individuals. Int Arch Otorhinolaryngol. 2011; 15:468–474

[15] Tyler RS, Baker LJ. Difficulties experienced by tinnitus sufferers. J Speech Hear Disord. 1983; 48(2):150–154

[16] Tyler RS, Pienkowski M, Roncancio ER, et al. A review of hyperacusis and future directions: part I. Definitions and manifestations. Am J Audiol. 2014; 23(4):402–419

[17] Ke J, Du Y, Tyler RS, Perreau A, Mancini PC. Complaints of people with hyperacusis. J Am Acad Audiol. 2020; 31(8): 553–558

[18] Blomberg S, Rosander M, Andersson G. Fears, hyperacusis and musicality in Williams syndrome. Res Dev Disabil. 2006; 27(6):668–680

[19] Hallberg LRM, Hallberg U, Johansson M, Jansson G, Wiberg A. Daily living with hyperacusis due to head injury 1 year after a treatment programme at the hearing clinic. Scand J Caring Sci. 2005; 19(4):410–418

[20] Khalfa S, Bruneau N, Rogé B, et al. Increased perception of loudness in autism. Hear Res. 2004; 198(1–2):87–92

[21] Pienkowski M, Tyler RS, Roncancio ER, et al. A review of hyperacusis and future directions: part II. Measurement, mechanisms, and treatment. Am J Audiol. 2014; 23(4):420–436

[22] Gothelf D, Farber N, Raveh E, Apter A, Attias J. Hyperacusis in Williams syndrome: characteristics and associated neuroaudiologic abnormalities. Neurology. 2006; 66(3): 390–395

[23] Gordon AG. "Hyperacusis" and origins of lowered sound tolerance. J Neuropsychiatry Clin Neurosci. 2000; 12(1): 117–119

[24] Hwang JH, Chou PH, Wu CW, Chen JH, Liu TC. Brain activation in patients with idiopathic hyperacusis. Am J Otolaryngol. 2009; 30(6):432–434

[25] Zeng FG. An active loudness model suggesting tinnitus as increased central noise and hyperacusis as increased nonlinear gain. Hear Res. 2013; 295:172–179

[26] Hazell JWP. Tinnitus masking therapy. In: Hazell JWP, ed. Tinnitus. London: Churchill Livingston; 1987

[27] Brandy WT, Lynn JM. Audiologic findings in hyperacusis and nonhyperacusic subjects. Am J Audiol. 1995; 44:46–51

[28] Gu JW, Halpin CF, Nam EC, Levine RA, Melcher JR. Tinnitus, diminished sound-level tolerance, and elevated auditory activity in humans with clinically normal hearing sensitivity. J Neurophysiol. 2010; 104(6):3361–3370

[29] Meeus OM, Spaepen M, Ridder DD, Heyning PH. Correlation between hyperacusis measurements in daily ENT practice. Int J Audiol. 2010; 49(1):7–13

[30] Nelson JJ, Chen K. The relationship of tinnitus, hyperacusis, and hearing loss. Ear Nose Throat J. 2004; 83 (7):472–476

[31] Aazh H, Moore BCJ. Effectiveness of audiologist-delivered cognitive behavioral therapy for tinnitus and hyperacusis rehabilitation: outcomes for patients treated in routine practice. Am J Audiol. 2018; 27(4):547–558

[32] Wallén MB, Hasson D, Theorell T, Canlon B. The correlation between the hyperacusis questionnaire and uncomfortable loudness levels is dependent on emotional exhaustion. Int J Audiol. 2012; 51(10):722–729

[33] Goebel G, Floetzinger U. Pilot study to evaluate psychiatric co-morbidity in tinnitus patients with and without hyperacusis. Audiol Med. 2008; 6:78–84

[34] Jüris L, Andersson G, Larsen HC, Ekselius L. Psychiatric comorbidity and personality traits in patients with hyperacusis. Int J Audiol. 2013; 52(4):230–235

[35] Aazh H, Moore BCJ. Usefulness of self-report questionnaires for psychological assessment of patients with tinnitus and hyperacusis and patients' views of the questionnaires. Int J Audiol. 2017; 56(7):489–498

[36] Khalfa S, Dubal S, Veuillet E, Perez-Diaz F, Jouvent R, Collet L. Psychometric normalization of a hyperacusis questionnaire. ORL J Otorhinolaryngol Relat Spec. 2002; 64(6):436–442

[37] Nelting M, Rienhoff NK, Hesse G, Lamparter U. The assessment of subjective distress related to hyperacusis with a self-rating questionnaire on hypersensitivity to sound. Laryngorhinootologie. 2002; 81(5):327–334

[38] Tyler RS, Bergan C, Preece J, Nagase S. Audiologische Messmethoden de Hyperakusis. In: Nelting M, ed. Hyperakusis. Stuttgart: Georg Thieme Verlag; 2003

[39] Tyler RS, Noble W, Coelho C, Haskell G, Bardia A. Tinnitus and hyperacusis. In: Katz J, Burkard R, Medwetsky L, Hood L, eds. Handbook of clinical audiology, 6th ed. Baltimore, MD: Lippincott Williams and Wilkins; 2009

[40] Elgandy MS, Tyler RS. Relief Strategies for Hyperacusis. Ainosco Press. 2018; 39:1-13. DOI:10.6143/JSLHAT.201812_39.0001

[41] Jastreboff PJ, Jastreboff MM. Tinnitus retraining therapy for patients with tinnitus and decreased sound tolerance. Otolaryngol Clin North Am. 2003; 36(2):321–336

[42] Katzenell U, Segal S. Hyperacusis: review and clinical guidelines. Otol Neurotol. 2001; 22(3):321–326, discussion 326–327

[43] Tyler RS, Gehringer AK, Noble W, Dunn CC, Witt SA, Bardia A. Tinnitus activities treatment. In: Tyler RS, ed. Tinnitus treatment: clinical protocols. New York: Thieme Medical Publishers; 2006

[44] Tyler RS, Gogel SA, Gehringer AK. Tinnitus activities treatment. Prog Brain Res. 2007; 166:425–434

[45] Coelho CB, Sanchez TG, Tyler RS. Hyperacusis, sound annoyance, and loudness hypersensitivity in children. Prog Brain Res. 2007; 166:169–178

[46] Perreau AE, Tyler RS, Mancini PC, Witt S, Elgandy MS. Establishing a group educational session for hyperacusis patients. Am J Audiol. 2019; 28(2):245–250

[47] Dillon H, James A, Ginis J. Client Oriented Scale of Improvement (COSI) and its relationship to several other measures of benefit and satisfaction provided by hearing aids. J Am Acad Audiol. 1997; 8(1):27–43

[48] Tyler RS, Noble W, Coelho C, Roncancio ER, Jun HJ. Tinnitus and hyperacusis. In: Katz J, ed. Handbook of clinical audiology. 7th ed. Baltimore, MD: Lippincott Williams & Wilkins; 2015:647–658

[49] Formby C, Sherlock LP, Gold SL. Adaptive plasticity of loudness induced by chronic attenuation and enhancement of the acoustic background. J Acoust Soc Am. 2003; 114(1):55–58

[50] Hazell JWP, Sheldrake JB. (1992). Hyperacusis and tinnitus. In: Aran J-M, Dauman R, eds. Tinnitus '91. Proceedings of the Fourth International Tinnitus Seminar. Amsterdam: Kugler Publications

[51] Formby C, Gold SL. Modification of loudness discomfort level: evidence for adaptive chronic auditory gain and its clinical relevance. Semin Hear. 2002; 23(1):21–34

[52] Formby C, Gold SL, Keaser ML, Block KL, Hawley ML. Secondary benefits from tinnitus retraining therapy (TRT): clinically significant increases in loudness discomfort level and in the auditory dynamic range. Semin Hear. 2007; 28(4):276–294

[53] Formby C, Hawley M, Sherlock L, et al. Intervention for restricted dynamic range and reduced sound tolerance. J Acoust Soc Am. 2008; 123:37

[54] Formby C, Hawley M, Sherlock LP, et al. Intervention for restricted dynamic range and reduced sound tolerance: clinical trial using a tinnitus retraining therapy protocol for hyperacusis. Proc Meet Acoust. 2013; 19:050083

[55] Vernon JA. Pathophysiology of tinnitus: a special case—hyperacusis and a proposed treatment. Am J Otol. 1987; 8 (3):201–202

[56] Vernon JA, Press L. Treatment for hyperacusis. In: Vernon JA, ed. Tinnitus treatment and relief. Boston, MA: Allyn & Bacon; 1998:223–227

[57] Tyler RS. The psychoacoustical measurement of tinnitus. In: Tyler RS, ed. Tinnitus handbook. San Diego, CA: Singular Publishing Group; 2000:149–179

[58] Sammeth CA, Preves DA, Brandy WT. Hyperacusis: case studies and evaluation of electronic loudness suppression devices as a treatment approach. Scand Audiol. 2000; 29(1):28–36

Suggested Reading

Iowa Hyperacusis Website. https://uiowa.qualtrics.com/SE/?SID=SV_22YHczpQkvXNHsE

Appendix 13.1 Hyperacusis Problems Questionnaire

Patient Name: _____

Date: _____

Hyperacusis is a condition where moderately loud or loud sounds are heard as *very* loud, or even painfully loud.

Please list the problems that you experience because of your **hyperacusis**. List as many as you can. List them in order of importance.

  1

  2

  3

  4

  5

  6

  7

  8

  9

10

11

12

Appendix 13.2 Hyperacusis Intake Questionnaire

Patient Name: _____

Date: _____

Some people report that many sounds are too loud for them; however, these same sounds do not appear too loud to others. This is called hyperacusis.

For questions that ask you to rate on a scale from 0 to100, 0 = strongly disagree and 100 = strongly agree.	

1. Sounds that others believe are moderately loud are **too loud** to me. _____ (0–100)

2. Which ear(s) seems to be affected by the hyperacusis? (circle one) Left Right Both

3. How long have you had hyperacusis? _____ months OR _____ years

4. What do you think originally caused your hyperacusis? (Please choose only ONE answer)

   a) Accident
   b) Aging
   c) Infection/virus
   d) Hearing loss (long term)
   e) Hearing loss (sudden)
   f) Medications

   a) Meniere's Disease
   b) Noise exposure-continuous
   c) Noise exposure-impulsive
   d) Surgery
   e) I don't know
   f) Other _____

5. Has it gotten worse, better, or stayed the same since it first started? (circle one) Same Better Worse

6. Which of the following sounds or events are often **too loud** for you?

   a) Baby crying/children squealing
   b) Crowds/large gatherings
   c) Dishes being stacked
   d) Dog barking
   e) High pitch voices/screaming
   f) Lawnmower
   g) Music (loud rock concerts)
   h) Music (religious service)
   i) Music (symphony, quartet, etc.)

   a) Power tools
   b) Restaurants
   c) Sporting events
   d) Telephone ringing
   e) TV/radio
   f) Vacuum cleaner
   g) Whistle/horn/siren
   h) Other _____

7. Which of the following sounds or events are those that you are **annoyed** by?

   a) Baby crying/children squealing
   b) Crowds/large gatherings
   c) Dishes being stacked
   d) Dog barking
   e) High pitch voices/screaming
   f) Lawnmower
   g) Music (loud rock concerts)
   h) Music (religious services)
   i) Music (symphony, quartet, etc.)

   a) Power tools
   b) Restaurants
   c) Sporting events
   d) Telephone ringing
   e) TV/radio
   f) Vacuum cleaner
   g) Whistle/horn/siren
   h) Other _____

8. Which of the following sounds or events are those that you would **fear attending or being around** because of your reaction to those sounds?

   a) Baby crying/children squealing
   b) Crowds/large gatherings
   c) Dishes being stacked
   d) Dog barking
   e) High pitch voices/screaming
   f) Lawnmower
   g) Music (loud rock concerts)
   h) Music (religious services)
   i) Music (symphony, quartet, etc.)

   a) Power tools
   b) Restaurants
   c) Sporting events
   d) Telephone ringing
   e) TV/radio
   f) Vacuum cleaner
   g) Whistle/horn/siren
   h) Other _____

9	How often do you experience headaches?	_____ #/month
10	Rate the severity of these headaches from 0 to 100.	_____ (0–100)
11	How often do you experience balance problems?	_____ #/month
12	Rate the severity of your balance problems from 0 to 100.	_____ (0–100)
13	How often do bright lights bother you?	_____ #/month
14	Rate the severity of how bothersome bright lights are from 0 to 100.	_____ (0–100)
15	How often do you experience smell problems?	_____ #/month
16	Rate the severity of these smell problems from 0 to 100.	_____ (0–100)

17   Are you bothered by strong smells?   Yes No
     If yes, please circle those below that bother you.

a) Bleaches, ammonia, cleaning solvents   a) Paint
b) Car exhaust   b) Perfume
c) Cigarette smoke   c) Pesticides/insecticides
d) Coffee   d) Spices
e) Farm odors   e) Other _____

18   Are you bothered by certain tastes?   Yes No
     If yes, please circle those below that bother you.

a) Cheese   a) Sour foods (e.g., Vinegar)
b) Coconut   b) Spices
c) Peppers   c) Sweet foods
d) Salty foods   d) Other _____

19   Are you bothered by touch?   Yes No

20   What makes your hyperacusis worse?

a) Being in complete silence   a) Loud voices
b) Dog barking   b) Medications
c) Changes in pressure & humidity   c) Sharp noises
d) Lack of sleep, fatigue   d) Stress/tension
e) Large crowds   e) TV/radio
f) Lawnmower/snow blower   f) Whistle/horn/siren
g)   g) Other _____

21   What makes your hyperacusis better?

a) Being alone or with few others   a) Removing self from noise
b) Being in a quiet environment   b) Soft music/TV
c) Being relaxed   c) Stress reduction exercises
d) Getting a good night's sleep   d) Wearing ear plugs/ear muffs
e) Low constant sounds (fan, car)   e) Wearing noise generators
f) Medications   f) When I wake up in the morning
g) Reading   g) Other _____

22.   In which ear do you wear hearing aids?   a. Left
                                                      b. Right
                                                      c. Both
                                                      d. None

23.   Do you suffer from tinnitus?   a. Yes
                                            b. No

Pain

24   **Which of the following sounds or events cause pain in your ears?**

a   Baby crying/children squealing

b   Crowds/large gatherings

c   Dishes being stacked

d   Dog barking

e   High pitch voices/screaming

f   Lawnmower

g   Music (loud rock concerts)

h   Music (religious services)

i   Music (symphony, quartet, etc.)

j   Power tools

k   Sporting events

l   Restaurants

m   Telephone ringing

n   TV/radio
             Vacuum cleaner

o   Whistle/horn/siren

p   Other _____

Appendix 13.3 Hyperacusis Disability and Handicap Scales

Part 1

Some everyday sounds are loud and some are soft. Some everyday sounds are annoying and some are not. Please rate the **loudness, annoyance, fear, and pain** of the following sounds. Do not consider the annoyance or fear when rating the loudness, do not consider the loudness or fear when rating the annoyance, do not consider the annoyance or loudness when rating the fear, and do not consider the annoyance or loudness or fear when rating the pain. For example, a sound might be very loud, but you might not be annoyed or afraid of it. Likewise, a sound might be very annoying, but it might not be loud or evoke fear.

Rate the sounds using a scale from 0 (not loud/annoying/fearful) to 100 (unbearably loud/annoying/fearful).

	Loudness	Annoyance	Fear	Pain
1. Standing next to a dog barking				
2. Someone stacking dishes in the same room				
3. Hearing music on the radio in a car when the volume is adjusted for normal-hearing listeners				
4. Hearing music on the radio in a quiet room when the volume is adjusted for normal-hearing listeners				
5. Telephone ringing in the same room				
6. Television in the same room when the volume is adjusted for normal-hearing listeners				
7. Standing next to a lawnmower				
8. Standing next to a car door closing				
9. Talking with someone in a noisy restaurant				
10. Baby crying in the same room				

Part 2

The following questions relate to hearing loss, tinnitus, and loudness hyperacusis. Loudness hyperacusis is when sounds that are moderately loud for other people are too loud for you.

Please rate your agreement/disagreement with the following statements, using a scale from 0 (completely disagree) to 100 (completely agree):

	Because of your hearing loss	Because of your tinnitus	Because some sounds are too loud
1. You avoid shopping			
2. You do not go out with your friends			
3. You have given up some hobbies			
4. You do not go to restaurants			
5. You avoid being in crowds			
6. You feel depressed			
7. You feel anxious			
8. You are not able to concentrate			
9. Your quality of life is poor			
10. You are not able to perform tasks or jobs as well			

Appendix 13.4 Life too Loud? Let's Talk Hyperacusis

What Is Hyperacusis?

Hyperacusis varies in its definitions, but it is essentially the phenomenon of experiencing soft or moderately loud environmental sounds as uncomfortably loud, and includes hypersensitivity and even intolerance of sounds.[1] There are four main categories of hyperacusis:

1. Loudness hyperacusis: preceiving moderately loud sounds as very loud.
2. Annoyance hyperacusis: creating a pervasive negative response, such as irritation or anger.
3. Fear hyperacusis: anticipating being uncomfortable, may lead to avoiding certain situations.
4. Pain hyperacusis: percieving sounds as very loud and causing pain.

Common trigger sounds include:
- Baby crying, children squealing, high pitched voices and / or screaming.
- Crowds, large gatherings, restaurants and / or sporting events.
- Music (e.g., loud rock concerts, orchestra, and / or religious services).
- Dishes being stacked, dog barking, lawnmower, telephone, vacuum, power tools, and / or TV, radio.
- Whistle/horn/siren, loud vehicles.

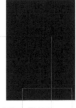

References

[1] Tyler RS, Pienkowski M, Roncancio ER, et al. A review of hyperacusis and future directions: part I. Definitions and manifestations. Am J Audiol. 2014; 23(4):402–419

[2] Park JM, Kim WJ, Ha JB, Han JJ, Park SY, Park SN. Effect of sound generator on tinnitus and hyperacusis. Acta Otolaryngol. 2018; 138(2):135–139

[3] Baguley DM. Hyperacusis: An Overview. Semin Hear. 2014; 35(2): 74–83

[4] Read "Counseling for Patients with Hyperacusis" on Augustana's Digital Commons at https://digitalcommons.augustana.edu/cgi/preview.cgi?article=1002&context=commstudent

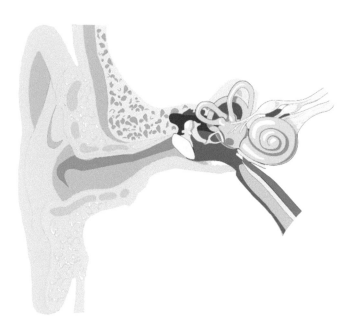

Custom Ear Plugs

Wearing hearing protection at all times can make hyperacusis worse. We recommend earplugs made for musicians to provide comfort in noisy environments, while still being able to understand speech.

Sound Therapy

Use background noise such as a fan, music, or white noise to distract from a trigger sound. Gradually increase this background sound over time to "desensitize" the brain.[2] There are also devices that can be worn like a hearing aid that generate background sound to achieve the same goal.

Mindfulness and Relaxation

Mindfulness is one strategy that can help you manage your hyperacusis. Activities such as meditations or progressive muscle relaxation can be an effective ways to manage annoyance hyperacusis or to help tune out loud sounds in certain situations.

Education and Counseling

Living with hyperacusis may disrupt daily activities and may co-occur with anxiety and depression.[3] Stay knowledgeable about your triggers and difficulties, and it will be easier to manage your hyperacusis. Talk to your audiologist about technology available and advancements in research.

How/Why Does Hyperacusis Occur?

First, it helps to understand the basic hearing mechanism. Sound travels through the air into the outer ear, through the middle ear, and changes from mechanical energy to chemical energy in the inner ear before it travels to the brain to be analyzed. The prevailing theory behind how hyperacusis occurs is that the brain codes all sounds as loud, regardless of how loud or soft they are.

There are many potential causes of hyperacusis. These include frequent migraines, noise exposure, head injuries, genetic disorders, Bell's Palsy, and Meniere's disease.

What Can We Do to Help?

Our clinic offers hyperacusis evaluation, counseling, and treatment for children and adults with hyperacusis. Our audiologists have worked in collaboration with Dr. Richard S. Tyler from the University of Iowa to provide the Hyperacusis Activities Treatment. We use picture-based counseling materials to make learning about hyperacusis easy, we review your experiences with hyperacusis, and we review different management strategies. To provide comprehensive care, we will partner with other professionals including psychologists, ear nose and throat specialists, and school-based personnel depending on the needs of the patient.

Management Solutions

Unfortunately, there is no cure for hyperacusis. However, there are multiple strategies for managing your hyperacusis. Remember, some strategies may work better than others depending on your particular symptoms. Take the time to find what works best for you. Medications can also be prescribed and used to manage anxiety and depression which might impact your hyperacusis.

Appendix 13.5 Hyperacusis Activities Treatment

Hyperacusis activities treatment

Richard S. Tyler, PhD, CCC-A
University of Iowa

Ann Perreau, PhD, CCC-A
Augustana College

THE UNIVERSITY OF IOWA

Hyperacusis Activities Treatment is a counseling program that includes education about hyperacusis, counseling on reactions to hyperacusis, and treatments to relieve symptoms such as sound therapy, medications, and relaxation exercises. The activities treatment is modified from Tinnitus Activities Treatment.

Hyperacusis Activities Treatment uses picture-based counseling and has several advantages for hyperacusis management, including:
• The session proceeds in an orderly fashion.
• The clinician does not overlook important concepts.
• It is easier for the patient to understand concepts.
• Treatment can be easily used by other clinicians.
• Sessions can be adapted to the needs and interests of the patient.
• These slides can be presented in one 1-hour session, or presented over several sessions. We typically begin therapy for a new patient with hyperacusis in one session and review as needed.

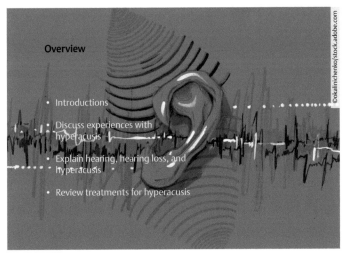

(Source: ©okalinichenko/stock.adobe.com)

The best place to start is with introductions either with the therapy group or if it is a one-on-one session, with the patient. Get to know them better by discussing their experience with hyperacusis, what brought them to the clinic, and what they are expecting out of treatment. A general explanation of how hearing works, as well as hearing loss and hyperacusis will also benefit the patient(s). Discussing treatments such as sound therapy, counseling, relaxation, and medication that could be used to decrease hyperacusis symptoms is also important to discuss, giving the patient(s) a sense of hope that their symptoms can be improved.

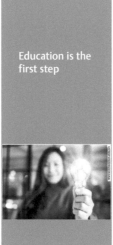

Education is the first step

- Knowledge is the first step to successful management of your hyperacusis
  - How does hyperacusis affect you, in what environments it is most problematic, etc.?
  - What strategies are effective for managing emotions and stressful situations?
- Be confident in communicating your needs to others

(Source: ©Farknot Architect/stock.adobe.com)

The famous Francis Bacon quote "knowledge is power" holds true with hyperacusis. Educating patients on the condition is the first step for them in understanding and managing their hyperacusis. Addressing questions such as:
- How does hyperacusis affect you and in what environments?

- What strategies are effective?

Will build confidence in your patient that they will be able to communicate their needs and manage their hyperacusis and start to regain control again.

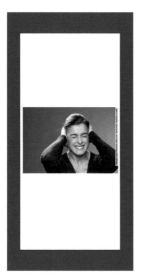

What is hyperacusis?

- Reactions to moderately loud sounds are too loud, annoying, fearful, and/or painful
  - Four types
- Affectes 6 to 17% of general population
- Similar terms:
  - Misophonia
  - Select sound sensitivity

(Source: ©Studio Grand Web/stock.adobe.com. Stock photo. Posed by a model.)

Hyperacusis emphasizes reactions to moderately loud sounds as very loud, annoying, fearful, and/or painful.

Hyperacusis affects approximately 6 to 17% of the general public.

Misophonia and select sound sensitivity are other terms that have been used to describe hyperacusis. Hyperacusis is a more general term and typically easier to interpret.

Types of hyperacusis
Loudness hyperacusis
Annoyance hyperacusis
Fear hyperacusis
Pain hyperacusis

Four categories of hyperacusis can be used to differentiate the perceptions and reactions of patients with hyperacusis. In our experience, most patients will report one or more types, though not all:
- Loudness hyperacusis—perceiving moderately loud sounds as very loud.
- Annoyance hyperacusis—having a negative response such as irritation or anger to sound.
- Fear hyperacusis—anticipating sounds that are uncomfortable and cause fear.

- Pain hyperacusis—perceiving pain in ear or head with sound exposure.

Using these categories can be helpful to learn how to manage hyperacusis. For example, patients with loudness hyperacusis may use an ear-level sound generator to gradually increase their exposure to sound. Patients with fear hyperacusis may need to work with a psychologist to change their aversions to sound through behavioral modifications.

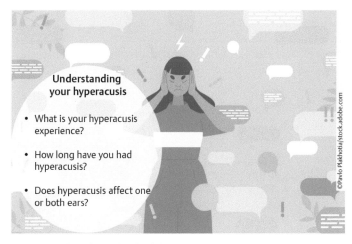

(Source: ©Pavlo Plakhotia/stock.adobe.com)

We begin sessions by getting to know our patients and establishing rapport with them. You might begin by asking these questions:

- What is your hyperacusis experience?
- How long have you had hyperacusis?
- Does hyperacusis affect one or both ears?

Your reactions to sounds

- Are there any sounds that are too loud?

- Are there any sounds that are annoying?

- Are there any sounds that cause fear?

- Are there any sounds that create pain?

(Source: ©Pixsooz/stock.adobe.com)

In the process of getting to know and better understand each patient, asking the following questions will give you a better idea of the impact hyperacusis has on their life:

Are there any sounds that...
- Are too loud?
- Are annoying?
- Cause fear?

- Create pain?

Patients might respond to any of the above with noises such as babies crying, telephone ringing, or doors slamming.

You can also use an intake questionnaire to gather this information about trigger sounds for hyperacusis.

Your daily experience with hyperacusis

- Are there times during the day when you are particularly bothered?

- Are there times during the day when you are not bothered?

- How long do the episodes typically last after the triggering event?

We inquire how often patients are bothered by their hyperacusis and their daily experience with it.

Patients will be different in how the hyperacusis affects them after a triggering event.

To determine their daily experience with hyperacusis, you might ask when they are or are not bothered during the day, and how long the episodes last after the trigger event.

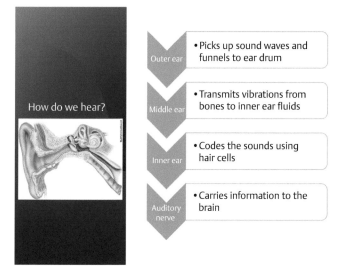

How do we hear?

Outer ear
• Picks up sound waves and funnels to ear drum

Middle ear
• Transmits vibrations from bones to inner ear fluids

Inner ear
• Codes the sounds using hair cells

Auditory nerve
• Carries information to the brain

(Source: ©Judith/stock.adobe.com)

There are two main body systems that are involved in the process of hearing. The peripheral system is composed of the outer, middle, and inner ear structures. Sound waves travel through the outer ear across the tympanic membrane (eardrum), passing through the middle ear to the inner ear and the cochlea. Within the cochlea there are small hair cells where the sound waves are converted into neural impulses. This marks the start of the central auditory system. The neural impulses are then carried up through the auditory nerve to the brain where they are processed.

There are two types of hair cells in the cochlea, located on the basilar membrane:
• Inner hair cells numbering 3,500.
• Outer hair cells numbering 12,000.

The hair cells are stimulated by the movement of fluids in the cochlea and activate the hearing nerve.
• Vibration of bones causes fluid in cochlea to move.
• This causes tiny hairs on top of cell to move.
• There is a chemical reaction between the hair cell and the nerves which causes the nerves to become active.
• The nerve activity goes to brain.
• Brain interprets nerve activity as sound.
• Loud sounds activate more nerves than soft sounds.
• The vertical lines indicate nerve impulses that are sent up to the brain.

Spontaneous activity on hearing nerves

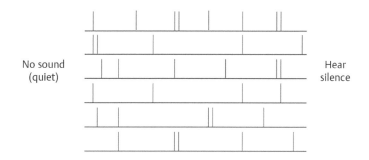

No sound (quiet)

Hear silence

- Even when there is no sound, there is nerve activity.
- This nerve activity can be measured even when you don't know it is happening.

- This nerve activity is called random spontaneous activity.
- No specific pattern to activity.
- Ignored by brain thus not perceived as sound.

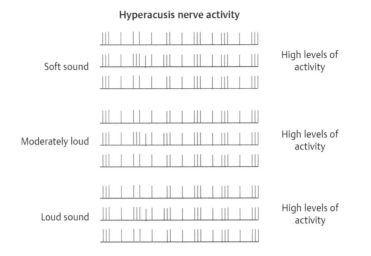

The amount of nerve activity for a person with hyperacusis. Note that there is no change in the nerve activity among the three examples.

In patients with hyperacusis, the nerve activity will be high for all sounds, regardless of the input sound level.

Sounds that are soft, moderately loud, and loud will all be interpreted as loud by the brain.

Some patients with hyperacusis also have hearing loss, but not all.

Having hearing loss does not mean you have hyperacusis or vice versa.

There are many different causes of hyperacusis

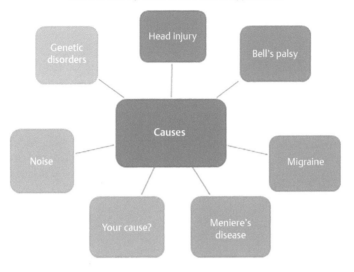

Hyperacusis has similar causes to hearing loss such as excessive noise exposure, Meniere's disease, and head injury.

Other causes of hyperacusis include Bell's palsy, migraines, and genetic disorders.

Reactions to hyperacusis
(Tyler et al., 2014)

- Emotional well-being

- Hearing and communication

- Sleep

- Concentration

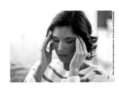

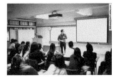

(Source: *Bottom left*: ©BullRun/stock.adobe.com. Stock photo. Posed by a model; *bottom center*: ©StockPhotoPro/stock.adobe.com. Stock photo. Posed by a model; *top right*: ©Von Syda Productions/stock.adobe.com. Stock photo. Posed by a model; *bottom right*: ©ibravery/stock.adobe.com)

Hyperacusis affects four areas that can result in functional impairments such as work or social problems:
- Emotional wellbeing, causing distress, depression, anxiety, in response to a sound exposure:

- Communication and hearing difficulties because it can be hard to focus on what people are saying.
- Sleep disturbances.
- Impacts concentration due to anticipation of being exposed to a sound.

Options to treat hyperacusis

- Counseling (hyperacusis activities treatment)
- Ear plugs and sound therapy
- Relaxation exercises
- Medications

There are several treatment options that show positive results for patients with hyperacusis. Research is still emerging about the effectiveness of these therapy approaches:

1. Counseling using Hyperacusis Activities Treatment, CBT, or others.
2. Ear plugs to reduce sound exposure and sound therapy using background sound to reduce annoyance and/or increase sound tolerance.
3. Relaxation exercises to provide coping strategies, lessen fear and anxiety.
4. Medications to manage anxiety, depression, sleep problems.

Hearing protection

- Ear plugs reduce noise exposure
  - Wear only in noisy environments
- Using ear plugs every day causes communication difficulties, worsens hyperacusis
- Ear plugs allow you to stay active, not be reclusive

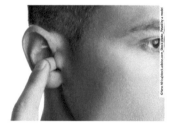

(Source: ©New Africa/stock.adobe.com. Stock photo. Posed by a model.)

- Musician earplugs should be recommended to patients with hyperacusis.
- Ear plugs will help in noisy environments to reduce noise exposure:
  - There is limited effectiveness in using them continually, including communication difficulties.
  - There are also negative consequences to wearing ear plugs daily, such as making hyperacusis worse as sound exposure lessens.
  - However, many hyperacusis patients find relieve for noisy situations. It allows you to stay active, not be reclusive.

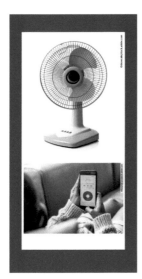

Sound therapy

- Used to reduce annoyance and/or increase sound tolerance

- Options include non wearable and ear-level sound generators

- Will take time for results

(Source: *Top*: ©showcake/stock.adobe.com; *bottom*: ©Rawpixel.com/stock.adobe.com)

Sound therapy, or the use of background sound, can be helpful for patients with loudness or annoyance hyperacusis.

Sound therapy options include nonwearable sound generators and ear level noise generators.

Will take time to treat hyperacusis. It is not unexpected for patients to show benefit from sound therapy after 6 to 18 months of treatment.

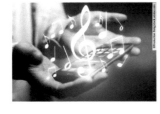

Sound therapy options

- Nonwearable sound generators
  - Sound pillow
  - Sound generators
  - Smartphone apps
  - CDs, radio, etc

- Wearable, ear-level sound generators
  - Tinnitus masking devices

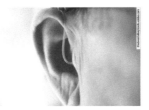

(Source: *Top*: ©Production Perig/stock.adobe.com; *bottom*: ©edwardolive/stock.adobe.com)

Sound therapy options include nonwearable sound generators:
- Sound Pillow ($50–150, www.soundpillow.com).
- Sound Generators ($20–50, www.amazon.com).
  - Marpac Dohm Classic White Noise Sound Machine.
- Smartphone apps for tinnitus relief (free).
  - Starkey, Phonak, GNResound, Oticon.
- CDs, radio, etc, to fill a quiet room.

Ear-level sound generators include tinnitus masking devices:

- GHI offers tinnitus masking devices.
- Neuromonics uses music that is customized for the patient to mask tinnitus.
- Desyncra has neuromodulation that creates therapeutic tones matched to patient's tinnitus.
- Widex uses (ZEN) fractal tones.
- GN Resound offers a combination unit for amplification and masking tinnitus.
- Signia has tinnitus sounds (modulated ocean waves + static sounds) and notch therapy.

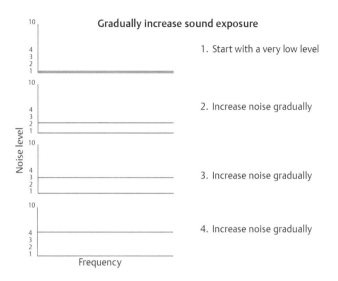

Gradually increase sound exposure

1. Start with a very low level

2. Increase noise gradually

3. Increase noise gradually

4. Increase noise gradually

For patients with loudness hyperacusis, the principle of successive approximations may be applicable. The patient listens to a low-level background sound for a prescribed time every day and increases their exposure gradually. Increasing sound exposure gradually over several weeks to make ears more tolerant of sound, and lessen bothersome reactions.

Background sound partially masks a barking dog

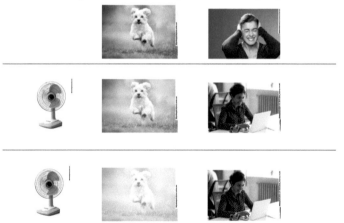

(Source: *Left*: ©showcake/stock.adobe.com; *center*: ©Dyrefotografi.dk/stock.adobe.com; *top right*: ©Studio Grand Web/stock.adobe.com. Stock photo. Posed by a model; *center and bottom right*: ©fizkes/stock.adobe.com. Stock photo. Posed by a model.)

For patients with annoyance hyperacusis, a background sound can partially mask the unwanted sound we hear.

Here, a barking dog is the unwanted sound, and the fan is the background sound.

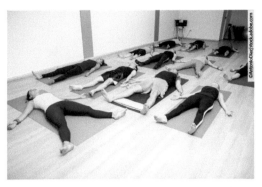

Progressive muscle relaxation	• Learn to systematically tense and relax groups of muscles • With practice, you will recognize a tensed muscle versus a relaxed muscle • This skill allows you to produce physical muscular relaxation at the first signs of tension

(Source: ©AntonioDiaz/stock.adobe.com)

Relaxation activities help manage stress and anxiety that is in response to environmental sounds. Progressive muscle relaxation is one method of practicing relaxation. It requires the patient to focus on tensing and relaxing groups of muscles. The goal is to be able to initiate muscular relaxation whenever tension arises.

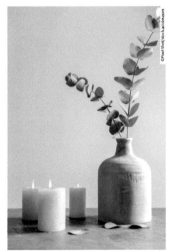

Progressive muscle relaxation

Completed in two steps:
1. Deliberately apply tension to certain muscle groups
2. Stop the tension and focus on how the muscles feel as they relax

(Source: ©Pixel-Shot/stock.adobe.com)

There are two parts to progressive muscle relaxation. First, one must tense a specific muscle group, then release the tension and focus on how the muscles are relaxing.

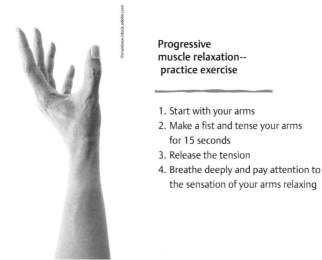

Progressive muscle relaxation-- practice exercise

1. Start with your arms
2. Make a fist and tense your arms for 15 seconds
3. Release the tension
4. Breathe deeply and pay attention to the sensation of your arms relaxing

(Source: ©mantinov/stock.adobe.com)

First, sit or lay in a comfortable position. Then begin to tense certain muscle groups, starting with one's arms. Make a fist and contract your arm muscles for 15 seconds. Then release the tension and focus in how the muscles feels as they start to relax. Take a deep breath and continue to breathe deeply.

Practice exercise (continued)

5. Continue tensing and relaxing the following muscle groups:
   - Face
   - Shoulders
   - Stomach
   - Legs and feet
6. When finished, release any remaining tension in your body

Repeat this process of tensing and relaxing with different muscle groups, one at a time. First with your face, then shoulders, working your way down to your stomach, then finally to your legs and feet.

The last step in progressive muscle relaxation is to finally release any remaining tension in the body.

This technique will allow the patient to release tension in any part of the body whenever it arises.

Deep breathing exercises

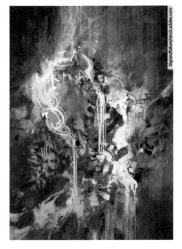

- Sit or lie flat in a comfortable position
- Put one hand on your belly just below your ribs and the other hand on your chest
- Take a **deep** breath in through your nose, and let your belly push your hand out
- **Breathe** out through pursed lips as if you were whistling
- Repeat 3 to 10 times

(Source: ©grandfailure/stock.adobe.com)

Deep breathing exercises are also useful relaxation techniques. To start, you find a comfortable position either sitting or lying down. Place one hand (or a small item such as a rubber ducky) on your belly just below your ribs. Place your other hand on your chest.

Take a deep breath. In through your nose and fill your belly up. Let it push your hand or small object up. Make sure you are not filling your chest up and your other hand on your chest does not move up too.

To breathe out, slowing blow the air out of your mouth, like you are blowing out a candle or blowing up a balloon.

Repeat this exercise anywhere 3 to 10 times; make sure to take a few normal breaths inbetween repetitions.

This is also a tool you can use to slow your thoughts down or take a little break where ever you are to calm yourself down.

Visual imagery

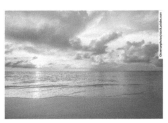

- Similar to daydreaming
- Attention is focused on some type of sensory experience
  - Creating novel mental images
  - Recalling past places and events

(Source: ©icemanphotos/stock.adobe.com)

Visual imagery can also be used as a relaxation tool. It is somewhat similar to daydreaming but your attention is focused on a particular sensation. The goal is to create a story of sensations that will help ground your body. This is most commonly a peaceful image or place that calms you down.

This could be equivalent to "going to your happy place."

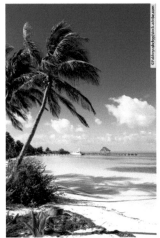

Visual imagery - practice exercise

1. Close your eyes
2. Think of a relaxing scene (the beach)
3. Try to imagine the scene as clearly as you can
4. The smell of the water, warm sand on feet, sound of ocean
5. Allow yourself to relax as you imagine the location in your mind

(Source: ©Pakhnyushchyy/stock.adobe.com)

We are going to do a practice visual imagery exercise. First close your eyes. Get comfortable in your seat or lay down. We are going to start by thinking of a relaxing scene. For this particular example, we will use the beach. Try to imagine the scene as clearly as you can, maybe a particular beach that you visited recently or as a child. Note the smell of the air around you, the smell of the salt water. Then focus your attention to your feet. They are in the warm sand, move your feet around, dig them into the sand. Notice the feel of the sand as it moves across your feet, notice the warmth. Listen to the sound of the waves crashing, of the birds that are flying or the noises of other activities going on. Allow yourself to relax as you explore the location in your mind, making special note of the sensory sensations around you.

When you are ready to return, slowly open your eyes again. Take a moment to reorient yourself to your surroundings.

One important note for this exercise is do not create a "to do" list or let your mind drift to your worries. If this happens, gently redirect your attention back to a specific sensory sensation. Make sure to not be upset at yourself or feel guilty if this happens. As you practice more, it will become easier to maintain your focus on the situation.

Medications

- Currently no drug or surgery can reliably eliminate the source of hyperacusis
- There are effective drugs for:
  - Sleep, anxiety, and depression

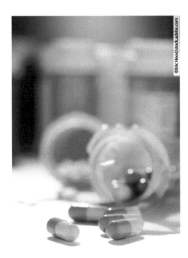

(Source: ©Eric Hood/stock.adobe.com)

- At this time, there are no widely accepted cures, including drugs or surgeries for hyperacusis. Medications can be helpful to relieve related symptoms.

- Medications for sleep problems, depression, or anxiety can be helpful.
- Work closely with psychiatrist or psychologist.

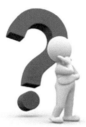

Questions?

This is a good opportunity to discuss any remaining questions with the patient.

You might do the following to support your patient:

- Set three goals for the counseling sessions.

- Teach the patient a mantra, such as "I am ok" or "This is ok" to start countering negative thoughts.
- Recognize the individual differences among patients.

Appendix 13.6 Sound Therapy Treatment Protocol for Hyperacusis

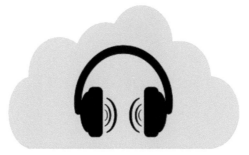

The information provided below will assist you in following the treatment protocol for hyperacusis.

Selecting the Sound

You will have the option of listening to noise or music during the course of your treatment. This can be presented through a stand-alone sound generator or using ear-level sound generators. The key is to have relaxing and enjoyable music, nature sounds, or other noise that you will find pleasant to listen to for an extended time every day.

Length of Time to Listen

You should try to play the sound for several hours at a time. This can be done either while you are sleeping or during the day. If you listen while you are asleep and you are unable to tolerate having the noise or music on all night, try to listen for at least 4 hours a night. During the day, try to play the music for at least 2 hours each day.

Setting the Volume

You should be listening to sound set at a loudness level that is comfortable for you. Do not force yourself to listen to anything set at a volume that is uncomfortable for you. Start by finding a low level that you can comfortably listen to for the whole listening period. After a period of 4 days, raise the level of the sound a little. Be sure the sound remains comfortable for you. If the new level becomes uncomfortable, turn it down slightly so that it is once again comfortable. Continue to increase the volume every 4 days during treatment, keeping in mind that you should not set it to a level that is uncomfortable or interferes with your ability to sleep if you are using it at night.

Keeping Track of Your Progress

Please use the diary we have provided to keep track of your progress with the listening protocol. Every day you should write down what sound you used, how many hours you listened, and what your reaction was to that particular sound and its loudness level. You may also want to write down any other comments that would be helpful for us to understand your experiences with this treatment protocol.

Please let us know if you have any questions or concerns at any time.

Appendix 13.7 Hyperacusis Listening Diary Example Case

Hyperacusis Listening Diary for_____

Day of week	Date	How long you listened	Sound used
Sunday Example	2/1/19	15 minutes	White noise from air purifier
Your Reaction			
It made annoying sounds like the refrigerator less noticeable immediately after the session.			
Monday			
Your Reaction			
Tuesday			
Your Reaction			
Wednesday			
Your Reaction			
Thursday			
Your Reaction			
Friday			
Your Reaction			
Saturday			
Your Reaction			

Hyperacusis Listening Diary for_____

Day of week	Date	How long you listened	Sound used
Sunday			
Your Reaction			
Monday			
Your Reaction			
Tuesday			
Your Reaction			
Wednesday			
Your Reaction			
Thursday			
Your Reaction			
Friday			
Your Reaction			
Saturday			
Your Reaction			

14 Navigating Future Directions in Tinnitus Treatment

Fatima T. Husain

Abstract

This chapter reviews current evidence regarding experimental methods for treating tinnitus, namely, neuromodulation, neurofeedback, and neurostimulation. Such methods rely on our increasing knowledge about neural mechanisms of tinnitus, specifically regarding several neural networks subserving tinnitus. The experimental methods, which are still in a development and testing phase, have the potential of being successful in treating one or more subtypes of tinnitus when fully validated. At the same time, they have the capability to test various theories and models of tinnitus, and improve our understanding of the variability and heterogeneity of the tinnitus patient population by linking them to different neural mechanisms.

Keywords: treatment, fMRI, neurofeedback, EEG, neuromodulation, neurostimulation

14.1 Introduction

An easy prediction to make about the future of tinnitus treatments and management strategies is that there will be several new interventions in the coming years. Not surprising given the fact that as we learn more about the neural mechanisms of chronic tinnitus and better understand an individual's psychological and physiological reaction to it, newer interventions will be tested in labs and clinics. Because there are several different causes of tinnitus, and likely several different subtypes,[1] it is unlikely there will be a single "cure." The best management strategy is and will continue to be customized care for each individual patient.

However, it is also inevitable that some interventions will fail to move beyond the bench and will not be adopted in the clinic. Nevertheless, reports in popular media often bring awareness to these potential interventions, and audiologists and other health care providers will be asked by tinnitus patients about these (as yet) unproven solutions.

The treatment methods reviewed in this chapter rely on our increasing knowledge about neural mechanisms to tinnitus, specifically of one or more neural networks subserving tinnitus. The more popular of these networks are shown in ▶ Fig. 14.1 and include the auditory network, the attention

network, the default mode network, and the emotion processing network. The **auditory network** is comprised of the bilateral primary and secondary auditory cortices; some investigators also include parts of the central auditory pathways in this network. The **attention network** is often divided into two pathways: the dorsal pathway (Dorsal Attention Network [DAN]) and ventral pathway (Ventral Attention Network [VAN]), each dedicated to somewhat different tasks, yet interacting with each other at various crossing points.[2] In this formulation, the dorsal attention network is comprised of bilateral frontal eye fields and intraparietal sulci, and is involved with top-down, goal-directed attention to certain features and locations of incoming stimuli. The **ventral attention network** includes the temporoparietal junction and the ventral frontal cortex; its functions include detecting novel or unexpected stimuli and focusing attention on them. A primary driver of processing emotions in the brain is the limbic system, including areas in the cortex such as the orbitofrontal cortex and subcortical regions such as the hippocampus and the amygdala.[3] Recent advances in imaging have focused on the brain at "rest," when it is not participating in any goal-directed activities. A neural network that become preferentially active during rest is the default mode network, comprising the posterior cingulate, precuneus, and the medial prefrontal cortex.[4]

These regions feature prominently in several theories of tinnitus and are the target for better understanding and reducing tinnitus-related distress. The Psychological Model, proposed by Tyler et al,[5] suggested that the overall annoyance of tinnitus was a result of the (1) tinnitus characteristics and the (2) psychological makeup of each individual patient. Several parts of the brain will be involved in the representation of the tinnitus and of the reactions to the tinnitus. The hippocampus and parahippocampal regions have been associated with retention of events and memory formation, specifically related to tinnitus.[6]

14.1.1 What Should a Clinician Tell a Patient About Novel Treatment Methods?

As our recent survey[7] suggests, some patients approach treatment with an unrealistic expectation

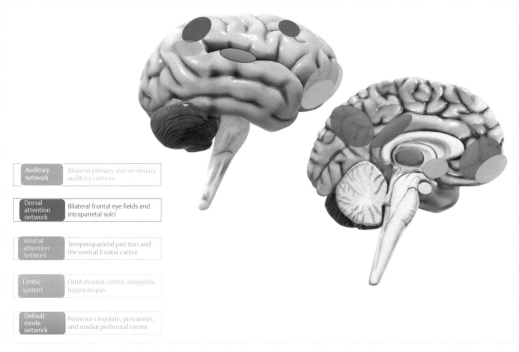

Auditory network	Bilateral primary and secondary auditory cortices
Dorsal attention network	Bilateral frontal eye fields and intraparietal sulci
Ventral attention network	Temporoparietal junction and the ventral frontal cortex
Limbic system	Orbitofrontal cortex, amygdala, hippocampus
Default mode network	Posterior cingulate, precuneus, and medial prefrontal cortex

Fig. 14.1 The major neural networks discussed in this chapter that possible mediate the tinnitus percept and its impact on the patient.

Table 14.1 Evaluation of novel treatment methods

Technique	Invasiveness	Cost	Strength of evidence	Efficacy
Neurofeedback-EEG	Noninvasive	$	C	Insufficient evidence
Neurofeedback-fMRI	Noninvasive	$$	C	Insufficient evidence
VNS	Invasive	$$$	C	Insufficient evidence
tVNS	Noninvasive	$	C	Insufficient evidence
tDCS	Noninvasive	$	C	Insufficient evidence
rTMS	Noninvasive	$	B	Recommended against for routine treatment

Abbreviations: VNS, vagus nerve stimulation; tVNS, transcutaneous vagus nerve stimulation; rTMS, repetitive transcranial magnetic stimulation.

of a "cure" for their tinnitus. Tyler[8] noted that most want a pill, and many would accept a brain implant! A clinician who is unaware of such expectations may provide less than satisfactory outcomes for their patients, even when there are declines in tinnitus-related distress. Elsewhere in this book, the reader will be able to better understand and evaluate interventions currently being used in the clinic. In this chapter, we review recent interventions that are being tested currently in the lab and discuss their potential in alleviating the sound of tinnitus itself

and its related psychological reaction. We also discuss the relative cost-benefits of these interventions, in terms of their invasiveness, cost, and efficacy (see ▶ Table 14.1). ▶ Table 14.2 provides an explanation of the quality and type of evidence necessary for the grades noted in ▶ Table 14.1. Due to their recent development, some of these treatment methods have not accumulated a body of evidence sufficient for us to comprehensively evaluate their efficacy. Over the next decade or two, some of these interventions may be refined further and their efficacy

Table 14.2 Methodological efficacy explanations

Grade	Quality of evidence for treatment and harm
A	Well-designed randomized controlled trials performed on a population similar to the guideline's target population
B	Randomized controlled trials; overwhelmingly consistent evidence from observational studies
C	Observational studies (case control and cohort design)

Source: Adapted from Tunkel et al,[19] which is in turn adapted from OCEBM Levels of Evidence Working Group. The Oxford Levels of Evidence 2. Oxford Centre for Evidence-Based Medicine. https://www.cebm.net/index.aspx?o=5653.

validated sufficiently that they migrate to the clinic. However, others will not.

14.2 Neuromodulation— Magnetic Stimulation, Electric Stimulation

Neuromodulation is a broad term referring to the causation of changes in the brain due to an electric or magnetic device placed outside the skull. The idea behind using neuromodulation in treating tinnitus is to somehow "reset" the brain such that the pathophysiology underlying tinnitus is reduced or eliminated. Neuromodulation can modulate brain activity because communication in the brain is via chemical and electrical transmission. When it is the latter, the tiny electrical impulses necessary for neuronal information transfer over axons also create their own magnetic fields, which are then susceptible to alteration based on external magnetic or electrical fields.

14.2.1 What Is Magnetic Neuromodulation?

In transcranial magnetic stimulation (TMS), a magnet is placed near the scalp and creates a magnetic field that induces a short duration electric current that stimulates principally cortical neurons, both at the site of interest and connected brain regions. The TMS pulse, if of sufficient amplitude, can induce brief excitation followed by longer-term inhibition, disrupting sensory, motor, and cognitive processes and causing a temporary "virtual lesion."[9] Repetitive pulses of subthreshold intensities may affect brain activity by inducing noise in the system,

while brain activity continues. The most often used repetition rate is 1 Hz, and has been found to have inhibitory effects, which are considered to be therapeutic for treating depression, although higher frequencies that are more excitatory in nature are also being studied.[10]

The popularity for rTMS is due to its success in treating intractable depression and other mood disorders. In fact, the US Food and Drug Administration (FDA) has approved rTMS for treatment for major depressive disorder in 2008 and more recently of obsessive compulsive disorder in 2018 (https://www.fda.gov/newsevents/newsroom/pressannouncements/ucm617244.htm).

The magnet approved for human experiments does not cause seizures and the intervention is considered to be noninvasive. In randomized controlled experimental studies using rTMS, a control condition is created by using "sham" stimulation, which reproduces the sounds and somatosensory effects of rTMS without the neural changes.

14.2.2 Magnetic Stimulation and Tinnitus

Studies using TMS as tinnitus intervention have either one or both goals, namely elimination of the tinnitus percept and reduction of tinnitus-related distress. The earlier studies were primarily concerned with the first goal (with not much success), while later studies have generally moved on to reducing subjective tinnitus distress.

Various brain regions have been employed as the foci for magnetic stimulation. Initially studies targeted the primary auditory cortex, with the intention of reducing any tinnitus-related hyperactivity.[11] Later studies have incorporated other sites such as the prefrontal cortex[12] and the temporoparietal junction.[13] In a 2014 review article about usage of rTMS to treat different disorders,[14] the authors supported a C-level evidence for the intervention, meaning possible efficacy for rTMS using 1-Hz stimulation of the left temporal or temporoparietal cortices, based on studies with smaller sample sizes and inconsistent standards.

A majority of small-scale studies (e.g., fewer than 20 subjects) suggest that rTMS might help some individuals with tinnitus. However, two well-controlled studies[15,16] did not find this to be true. In one study,[16] pulses of 1 Hz in frequency were applied to the left temporoparietal junction, for periods of about 43 minutes, 5 days a week, for 4 weeks. This was a crossover, double-blind, randomized controlled trial, with the control condition being a sham stimulation, with the magnet shielded but replicating all sensory and somatosensory effects of rTMS. Those who had at least a moderate tinnitus handicap (defined as having scores greater than 36 on the Tinnitus Handicap Inventory) were recruited into the study (data were obtained from 14 subjects, with 13 completing both arms of the study). Subjects in both the sham and active stimulation groups showed declines in THI scores, on average 6 and 10 points, respectively. Because the declines were not statistically significant, this particular experimental paradigm was not successful or better than the placebo effect.

Several large-scale studies (typically having at least 100 subjects in the study) have attempted to parse out the relative efficacy of different rTMS paradigms, without much success. In a recent multicenter trial[17] with about 75 subjects in each of the active and sham stimulation groups, no statistically significant changes in tinnitus handicap were found, either with respect to their own baseline condition or when compared across groups. Subjects underwent 10 sessions of active or sham stimulation over the left temporal cortex.

One reason for the lack of success can be that the optimal brain region was not targeted. Some studies have found success in temporarily suppressing the tinnitus-related distress when frontal sites[12] or parietal sites[13] were targeted. Other studies have not found any advantage for stimulating these locations or in targeting multiple foci of stimulation versus one.[18]

In 2014, Tunkel and 22 colleagues, including leading audiologists and ENT physicians, published guidelines on usage and efficacy of interventions for tinnitus management at the direction of the American Academy of Otolaryngology—Head and Neck Surgery Foundation (AAO-HNSF).[19] The authors evaluated the evidence for various interventions currently being employed to treat tinnitus and found the most support for cognitive behavioral therapy and hearing aid evaluation, with an option for sound therapy. Of the interventions discussed in this chapter, the only one reviewed by Tunkel et al[19] was rTMS. The authors recommended against routine usage of rTMS for treating chronic, bothersome tinnitus while acknowledging that clinicians and patients may deviate from this recommendation on a case-by-case basis. They based their recommendation on the lack of evidence from randomized controlled trials and a lack of long-term benefit of TMS. We concur with this recommendation regarding using TMS to reduce tinnitus-related distress.

14.2.3 Caveats

While small-scale trials of rTMS have suggested some success, these successes have not translated into large-scale studies. Further, it is unclear at this time whether heterogeneity of the patient population or of the experimental paradigm (e.g., different types of stimulation devices, settings, or site of stimulation) is most likely to have resulted in the discrepant findings. Another caveat is that tinnitus is listed as a side effect of rTMS because the noise produced by the magnet as it sends in the pulses can result in some hearing damage, and adequate hearing protection must be worn during treatment.[20]

14.2.4 Electric Stimulation

Transcranial direct current stimulation, or tDCS, is a noninvasive method used to alter the electrical firings of certain brain regions. In tDCS, two electrodes are placed over the head, one electrode being a cathode (negative) and the other an anode (positive) with the brain completing the circuit. A low-intensity, constant current flowing between the electrodes serves to modulate neuronal activity in two ways: in anodal stimulation, neuronal activity is enhanced, while in cathodal stimulation, it is inhibited.

Currently, tDCS is not FDA approved, but it has garnered some success in treating conditions like mood disorders and Parkinson disease, as an off-label device. Its appeal lies in being cheap, noninvasive, and easy to set up and the ability to use the device without supervision by medical professionals. Like rTMS, in tDCS active stimulation can be contrasted easily with sham conditions without knowledge of participants, thus allowing for randomized controlled trials. In the sham condition, active stimulation is delivered for the first few and last few seconds of the stimulation paradigm, to mimic the onset and offset effects with the current remaining off for the great majority of the time.[21]

14.2.5 Electric Stimulation and Tinnitus

In the case of tinnitus, the goal of tDCS is to balance the excitation and inhibition in the brain regions; here, the underlying assumption is that there is an imbalance in the case of tinnitus as manifested by hyperactivity (or noise in the system). Similar to studies employing rTMS, the main foci of stimulation in tDCS are the dorsolateral prefrontal cortex and the auditory cortex. Typically, up to 10 sessions are conducted as part of the intervention, with each session about 20 minutes in duration and with current intensities between 1 and 2 mA. Shekhawat et al[22] conducted a feasibility study of different intensities of the electric current targeting the temporoparietal area and the dorsolateral prefrontal cortex. Out of the 27 participants, 21 reported a minimum reduction of 1 point on subjective tinnitus loudness and annoyance scales. Higher intensity (2 mA) and longer duration (20 min) were more effective, although there was no interaction between location, intensity, and duration of stimulation. The primary benefit of tDCS appears to be in reducing tinnitus-related distress, including associated depression and anxiety.[23]

14.2.6 Caveats

Whereas tDCS is cheaper than rTMS, its lack of focused stimulation compared to rTMS has led to smaller effect sizes. Like rTMS, the variability in the devices, stimulation protocols, and the brain regions being targeted have led to ambiguous results. However, there exists the potential to develop tDCS as an adjunct to treatment of severe or bothersome tinnitus, complimenting other therapies.

14.3 Vagus Nerve Stimulation

The vagus nerve is a cranial nerve connecting the brainstem with various parts of the body. It regulates some sensory, motor, and parasympathetic nervous functions. The parasympathetic along with the sympathetic nervous system constitutes the autonomic nervous system and, in the case of the vagus nerve, regulates heart rate, breathing, and gastrointestinal function.

The FDA has approved the use of vagus nerve stimulation (VNS) for reducing the severity of depression or reducing or eliminating seizures from refractory epilepsy. To stimulate the nerve, a small wire is threaded from a small electrical device, much like a pacemaker, into the nerve. The device is placed on the chest and the wire threaded via surgery under general anesthesia. In the case of epilepsy, electrical impulses are sent at regular intervals, via the vagus nerve to the brain, which helps reduce seizure activity.

14.3.1 Vagus Nerve Stimulation and Tinnitus

Kilgard and colleagues[24] were the first to use VNS as a potential method to eliminate the percept of tinnitus. Their first study[24] paired VNS with pure tones in an animal model of tinnitus and, per the authors, "completely eliminated the physiological and behavioral correlates of tinnitus in noise-exposed rats." This study also served to test the hypothesis of the underlying pathophysiology that may have caused tinnitus, namely neuroplasticity due to sensory deprivation resulting in tinnitus. Resetting this neuroplasticity via VNS and sound stimulation was thought to eliminate tinnitus.

However, subsequent human studies of VNS from Kilgard's group and other groups have not proven to be as successful. In a 2014 feasibility study,[25] 10 patients with bothersome chronic tinnitus received an implant in their left vagus nerve and were stimulated with tones and brief electrical pulses for 2.5 hours per day. All patients tolerated the procedure and electrical stimulation. Out of the 10 patients, 4 showed reduction in tinnitus handicap as well as in the loudness of the percept. Five patients did not show any improvement, possibly due to the mood altering medications they were taking during the trial, which may inhibit plasticity and reduce the efficacy of VNS, as the authors speculate. A larger study, over multiple centers[26] showed significant improvement in one subgroup of patients, mostly those who had tonal and nonblast-induced tinnitus. Note that none of the patients reported by Tyler et al[26] were on medications.

More recently, studies have been conducted using transcutaneous VNS, where stimulation of different branches of the vagus nerve via the pinna of the ear or the interior of the auditory canal is thought to be sufficient and no invasive procedures are performed. There is as yet no consensus regarding which branch and intensity of stimulation is optimal in reducing tinnitus-related distress. One pilot study[27] paired transcutaneous VNS with sound stimulation and found a reduction in tinnitus-related distress for 10 subjects. Simultaneously, the responses of the auditory cortex decreased when measured via magnetoencephalography for the small group of subjects.

14.3.2 Caveats

Currently, VNS remains in the lab and the sample size of all the studies conducted thus far has been small. Transcutaneous VNS, which is noninvasive, appears to have a better cost-benefit ratio than the more invasive VNS. But in all cases, the effect size remains small and the studies have been open-label, often without a control condition (except wait-list).

14.4 Neurofeedback

Neurofeedback is a type of biofeedback used to teach participants to control aspects of their brain activity. In a typical neurofeedback experimental setting, subjects are seated with an EEG cap and their brain waves are continuously recorded. Subjects receive feedback about their brain activity using video or audio input, often in the form of the movement of an object on the screen (see ▸ Fig. 14.2). The movement of the object on the screen is controlled by the software that tracks their brain waves in real time. In EEG (sometimes called quantitative EEG), different power bands can be calculated from the frequency associated with the neuronal electrical activity and picked up by the electrodes. These range from 0 to 4 Hz (delta), 4 to 8 Hz (theta), 8 to 12 Hz (alpha), 12 to 40 Hz (beta), and above 40 Hz (gamma). The investigator can set up the system such that one or more of these EEG waves control the object's movement. For instance, if the goal is to make the subject relax, the desired movement of the object will be linked to their alpha waves, which are thought to be a marker for relaxation. As subjects relax, the object moves in the appropriate direction. Note that the subjects are not given explicit directions on what to do; in the relaxation scenario, they are told to move the object on the screen in a particular direction. Over the period of one or two sessions, they learn what is necessary for the object to move. In terms of creating a sham condition, placebo feedback is provided from an unrelated brain region, or via frequency bands that are not being used to provide active feedback.

14.4.1 Neurofeedback and Tinnitus

Two different types of neurofeedback have been used in tinnitus treatment—one relies on accurately mapping brain activity using EEG and the other on real-time fMRI. As early as 2000, biofeedback, including "Electroencephalographic Training," was noted as a potential treatment for tinnitus.[28] Starting in the early to mid-2000s, EEG was used to train participants in becoming calmer and thereby reducing their attention and focus on distressing tinnitus. Here, the pathophysiology is thought to be abnormal oscillatory brain activity and modifying it to have a more "normal" profile was said to reduce

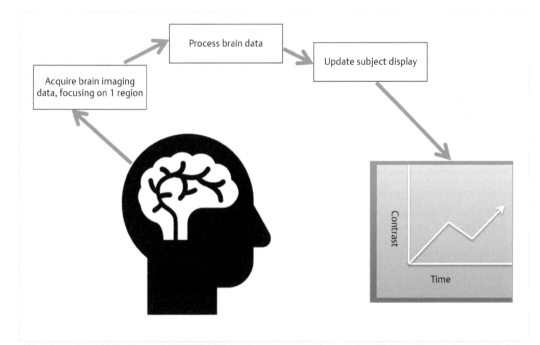

Fig. 14.2 The standard approach to neurofeedback. The brain imaging data can be obtained from EEG or fMRI and is used to control a display that the subject sees. Over the duration of the experiment, the subject learns to change their own brain activity based on the display.

tinnitus-related distress. In a series of experiments by Weisz and colleagues,[29,30] the main markers of effective treatment were enhanced alpha activity and reduced delta activity. Participants who modified the ratio the most between the alpha and delta activity achieved the best results. However, in the next decade, the number of new studies regarding neurofeedback and tinnitus decreased until more recently there was a resurgence of interest in neurofeedback because of the newer tool of real-time fMRI.

In terms of the task in real-time fMRI, the goals remain the same as in the earlier EEG studies. The primary differences are that subjects are in an MRI scanner, functional MRI signals are decoded, and the visual displays are changed based on activation or correlation patterns of the brain's fMRI activity.[31] While the temporal resolution of the fMRI signal is quite poor compared to the EEG signal, it does have the benefit of obtaining signals from deeper brain structures that are implicated in tinnitus. A pilot study[32] found that activity in the auditory cortex reduced with feedback; however, only two of the six participants reported a reduction in the tinnitus handicap. Similar results were obtained in follow-up study[33] that compared intermittent with continuous feedback to changes in TFI scores. The authors found changes to the brain connectivity patterns and the authors concluded that continuous neurofeedback is superior to intermittent feedback in down-regulating auditory cortex activity.

14.4.2 Caveats

Whereas neurofeedback is beginning to show results for disorders, such as major depressive disorder,[34] in the context of tinnitus, it remains experimental. More data are needed about the neural mechanisms of tinnitus persistence, in particular, specific brain regions whose activity modulate tinnitus severity.

14.5 Conclusions

The intervention methods reviewed in this chapter rely on our improving understanding of the neural mechanisms of tinnitus and its variable impact on a person. The different approaches mentioned might also be a means to test various theories of such neural mechanisms. Although they are firmly experimental at the moment, even were they to

fail, these novel interventions improve our understanding of the heterogeneity in the tinnitus population by linking such variability to specific neural mechanisms. They also have the potential for being successful as they are refined.

Acknowledgments

The author is grateful to Rafay Khan and Jenna Vangalis for reading drafts of the chapter and assistance with the figures.

References

[1] Tyler R, Coelho C, Tao P, et al. Identifying tinnitus subgroups with cluster analysis. Am J Audiol. 2008; 17(2):S176–S184

[2] Vossel S, Geng JJ, Fink GR. Dorsal and ventral attention systems: distinct neural circuits but collaborative roles. Neuroscientist. 2014; 20(2):150–159

[3] Morgane PJ, Galler JR, Mokler DJJPIN. A review of systems and networks of the limbic forebrain/limbic midbrain. Prog Neurobiol. 2005; 75(2):143–160

[4] Schmidt SA, Carpenter-Thompson J, Husain FT. Connectivity of precuneus to the default mode and dorsal attention networks: A possible invariant marker of long-term tinnitus. Neuroimage Clin. 2017; 16:196–204

[5] Tyler RS, Aran JM, Dauman R. Recent advances in tinnitus. Am J Audiol. 1992; 1(4):36–44

[6] De Ridder D, Fransen H, Francois O, Sunaert S, Kovacs S, Van De Heyning P. Amygdalohippocampal involvement in tinnitus and auditory memory. Acta Otolaryngol Suppl. 2006; 556(556) Suppl:50–53

[7] Husain FT, Gander PE, Jansen JN, Shen S. Expectations for tinnitus treatment and outcomes: a survey study of audiologists and patients. J Am Acad Audiol. 2018; 29(4): 313–336

[8] Tyler RS. Patient preferences and willingness to pay for tinnitus treatments. J Am Acad Audiol. 2012; 23(2):115–125

[9] Siebner HR, Rothwell J. Transcranial magnetic stimulation: new insights into representational cortical plasticity. Exp Brain Res. 2003; 148(1):1–16

[10] Pohar R, Farrah K. Repetitive transcranial magnetic stimulation for patients with depression: a review of clinical effectiveness, cost-effectiveness and guidelines—an update [Internet]. Ottawa, ON: Canadian Agency for Drugs and Technologies in Health; 2019 Jun 28. http://www.ncbi.nlm.nih.gov/books/NBK545105/ PubMed PMID: 31433608

[11] Kleinjung T, Eichhammer P, Langguth B, et al. Long-term effects of repetitive transcranial magnetic stimulation (rTMS) in patients with chronic tinnitus. Otolaryngol Head Neck Surg. 2005; 132(4):566–569

[12] De Ridder D, Song JJ, Vanneste S. Frontal cortex TMS for tinnitus. Brain Stimul. 2013; 6(3):355–362

[13] Khedr EM, Abo-Elfetoh N, Rothwell JC, El-Atar A, Sayed E, Khalifa H. Contralateral versus ipsilateral rTMS of temporoparietal cortex for the treatment of chronic unilateral tinnitus: comparative study. Eur J Neurol. 2010; 17(7):976–983

[14] Lefaucheur JP, André-Obadia N, Antal A, et al. Evidence-based guidelines on the therapeutic use of repetitive transcranial magnetic stimulation (rTMS). Clin Neurophysiol. 2014; 125 (11):2150–2206

[15] Piccirillo JF, Garcia KS, Nicklaus J, et al. Low-frequency repetitive transcranial magnetic stimulation to the temporoparietal junction for tinnitus. Arch Otolaryngol Head Neck Surg. 2011; 137(3):221–228

[16] Piccirillo JF, Kallogjeri D, Nicklaus J, et al. Low-frequency repetitive transcranial magnetic stimulation to the temporoparietal junction for tinnitus: four-week stimulation trial. JAMA Otolaryngol Head Neck Surg. 2013; 139(4):388–395

[17] Landgrebe M, Hajak G, Wolf S, et al. 1-Hz rTMS in the treatment of tinnitus: A sham-controlled, randomized multicenter trial. Brain Stimul. 2017; 10(6):1112–1120

[18] Lehner A, Schecklmann M, Greenlee MW, Rupprecht R, Langguth B. Triple-site rTMS for the treatment of chronic tinnitus: a randomized controlled trial. Sci Rep. 2016; 6:22302

[19] Tunkel DE, Bauer CA, Sun GH, et al. Clinical practice guideline: tinnitus. Otolaryngol Head Neck Surg. 2014; 151 (2) Suppl:S1–S40

[20] Tringali S, Perrot X, Collet L, Moulin A. Repetitive transcranial magnetic stimulation: hearing safety considerations. Brain Stimul. 2012; 5(3):354–363

[21] Thair H, Holloway AL, Newport R, Smith ADJFIN. Transcranial direct current stimulation (tDCS): a beginner's guide for design and implementation. Front Neurosci. 2017; 11:641

[22] Shekhawat GS, Sundram F, Bikson M, et al. Intensity, duration, and location of high-definition transcranial direct current stimulation for tinnitus relief. Neurorehabil Neural Repair. 2016; 30(4):349–359

[23] Yuan T, Yadollahpour A, Salgado-Ramírez J, Robles-Camarillo D, Ortega-Palacios R. Transcranial direct current stimulation for the treatment of tinnitus: a review of clinical trials and mechanisms of action. BMC Neurosci. 2018; 19(1):66

[24] Engineer ND, Riley JR, Seale JD, et al. Reversing pathological neural activity using targeted plasticity. Nature. 2011; 470 (7332):101–104

[25] De Ridder D, Vanneste S, Engineer ND, Kilgard MP. Safety and efficacy of vagus nerve stimulation paired with tones for the treatment of tinnitus: a case series. Neuromodulation. 2014; 17(2):170–179

[26] Tyler R, Cacace A, Stocking C, et al. Vagus nerve stimulation paired with tones for the treatment of tinnitus: a prospective randomized double-blind controlled pilot study in humans. Sci Rep. 2017; 7(1):11960

[27] Lehtimäki J, Hyvärinen P, Ylikoski M, et al. Transcutaneous vagus nerve stimulation in tinnitus: a pilot study. Acta Otolaryngol. 2013; 133(4):378–382

[28] Young DW. Biofeedback training the treatment of tinnitus. In: Tyler RS, ed. Tinnitus handbook. San Diego, CA: Singular Publishing Group; 2000: Ch. 12, 281–295

[29] Dohrmann K, Weisz N, Schlee W, Hartmann T, Elbert T. Neurofeedback for treating tinnitus. Prog Brain Res. 2007; 166:473–485

[30] Weisz N, Moratti S, Meinzer M, Dohrmann K, Elbert T. Tinnitus perception and distress is related to abnormal spontaneous brain activity as measured by magnetoencephalography. PLoS Med. 2005; 2(6):e153

[31] Stoeckel LE, Garrison KA, Ghosh S, et al. Optimizing real time fMRI neurofeedback for therapeutic discovery and development. Neuroimage Clin. 2014; 5:245–255

[32] Haller S, Birbaumer N, Veit R. Real-time fMRI feedback training may improve chronic tinnitus. Eur Radiol. 2010; 20 (3):696–703

[33] Emmert K, Kopel R, Koush Y, et al. Continuous vs. intermittent neurofeedback to regulate auditory cortex activity of tinnitus patients using real-time fMRI: a pilot study. Neuroimage Clin. 2017; 14:97–104

[34] Young KD, Zotev V, Phillips R, et al. Real-time FMRI neurofeedback training of amygdala activity in patients with major depressive disorder. PLoS One. 2014; 9(2):e88785

15 Establishing a Tinnitus and Hyperacusis Clinic

Patricia C. Mancini, Shelley A. Witt, Richard S. Tyler, and Ann Perreau

Abstract

Tinnitus is a common symptom among individuals with hearing loss, but specific treatment for tinnitus is not provided in most audiology clinics. Licensed audiologists generally have the essential training necessary to provide counseling and sound therapy to treat tinnitus and hyperacusis patients. This chapter provides an overview on structuring clinical services for tinnitus and hyperacusis patients. We usually initiate treatment with group educational sessions, and individual counseling sessions are provided for those patients who are more severely bothered by their tinnitus. Follow-up and referrals might be necessary in severe cases. Tinnitus and hyperacusis management typically involves some form of counseling and sound therapy. Tinnitus Activities Treatment (TAT) is an excellent approach that combines counseling and the use of partial masking therapy. In counseling, we provide information to the patient about tinnitus and related problems, consider the patient's overall well-being, and suggest appropriate coping strategies based on the issues that are especially important to each single patient. Sound therapy options are presented at the group session, and patients also have the opportunity to discuss and try a variety of wearable ear-level devices for tinnitus management in individual sessions. Tailoring the sessions to the patient's level of tinnitus severity (interested, concerned, or distressed) is important. We often include partners and significant others in group and individual sessions to help them understand tinnitus, and to suggest strategies that enable partners to help the patients cope with tinnitus. Similar to TAT, Hyperacusis Activities Treatment is a picture-based counseling and sound therapy treatment that targets the areas that are largely impacted by hyperacusis. The tinnitus and hyperacusis clinic must provide an individualized treatment, estimating the need for additional staff and resources, and providing reasonable reimbursement options.

Keywords: tinnitus, hyperacusis, outpatient care, counseling, therapy

15.1 Introduction

Although tinnitus is very common among individuals with hearing loss, specific treatment for tinnitus is not provided in most audiology clinics. In addition, patients who are distressed by hyperacusis are now seeking treatment by audiologists to alleviate their symptoms.[1,2,3] Tinnitus and hyperacusis patients often have difficulty finding adequate professional service. Some audiologists simply do not have a concrete plan on how to provide treatment. Others are simply unsure of what to do, and many lack experience. However, audiologists are good listeners, interact well with patients, and receive adequate training in hearing, hearing loss, and counseling that readily apply to the management of tinnitus and hyperacusis. Explanatory counseling, together with patient expectation nurturing, will help many.[4,5,6] In this chapter, we provide an overall view for establishing a tinnitus and hyperacusis clinic with an aim to encourage audiologists to expand their role in this important area of service.

15.2 Structuring Clinical Services

Tinnitus and hyperacusis are challenging to treat because there are no cures for these conditions. However, several forms of treatment are available. Audiologists should possess an in-depth knowledge of hearing loss, hearing measurement, and rehabilitation to provide an accurate evaluation and effective management plan for tinnitus and hyperacusis. Here, we advocate a flexible approach, meeting the individual needs of each patient that includes counseling, sound therapy, and collaboration with psychologists and physicians, when necessary.

A detailed clinical history is crucial to obtain important information about the patient's etiology and to help the physician select appropriate laboratory and radiologic exams, if needed. Audiologists should refer to an otologist when a patient presents for pulsatile tinnitus, sudden onset or worsening tinnitus, asymmetrical hearing, and other diseases of the auditory system.[7] If there is evidence of depression, anxiety, unrealistic thoughts or actions, or the patient talks about suicide, then these should be addressed with the patient and a referral to a mental health professional should be made. Our goal is to work together with mental health professionals.[8]

A full diagnostic hearing examination is important because most individuals with tinnitus have

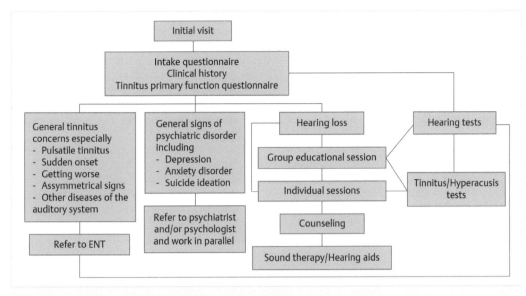

Fig. 15.1 Management of the tinnitus and hyperacusis patient.

some degree of hearing loss. We believe that everyone who experiences persistent tinnitus has experienced a change in their hearing function.

Tinnitus evaluation involves the measurement of its characteristics, as well as the reactions or negative consequences on a patient's life. The measurement of tinnitus can be helpful to confirm to the patient that their tinnitus is real, to provide insight on the possible mechanisms involved, to monitor changes in the tinnitus magnitude, and to aid in providing information for the fitting of a hearing or masking device, if indicated. The handicapping nature of tinnitus and hyperacusis can be assessed using several questionnaires designed to quantify the problems caused by each. These questionnaires are discussed in Chapters 12 and 13. Audiological measurement of tinnitus and hyperacusis does not need to be done first before services are started; rather, measurement of tinnitus and/or hyperacusis can be done as a separate session.

Our model of treating tinnitus and hyperacusis patients incorporates both group and individual educational sessions. We advocate that patients participate in a group session first. The group educational session is intended to provide general information and to educate patients on the possible causes and mechanisms of tinnitus and hyperacusis, their prevalence, and the available treatment options, including counseling and sound therapy. The individual sessions are planned for those patients who typically are more affected by their

tinnitus/hyperacusis, and are focused on each patient's individual needs. Our overall philosophy on tinnitus and hyperacusis treatment is to customize management for each individual patient that usually involves discrete steps as shown in ▶ Fig. 15.1. The order of the steps is adjusted to suit an individual's needs, and not all patients must complete all steps. A Tinnitus Treatment Fact Sheet may be available in the clinic waiting room with an explanation of these steps using accessible language to the patient and family members (see Appendix 15.3 Tinnitus Treatment Fact Sheet).

15.2.1 Group Educational Session

Group educational sessions have been offered to our tinnitus and hyperacusis patients because it is an efficient method for providing counseling in a busy clinical setting. In our clinic, patients are initially scheduled for the group educational session. The advantages of holding a group educational session to tinnitus and hyperacusis patients include[9,10]:

- It is cost and time efficient to clinicians because the information can be provided to more patients and their significant others in less time.
- It allows the patients to realize that they are not alone, and that there are other people suffering from tinnitus and hyperacusis as well.
- Some patients feel more comfortable in a group session.

- It is possible to include patients' partners and significant others.
- The group session promotes a supportive and safe environment to share experiences with other patients, learning how to cope, or not cope, with tinnitus/hyperacusis.
- Some patients are more likely to accept treatment beginning in a group setting.

However, the group setting also presents some disadvantages and concerns for which audiologists should recognize:

- The lack of opportunity to develop the one-on-one relationship with the patient.[9]
- Some distressed patients may dominate the session.[11]
- The control of the group size because a very large group will inhibit individual participation and a small group might reduce opportunities of interaction between participants.
- The ability to maintain the confidentiality and privacy of participants as much as possible.

We usually schedule 8 to 10 patients per group educational session. Partners and significant others are encouraged to attend and participate, if the patient feels comfortable with including a family member in this session. It is well known that individuals with tinnitus may experience difficulties with sleep, thoughts and emotions, concentration, and hearing.[10,12] These difficulties can also affect their significant others' lives, and can impact their relationship and activities of everyday life.[10,13,14] Partners are often the closest person to the patient and can play a significant role in tinnitus management. However, significant others usually have a limited knowledge regarding tinnitus and hyperacusis.[13,15] We believe that the inclusion of partners in counseling sessions allows patients and partners to find appropriate strategies for managing tinnitus and hyperacusis in the home and social environments, and can further help patients to cope.[15,16] Therefore, we suggest that partners participate in counseling provided to tinnitus and hyperacusis patients as part of treatment. This could be included in both group and individual sessions.

Attendees at the group educational sessions are asked to bring a copy of their audiogram if they have one and/or are encouraged to have their hearing tested prior to the session. We also have attendees complete the Tinnitus Primary Functions Questionnaire (TPFQ) before the session[12] (see Chapter 4 supplemental materials), the Tinnitus Intake Questionnaire, and the Shared Medical Visit

Waiver (see Appendix 15.1 and 15.2 supplemental materials).

The group session proceeds in a progressive management approach to make it easier for the patients to understand important concepts while interacting with the clinician and participants. In addition, this approach is helpful because the clinician does not overlook important topics and concepts.

The main topics to be discussed at the group educational session include:

- Tinnitus and hyperacusis definitions.
- Normal and abnormal anatomy and physiology of the auditory system.
- Mechanisms and causes of tinnitus and hyperacusis.
- Hearing testing and hearing loss.
- Common reactions to tinnitus.
- Overview of available treatment options.
- Self-help strategies for tinnitus.
- Steps in treatment of tinnitus/hyperacusis offered in our clinic.

At the beginning of the group educational session, participants are invited to say their first name, what their tinnitus sounds like and/or what their experience with hyperacusis has been, and for how long they have had it. This is an opportunity for participants to realize that other people suffer from tinnitus and hyperacusis as well, that it appears in many different forms, and that time and/or duration can similarly vary among different people with tinnitus.

The human auditory system and its physiology are presented in a comprehensive manner. Our presentation is picture-based, making it easier for the patients to understand important concepts (see ▶ Fig. 15.2a–d). However, the discussions can be adapted to the needs and sophistication of each group.

We often include some explanation of the hearing examination, the audiogram and normal hearing thresholds, and the various degrees of hearing loss. Patients are invited to share their audiogram if they wish that helps many patients realize the perceptual consequences of their hearing loss. Particularly, we help them understand that some sounds that they once heard may be difficult to distinguish or may be no longer audible to them at all. For example, if patients have high-frequency hearing loss, they probably perceive people talking to them as "mumbling," and sounds with mostly high-frequency energy, like /s/, often will not be heard.

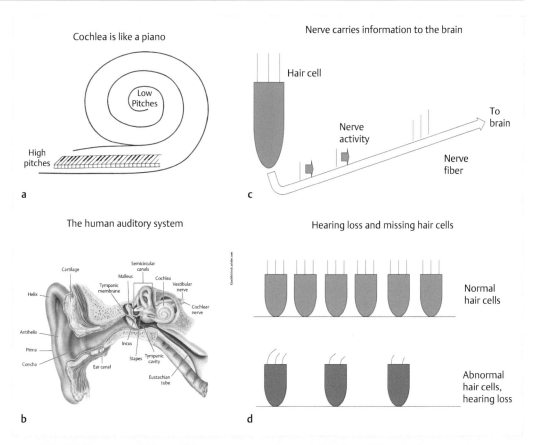

Cochlea is like a piano

Low
Pitches

High
pitches

a

Nerve carries information to the brain

Hair cell

Nerve
activity

To
brain

Nerve
fiber

c

The human auditory system

b

Hearing loss and missing hair cells

Normal
hair cells

Abnormal
hair cells,
hearing loss

d

Fig. 15.2 (a-d) Illustrations used to explain patients the anatomy and physiology of the human auditory system. (Source: *Bottom left*: ©Judith/stock.adobe.com)

Participants are also asked to tell in one sentence what they think caused their tinnitus. When all attendees answer the question, it becomes clear to patients and their partners that the same things that cause hearing loss can also cause tinnitus. The main causes of tinnitus and its prevalence are then discussed with attendees.

We also have the patients describe how tinnitus has affected their lives to learn about their specific problems. We usually ask attendees to make a list, in order of importance, of the difficulties that are associated with or caused by their tinnitus. At the moment when all patients explain their main difficulties, it becomes easy to identify the following four common areas that tinnitus may compromise[10]:

- Affects thoughts and emotions, causing distress, depression, anxiety, etc.
- Causes communication difficulties because it can be hard to focus on what people are saying over the tinnitus.

- Disturbs sleep—most common lifestyle problem reported by tinnitus patients.
- Impacts concentration.

When tinnitus affects thoughts and emotions, hearing, sleep, and concentration, patients can experience limitations in secondary activities such as socialization and work, as well as general quality of life.[12] Because tinnitus is almost always accompanied by hearing loss,[17,18,19] many patients who experience both tinnitus and hearing loss attribute their hearing difficulties to tinnitus, even if they have significant hearing loss.[20] Therefore, it is important to help patients understand and distinguish the difficulties that they may be experiencing due to their hearing loss compared to those that result from their tinnitus. We explain to participants that hearing loss can make some sounds seem distorted and other sounds almost completely inaudible, such as doorbell or bird song. Tinnitus can produce hearing difficulty because it may distract patients from listening.

In addition, the sound of the tinnitus might mask some sounds.[21] We also explain to our patients that tinnitus can cause difficulties in distinguishing one sound from another because it can be confused with other environmental sounds that have the similar pitch. In the group educational session, it is important for patients to understand that tinnitus does not cause a hearing loss, make someone deaf, lead to senility, or imply a sign of mental illness.

We encourage partners, significant others, and family members (e.g., daughter or son) to participate in our sessions. During the group session, we ask tinnitus patients "What is the most difficult thing to explain to others about your tinnitus?" and "What could others do to help you with your tinnitus?" The question for partners and significant others is "What have you been able to do to help your partner with their tinnitus?" These questions point to the current knowledge and misconceptions of patients and their partners about tinnitus. Providing information about hearing, hearing loss, and tinnitus to patients and partners (1) removes many of the unknowns, misconceptions, and fears; (2) helps patients realize they are not alone; and (3) assists them in developing realistic expectations.[10,20] We believe the group educational session is an opportunity for patients to better understand tinnitus and the reactions they may have to it, as well as for partners to learn some strategies to help patients to cope.

The group educational session also provides an overview of available treatment options for tinnitus and hyperacusis. Many patients report that they have tried various treatments to tinnitus. At this point, we provide realistic expectations for patients and their significant others stating that there are no widely accepted cures for tinnitus currently; there are no studies that have shown a cure for tinnitus using appropriate research designs, and that have been replicated by others. We also explain that currently no drug or surgery can reliably eliminate the source of tinnitus, but that there are effective drugs for sleep, anxiety, and depression. Furthermore, there are many excellent treatment options for tinnitus that have been researched and show positive results for some, but not all tinnitus patients. These treatment options include:

- Individualized counseling.
- Sound therapy.
- Wearable sound generators.
- Hearing aids.

Our individualized counseling is based on Tinnitus Activities Treatment[10] (TAT; see Chapter 4). TAT is a comprehensive tinnitus therapy approach for improving emotional reactions and thoughts, hearing and communication, sleep, and concentration abilities. For example, in thoughts and emotions section, patients are taught how their thoughts create emotions that may be influenced by tinnitus, and ways to change our negative thoughts into a more positive or neutral thoughts. In sleep, we teach normal patterns to sleep, and how patients can facilitate and prepare for sleep using relaxation techniques.

Sound therapy includes nonwearable sound generators, such as sound pillows, environmental sound generators, smartphone apps, radio, etc.; and wearable sound generators, including the tinnitus masking devices (see Chapters 7–9). In our group educational session, we give general information on the use and different types available, and provide a demonstration of some devices. We also provide information about hearing aids that help to improve hearing sounds and speech, and also reduce the amount of effort patients have to put into listening. Patients are informed that hearing aids also help with tinnitus because (1) patients hear better and are less stressed, facilitating positive reactions to tinnitus, and (2) the background noise amplified by the hearing aids provides partial masking of tinnitus.

The group session also provides information about self-help strategies for tinnitus. Sizer and Coles[22] recommend specific lifestyle changes that help tinnitus patients to improve their overall condition, reducing the severity of tinnitus until it is no longer a negative factor in the patient's life. These specific lifestyle changes include improving sleep patterns, reducing anxiety associated to tinnitus, addressing communication problems, reducing noise exposure, having a balanced diet and physical activity. If patients can be motivated to implement positive lifestyle changes, their overall condition will improve and the severity of their tinnitus will decrease (see Chapter 3). For those patients that will take responsibility for their own improvement and make concrete efforts to follow specific recommendations formulated by health care professionals, we also suggest reading "The Consumer Handbook on Tinnitus."[23]

Other materials and information given in the group session include the website of the American Tinnitus Association (www.ata.org), where patients can find information about tinnitus health providers, events, research, and new treatments. In addition, we inform the patients that regular conferences are available to audiologists and other health care professionals, as well as to tinnitus patients. We have provided the International Conference on the Management of the Tinnitus and Hyperacusis Patient one each year for the past 28 years (information available at: https://medicine.uiowa.edu/oto/education/conferences-and-events/international-conference-management-tinnitus-and-hyperacusis). See Appendix 15.3 for an example handout of services provided to tinnitus patients.

In summary, the counseling provided during the group educational session assures us that tinnitus patients and their partners understand the following:

- The mechanisms and causes of tinnitus and hyperacusis.
- Tinnitus is common.
- The reactions to tinnitus.
- Tinnitus is not life threatening.
- There is no universal cure to tinnitus and hyperacusis.
- Treatment does exist.

15.2.2 Individual Sessions

Individual sessions in our clinic are tailored to the individual needs of each patient and consist of counseling for patients that are concerned or distressed, sound therapy for those who want to try devices and/or treatment approaches for management, or a combination of these.

The optimal number and duration of counseling sessions will vary across patients. Some patients will require long-term follow-up visits. The optimum treatment duration depends on each patient because the primary goal of our tinnitus treatment protocol is to equip our patients with the necessary knowledge and tools to promote tinnitus relief by helping them overcome the physical, psychological, and social consequences of tinnitus/hyperacusis. For many patients, a 30-minute discussion will be sufficient. For others, much longer sessions will be necessary.[24]

Counseling Session

We use TAT as our primary counseling tool. The series of pictures in activities treatment provides a nice orderly fashion helping make sure that important concepts are not overlooked. It is an easy format to help people understand difficult concepts related to hearing and tinnitus. The pictures provide the basis for the sessions that incorporate opportunities to pause and open up collaborative

discussions, making the whole process patient-centered.

There is no right or wrong way to use the pictures, and there is no specific order. There are a few main topics, but the audiologist can pick and choose how to present them and in which order to present them. Techniques discussed in one area (e.g., sleep) can be used to help in other areas (e.g., thoughts and emotions). The area addressing thoughts and emotions is typically where audiologists will spend the most time. The concepts and techniques are not easy for everyone to incorporate into daily life. However, this section can be the most helpful and often is an underlying feature in all of the other primary areas.

The approach to TAT is evidence based. As discussed in Chapter 4, activities treatment incorporates cognitive behavior therapy techniques, relaxation techniques, imagery training as well as the concept of acceptance, ownership and Sensory Meditation for Tinnitus into the sessions.

Patients must take an active role in the process, must be willing to work together to make things better with regard to their own situation. It is important to have each patient set individual goals for these sessions. TAT provides a systematic method of helping patients move through the process of coming to terms with living with tinnitus.[10] Sessions allow patients to tell their story and feel validated about their journey. Many tinnitus patients have a hard time finding a professional who (1) has the time to listen to their unique situation and (2) acknowledges their struggles. TAT provides an opportunity for the patient to think about specific problems being experienced and to take a mental inventory to determine if it has been possible to change their thoughts and emotions and accept their tinnitus.

Sessions help patients determine if the issues are related to hearing and communication difficulties versus the patient's tinnitus. They also provide a clear explanation of the link between our thoughts and emotions. TAT helps patients focus on other areas of their life and, if possible, reduce the contrast between their tinnitus and background sound.

Sound Therapy Session

The purpose of this session is to provide patients with the opportunity to discuss and try a variety of sound therapy devices for tinnitus management. We typically schedule a single 3-hour sound therapy session. During this session, we fit the patient with a variety of wearable ear-level devices and discuss in detail current therapy techniques. We include in our sound therapy session a short trial with the following:

- Masking via ear-level noise generators (any manufacturer; can try various frequency shaped noise).
- Masking via amplification (any manufacturer; slight amplification even in the absence of hearing loss).
- Masking via amplification plus noise generators (any manufacturer).

During this session, the proper use of desktop devices, sleep pillows, and/or apps via a smart phone are demonstrated. Patients typically leave this session with a better understanding of the concept of masking and specific treatment milestones and expectations. If a patient wants to pursue a specific device/approach, the cost, milestones, treatment expectations, and follow-up schedule are reviewed. In addition, subsequent sessions are scheduled.

15.3 Different Treatment Levels for Different Tinnitus and Hyperacusis Patients

Because tinnitus and hyperacusis patients have many different experiences, thoughts, and emotions, it is important to find and address each patient's special needs and problems.

15.3.1 Tinnitus

During the first visit, it is helpful to determine if patients are curious, concerned, or distressed about their tinnitus (see ▶ Table 15.1[8,25]). Curious patients may have questions about their tinnitus, and much of their anxiety associated with tinnitus arises from uncertainty regarding its nature and consequences. These patients often need basic information on possible causes of tinnitus, its mechanisms, prevalence, consequences, and outcomes. Once the mystery of tinnitus is unveiled, their reaction is also largely resolved. These curious patients usually benefit from the group educational session and typically do not pursue individual sessions.

The concerned patients usually require more time to discuss specific problems and situations, and express themselves. This group of patients needs more detailed information regarding treatment options. In addition, a formal evaluation of tinnitus that includes questionnaires and psychoacoustical measurements, as discussed on Chapter 12, may be necessary. We also develop some self-directed management strategies (see Chapter 3). Sometimes more than one individual session is necessary as well as a referral to a psychologist or psychiatrist, depending on the level of concern.

Finally, the third group consists of distressed patients who present with more serious problems

Table 15.1 Levels of tinnitus patients and proposed treatment

Tinnitus patient	Treatment required	Session	Focus areas
Curious	Provide basic information	Group session	• Listen to the patient • Provide hearing aid referral if necessary • Provide general information about tinnitus and possible treatments • Determine if further treatment or referral is needed
Concerned	Provide basic information Review treatment options	Group session and individual sessions (if necessary)	• Listen to the patient • Provide more detail about tinnitus and possible treatments • Assess individual needs • Provide plan for self-treatment • Determine if further treatment or referral is needed
Distressed	Counseling and sound therapy Referral when appropriate	Group session and individual sessions	• Listen to the patient • Assess tinnitus handicap using established instruments • Measure psychoacoustic characteristics of tinnitus • Assess psychological well-being and determine if referral is needed • Provide information about treatments • Assess treatment plan options and decide on treatment(s)

Source: Adapted from Tyler et al.[25]

associated with their tinnitus. This group requires a more specific follow-up plan that includes formal assessment of tinnitus and handicap, and a systematic outline for treatment. Special attention should be given to the emotional consequences of tinnitus, and sometimes a referral to clinical psychology or psychiatric services should be made immediately if any concern exists. We usually devote a more comprehensive treatment plan that requires several individual sessions, depending on the distress level.

15.3.2 Hyperacusis

We currently offer group education sessions for patients with hyperacusis, as well as individual counseling sessions and sound therapy, where appropriate. Recently, our approach to establishing group educational sessions for hyperacusis patients was shared.[15] The group sessions utilize Hyperacusis Activities Treatment[8,15] that targets the areas that are largely impacted by hyperacusis: emotional well-being, hearing and communication, sleep, and concentration. In our group educational sessions, we emphasize five areas that include getting to know patients well and establishing rapport, understanding problems associated with hyperacusis, explaining the auditory system and the relationship of hyperacusis to hearing loss and tinnitus, describing the impact of hyperacusis on daily life, and discussing treatment options. Similar to tinnitus treatment, some patients will be helped by the group educational session and may not pursue additional counseling for their hyperacusis.[15] However, others will need more support, and then we begin individual counseling sessions and/or sound therapy devices as described earlier.

15.4 Billing for Tinnitus Services

At this time, the audiological measurement of tinnitus is the only billable service available to audiologists in the management of tinnitus patients. We are hopeful that reimbursement for tinnitus services will improve in the future. All services provided by our Tinnitus and Hyperacusis clinic, except the hearing examination and audiological tinnitus measurement examination, are an out-of-pocket expense. Reimbursement is available to audiologists for hearing assessment. Tinnitus evaluation is also billable in the United States and includes the measurement of tinnitus pitch, loudness, and masking level. This is currently the only billable procedure for tinnitus to the Centers of Medicare and Medicaid Services. The Current Procedural Terminology (CPT) code for Tinnitus Evaluation is #92625 and the billing description is "Tinnitus Evaluation (pitch, loudness, masking)."

In our clinic, patients are given a cost list for each service provided (i.e., group educational session, sound therapy session, and individual counseling session). Counseling sessions can be provided by an individual as needed cost or can be bundled for reduced cost. Counseling sessions can also be provided via telephone or internet if needed. If a patient pursues a particular tinnitus device, follow-up sessions can be bundled or unbundled. We also provide support letters to tinnitus patients, and they can pass on to their insurance companies.

Lack of appropriate coding is an impediment to the comprehensive treatment of the tinnitus patient, in view of the extensive time requirements necessary for these patients' treatment. The availability of appropriate CPT codes with associated adequate reimbursement could potentially facilitate the delivery of clinical services by audiologists to tinnitus patients. However, because we deliver high-quality services for the management of tinnitus and hyperacusis, patients are willing to pay out-of-pocket for these services. Some patients are hindered by the lack of insurance coverage, and we continue to advocate for change.

15.5 Conclusion

Patients with tinnitus and/or hyperacusis often seek help from audiologists when the effects lower their quality of life. In this chapter, we have provided an overview on structuring clinical services for tinnitus and hyperacusis patients. We usually start with group educational sessions, and individual counseling sessions are provided for those patients who are more severely bothered by their tinnitus. Audiologists receive adequate training in hearing, hearing loss, and counseling. When it comes to tinnitus, we can provide helpful counseling regarding the effects that tinnitus may have on sleep, concentration, hearing, thoughts, and emotions. If emotional consequences of tinnitus or hyperacusis become severe, we should and do refer to other mental health professionals.

Although some patients may choose to independently query information on tinnitus, many patients seek individualized, patient-centered care. TAT is an excellent approach that combines counseling and the use of partial masking therapy. In counseling, we provide information to the patient about tinnitus and associated problems, considering the patient's overall well-being, and suggesting appropriate coping strategies based on the issues that are especially important to each single patient. Tailoring the sessions to the patient's level of tinnitus severity (interested, concerned, or distressed) is important. We often include counseling to patients' partners and significant others to help them understand tinnitus, and to suggest strategies that enable partners to help the patient cope with tinnitus. Similar to TAT, Hyperacusis Activities Treatment is a picture-based counseling and sound therapy treatment that targets the areas that are largely impacted by hyperacusis. Through group and individual sessions, we hope to support and address the needs of our patients with tinnitus and hyperacusis.

References

[1] Andersson G, Strömgren T, Ström L, Lyttkens L. Randomized controlled trial of internet-based cognitive behavior therapy for distress associated with tinnitus. Psychosom Med. 2002; 64(5):810–816

[2] Hannula S, Bloigu R, Majamaa K, Sorri M, Mäki-Torkko E. Self-reported hearing problems among older adults: prevalence and comparison to measured hearing impairment. J Am Acad Audiol. 2011; 22(8):550–559

[3] Tyler RS, Noble W, Coelho C, Haskell G, Bardia A. Tinnitus and hyperacusis. In: Katz J, Burkard R, Medwetsky L, Hood L, eds. Handbook of clinical audiology. 6th ed. Baltimore, MD: Lippincott Williams & Wilkins; 2009:647–658

[4] Tyler RS, Stouffer JL, Schum R. Audiological rehabilitation of the tinnitus client. J Acad Rehabilitative Audiol. 1989; 22: 30–42

[5] Tyler RS. The use of science to find successful tinnitus treatments. In Proceedings of the Sixth International Tinnitus Seminar. London: The Tinnitus-Hyperacusis Center; 1999:3–9

[6] Tyler RS, Haskell G, Preece J, Bergan C. Nurturing patient expectations to enhance the treatment of tinnitus. Semin Hear. 2001; 22(1):15–21

[7] Perry BP, Gantz BJ. Medical and surgical evaluation and management of tinnitus. In: Tyler RS, ed. Tinnitus handbook. San Diego, CA: Singular; 2000:221–241

[8] Tyler RS, Noble W, Coelho C, Rocancio ER, Jun HJ. Tinnitus and hyperacusis. In: Katz J, ed. Handbook of clinical audiology. 7th ed. Philadelphia, PA: Lippincott Williams & Wilkins; 2015:647–658

[9] Newman CW, Sandridge SA. Incorporating group and individual sessions into a tinnitus management clinic. In: Tyler RS, ed. Tinnitus treatment: clinical protocols. New York, NY: Thieme; 2006:187–197

[10] Tyler RS, Gehringer AK, Noble W, Dunn CC, Witt SA, Bardia A. Tinnitus activities treatment. Chapter 9. In: Tyler RS, ed. Tinnitus treatment: clinical protocols. New York: Thieme; 2006:116–132

[11] Sweetow R. Cognitive behavior therapy for tinnitus. In: Tyler RS, ed. Tinnitus handbook. San Diego, CA: Singular; 2000:297–312

[12] Tyler R, Ji H, Perreau A, Witt S, Noble W, Coelho C. Development and validation of the tinnitus primary function questionnaire. Am J Audiol. 2014; 23(3):260–272

[13] Mancini PC, Tyler RS, Perreau A, Batterton LF, Ji H. Considerations for partners of our tinnitus patients. Int Tinnitus J. 2018; 22(2):113–122

[14] Tyler RS, Baker LJ. Difficulties experienced by tinnitus sufferers. J Speech Hear Disord. 1983; 48(2):150–154

[15] Perreau AE, Tyler RS, Mancini PC, Witt S, Elgandy MS. Establishing a group educational session for hyperacusis patients. Am J Audiol. 2019; 28(2):245–250

[16] Mancini PC, Tyler RS, Smith S, Ji H, Perreau A, Mohr AM. Tinnitus: how partners can help? Am J Audiol. 2019; 28(1): 85–94

[17] Kochkin S, Tyler RS. Tinnitus treatment and the effectiveness of hearing aids: hearing care professional perceptions. Hearing Rev. 2008; 15(13):14–18

[18] Kochkin S, Tyler R, Born J. MarkeTrak VIII: prevalence of tinnitus and efficacy of treatments. Hearing Rev. 2011; 18 (12):10–26

[19] Tyler RS. Neurophysiological models, psychological models, and treatments for tinnitus. In: Tyler RS, ed. Tinnitus treatment: clinical protocols. New York: Thieme; 2006b:1–22

[20] Tyler RS, Gogel SA, Gehringer AK. Tinnitus activities treatment. Prog Brain Res. 2007; 166:425–434

[21] Surr RK, Montgomery AA, Mueller HG. Effect of amplification on tinnitus among new hearing aid users. Ear Hear. 1985; 6 (2):71–75

[22] Sizer DI, Coles RRA. Tinnitus self-treatment. In: Tyler RS, ed. Tinnitus treatment: Clinical protocols. New York, NY: Thieme; 2006:23–28

[23] Tyler RS, ed. The consumer handbook on tinnitus. 2nd ed. Sedona, AZ: Auricle Ink Publishers; 2016

[24] Tyler RS, Erlandsson S. Management of the tinnitus patient. In: Luxon LM, Furman JM, Martini A, Stephens D, eds. Textbook of audiological medicine. London, England: Taylor & Francis Group; 2003:571–578

[25] Tyler RS, Haskell GB, Gogel SA, Gehringer AK. Establishing a tinnitus clinic in your practice. Am J Audiol. 2008; 17(1):25–37

Appendix 15.1 Shared Medical Visit Waiver

Date:
Patient Name:

I, _____, agree that the (**insert name of your clinic**) shall not be liable for any financial or other damages resulting from breach of confidentiality committed by members of the group session. I agree to protect other's privacy by not identifying patients or discussing their health problems outside of the group setting.

_____

Patient Signature

_____   _____

(Credentials and signature   (Credentials and signature
of supervising Audiologist)   of supervising Audiologist)

Appendix 15.2 Tinnitus Intake Questionnaire

The University of Iowa
Department of Otolaryngology–Head & Neck Surgery

1. What is your gender?   Female Male

2. What is your age?   _____ years

3. Please rate, using a scale from 0–100, whether sounds that others believe are   _____ (0–100)
    moderately loud are *too* loud to you. (0 = strongly disagree; 100 = strongly agree)
    Please list sounds that are too loud to you:

4. Where is your tinnitus? (Please choose only ONE answer.)

    a) Left ear   a) In the head, but no exact place
    b) Right ear   b) More in the right side of head
    c) Both ears, equally   c) More in the left side of head
    d) Both ears, but worse in left ear   d) Outside of head
    e) Both ears, but worse in right ear   e) Middle of head

> If you hear more than one sound or a different sound in each ear, answer the following questions with regard to the one most annoying sound.

5. Describe the most prominent *PITCH* of your tinnitus on a scale from 1 to 100,   _____ (1–100)
    where 1 is like a *VERY LOW* pitch fog horn, and 100 is like a *VERY HIGH* pitch
    whistle.

6. Does the *PITCH* of the tinnitus vary from day to day?   a. No
                                                                                         b. Yes

7. Describe the *LOUDNESS* of your tinnitus using a scale from 0–100. (0 = *VERY FAINT*; _____ (0–100)
    100 = *VERY LOUD*)

8. Does the *LOUDNESS* of the tinnitus vary from day to day?   No
                                                                                         Yes

9. Describe the typical *ANNOYANCE* of your tinnitus using a scale from 0–100.   _____ (0–100)
    (0 = *NOT ANNOYING AT ALL*; 100 = *EXTREMLY ANNOYING*)

10. Which of all these qualities *BEST* describes your tinnitus? (Please circle only ONE.)

    a) Ringing or whistling   a) Humming
    b) Cricket-like   b) Hissing
    c) Roaring, "Shhh," or rushing   c) OTHER, PLEASE SPECIFY:
    d) Buzzing   _____

11. During the time you are awake, what percentage of the time is your tinnitus present? For example, 100%
    would indicate that your tinnitus was present all the time, and 25% would indicate that your tinnitus was
    present ¼ of the time.
    _____% (Please write in a single number between 1 and 100.)

12. On the average, how many days per month are you bothered by your tinnitus?   _____ days

13.   How many months or years have you had tinnitus?   _____ months OR
                                                                           _____ years

14.   When you have your tinnitus, which of the following makes it *WORSE*?

a) Alcohol
b) Being in a noisy place
c) Being in a quiet place
d) Caffeine (coffee/tea/cola)
e) Drugs/medicine
f) Eye movement
g) Food (please specify) _____
h) Moving your head or neck
i) Physical activity
j) Relaxation
k) Touching your head

a) Wearing a hearing aid
b) When you first wake up in the morning
c) Being tired
d) During your menstrual period
e) Emotional or mental stress
f) Lack of sleep
g) Shooting guns, rifles, etc.
h) Smoking
i) Nothing makes it worse
j) OTHER, PLEASE SPECIFY

_____

15   Which of the following *REDUCES* your tinnitus?

a) Alcohol
b) Being in a noisy place
c) Being in a quiet place
d) Caffeine (coffee/tea/cola)
e) Drugs/medicine
f) Eye movement
g) Food (please specify) _____
h) Moving your head or neck

a) Physical activity
b) Relaxation
c) Touching your head
d) Wearing a hearing aid
e) When you first wake up in the morning
f) Nothing makes it better
g) OTHER, PLEASE SPECIFY

_____

16   What do you think originally caused your tinnitus? (Select up to THREE choices)

a) Aging
b) Autoimmune disease
c) Brain Tumor
d) Cochlear implant, after surgery
e) Cochlear implant, after switch on
f) Cochlear implant, unknown
g) Deafness from birth, genetic
h) Deafness from birth, syndromic
i) Deafness from birth, unknown
j) Diabetes
k) Electrical trauma
l) Head injury
m) Medication/drug
n) Ménière's Disease
o) Middle ear, blood vessel
p) Middle ear, muscle

a) Middle ear, unknown
b) Noise exposure
c) Noise exposure (non-gunfire, impulsive)
d) Noise exposure (hunting/gunfire)
e) Noise exposure (military service)
f) Otosclerosis
g) Problems with teeth or jaw
h) 8th nerve tumor (acoustic neuroma)
i) Sudden hearing loss
j) Surgery
k) Thyroid
l) Unknown
m) Other (please specify)_____

17   In which ear do you wear hearing aids?

a) Left
b) Right
c) Both
None

18   Do you have any legal action or compensation
claim pending in relation to your tinnitus, or are
you planning legal action?

a) No
b) Yes

Appendix 15.3 Tinnitus Treatment Fact Sheet

Do you experience ringing or buzzing in your ears? If so, you are not alone! Tinnitus is the perception of a sound when no external sound is present. Though there is no cure for tinnitus, there are many treatment options to help. We have outlined them below.

Step 1

- ○ Medical Consultation with ENT specialist
- ○ Hearing test

- Obtaining a medical consultation with an Ear, Nose, and Throat (ENT) specialist can be beneficial to determine the cause of your tinnitus.
- There are many ENTs locally area:
  - ○ Dr. Smith (insert information here)
  - ○ Dr. Johnson (insert information here)
- Testing your hearing regularly is important if you have tinnitus. At the Center, we provide comprehensive hearing testing for individuals of all ages. Changes in hearing ability can influence tinnitus, so have your hearing tested annually if you have tinnitus.

Step 2: Group Educational Session

- ○ We provide monthly group educational sessions to learn more about tinnitus, what causes it, and how to manage it. You will meet others with tinnitus to know you are not alone.
- ○ The cost is **$XX** to attend and family members or friends are encouraged to attend with no additional cost.

Step 3:

- ○ Counseling
- ○ Sound therapy devices
- ○ Counseling and sound therapy devices

- We offer individual counseling, and sound therapy devices to help you learn to cope and provide relief from tinnitus.
  - ○ The fee for individual counseling is **$XX** per session, and typically two sessions are required. We will provide comprehensive, customized therapy to help you manage your reactions to tinnitus.
- Hearing aids and tinnitus devices are available at the Center or from other audiologists in our area.
- We recommend everyone try sound therapy for tinnitus relief. Here are some suggestions:
  - ○ Sound Pillow ($50–150, www.soundpillow.com)
  - ○ Sound Generators ($20+, www.amazon.com)
  - ○ Smartphone applications for tinnitus relief (free): ReSound^{GN} Tinnitus Relief, Tinnitus Balance by Phonak, Starkey Relax, and Widex Zen; Tinnitus Management

Step 4: Individual tinnitus evaluation

- ○ To measure your tinnitus, you also might want an individual tinnitus evaluation. We will measure the pitch and loudness of your tinnitus, and how well it can be masked. We will discuss treatment options and administer several questionnaires. The fee is **$XX** which is billable to Medicare if a doctor referral is provided.

Finally, check out these self-help books and support networks for tinnitus:
- *Tinnitus: A Self-Management Guide for the Ringing in Your Ears* (Henry and Wilson, 2002).
- *The Consumer Handbook on Tinnitus* (Tyler, 2016).
- *American Tinnitus Association:* www.ata.org

For more information:
- Contact the clinic:

Index

Note: Page numbers set **bold** or *italic* indicate headings or figures, respectively.